# Therapeutic Uses of Botulinum Toxin

# Therapeutic Uses
# of Botulinum Toxin

Edited by

## *Grant Cooper,* MD

*Department of Physical Medicine and Rehabilitation*
*New York Presbyterian Hospital, The University Hospital*
*of Columbia and Cornell,*
*New York, NY*

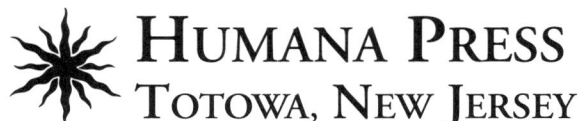

HUMANA PRESS
TOTOWA, NEW JERSEY

Due diligence has been taken by the publishers, editors, and authors of this book to assure the accuracy of the information published and to describe generally accepted practices. The contributors herein have carefully checked to ensure that the drug selections and dosages set forth in this text are accurate and in accord with the standards accepted at the time of publication. Notwithstanding, as new research, changes in government regulations, and knowledge from clinical experience relating to drug therapy and drug reactions constantly occurs, the reader is advised to check the product information provided by the manufacturer of each drug for any change in dosages or for additional warnings and contraindications. This is of utmost importance when the recommended drug herein is a new or infrequently used drug. It is the responsibility of the treating physician to determine dosages and treatment strategies for individual patients. Further it is the responsibility of the health care provider to ascertain the Food and Drug Administration status of each drug or device used in their clinical practice. The publisher, editors, and authors are not responsible for errors or omissions or for any consequences from the application of the information presented in this book and make no warranty, express or implied, with respect to the contents in this publication.

This publication is printed on acid-free paper. ∞
ANSI Z39.48-1984 (American Standards Institute) Permanence of Paper for Printed Library Materials.

Cover illustrations: Clockwise, top to bottom: Fig. 7, Chapter 3, "Radiation Fibrosis Syndrome: *Trismus, Trigeminal Neuralagia, and Cervical Dystonia*," by Michael D. Stubblefield (image courtesy of Michael D. Stubblefield, MD); Fig. 9, Chapter 10, "Cosmetic Applications," by Tara D. Miller and Isaac M. Neuhaus; Fig. 3, Chapter 12, "Urological Applications," by David E. Rapp and Gregory T. Bales; Fig. 10, Chapter 6, "Plantar Fasciitis," by Mary S. Babcock; and Fig. 2, Chapter 3 (image courtesy of Michael D. Stubblefield, MD).

Cover design by Nancy K. Fallatt.

Production Editor: Amy Thau

For additional copies, pricing for bulk purchases, and/or information about other Humana titles, contact Humana at the above address or at any of the following numbers: Tel.: 973-256-1699; Fax: 973-256-8314; E-mail: orders@humanapr.com, or visit our Website: http://humanapress.com

**Photocopy Authorization Policy:**

Printed in the United States of America. 10 9 8 7 6 5 4 3 2 1

eISBN 13: 978-1-59745-247-2
eISBN:     1-59745-247-5

Library of Congress Control Number:     200792705

# Dedication

*For Ana.*

# Preface

Justinius Kerner, a German medical officer and poet, was the first to realize that botulinum toxin potentially might be useful for therapeutic purposes. Kerner made this observation in 1822, but he did not call the toxin "botulinum toxin." Instead, Kerner called it the substance in "wirkenden stoffes," which translates to "bad sausages." Kerner realized that there was a "fat poison" or "fatty acid" within sausages that produced the toxic effects that we now know as botulism. Nearly a century would pass before the bacterium producing the toxin would be isolated and the toxin ultimately renamed "botulinum toxin." As farsighted as Kerner was, it is doubtful that even he could have predicted just how much potential therapeutic punch was packed within his wirkenden stoffes. It was not until 1978, more than a century and a half after Kerner's prediction, that Dr. Allan Scott received Food and Drug Administration approval to test botulinum toxin type A in human volunteers.

We do not yet have a comprehensive understanding of precisely how botulinum toxin works in the human body or how our bodies fully respond to the toxin. We do know that it temporarily paralyzes muscle by inhibiting the release of acetylcholine, and it also appears to inhibit the release of other neurotransmitters. Botulinum toxin's unique ability to temporarily paralyze muscle and potentially inhibit nociceptive neuropeptide release has stimulated physicians and scientists from a wide range of medical disciplines to seek to exploit it with the purpose of benefiting their respective patient populations. Although the temporary nature of the effects of botulinum toxin means that the injections must be repeated periodically, it also minimizes the impact of potential side effects.

The idea for this book occurred to me gradually as I continued to speak with colleagues from various disciplines, many of whom were, or had heard of, using botulinum toxin within their respective specialties. It is rare indeed to find one drug that can simultaneously help people suffering with headaches, speaking and swallowing difficulties, vision problems, back pain, spasticity, urinary problems, gastrointestinal problems, foot pain, shooting leg pains, and profuse sweating. Botulinum toxin does all of this while, at the same time, is able to help people get rid of unwanted wrinkles. This book aims to define our current state of knowledge of botulinum toxin and, in particular, how the use of this novel compound fits into the various overall treatment algorithms. There are still many questions related to botulinum toxin. Will resistance develop and become widespread with increased usage? Will the toxin be a cost-effective treatment in the long run? Will more subtypes of the toxin find therapeutic use? Clearly, as research continues and as we learn more about how botulinum toxin works, its role in current treatment algorithms will become better defined. At the same time, new algorithms for its use are likely to emerge.

I hope you find *Therapeutic Uses of Botulinum Toxin* enjoyable to read and useful for your practice. If you are a spine and musculoskeletal medicine doctor like me, ideally, you will be able to sit with this book over a cappuccino or a glass of wine and read about how our colleagues in other disciplines are using botulinum toxin for their patients. Similarly, I hope that no matter which medical or scientific discipline you practice, you will take the time to read all of the chapters. I encourage you to do so because first, each chapter is fascinating in its own right, and second, because learning how a drug is used in one patient population may awaken you to explore its use in novel ways in your own patients. It is my sincere hope that one of the benefits of this book will be to stimulate responsible research into how botulinum toxin can be used for the benefit of more patients in the future.

*Grant Cooper, MD*

# Acknowledgments

This book has been a true team effort. I would like to first acknowledge and thank its contributing authors. This book required the hard work of leading physicians from a broad range of medical specialties. It is their selfless dedication, experience, and expertise that made this book possible. I would like to also give a special acknowledgement and thank you to Humana Press, an outstanding publishing company to work with. Patrick Marton, Amy Thau, and Melissa Caravella are important team members that have made this book possible. Don Odom was instrumental in putting this book in motion. Richard Lansing has been a joy to work with and has ensured this book's success as it has passed through its different phases of development.

I would like to take this opportunity to also thank some of my early mentors who helped lay the foundation for all that I do. Without caring, insightful, and selfless teachers helping us along our journey, I don't think any of us would have the opportunity to reach our full potential. I would especially like to thank Dr. Roger Rossi for showing me how compassionate a physician can be; Dr. Roger Pine for teaching me cardiology, and for showing me what it means to carry oneself with grace, style, and humility; and Dr. Kevin Barry, my good friend and mentor, for showing me how to stand strong in the face of raging winds, and for always reminding me that common sense and perspective are our best friends. Thank you to Dr. Richard Meyer for shepherding me with kindness, patience, and wisdom through my medical school sub-internship in medicine. I learned more during that rotation than perhaps any other. Thank you to Dr. Robert Carty for showing me how a doctor can have a loving family, treat his patients with dignity and compassion, and still make time for medical students. Dr. Carty reached out and, through acts of everyday kindness, made a difference. Finally, it is my privilege to extend a very special thank you to Dr. Richard Holstein. Dr. Holstein's intelligence, fairness, commitment to excellence, and, above all, integrity is a source of continual inspiration.

This book would not have been possible without my wife, Ana. Her love, support, and close counsel make everything I do possible. I would also like to thank my parents for their continued unwavering support (for each of the steps I take, big or small).

# Contents

*xi*

# Contributors

MARY S. BABCOCK, DO, MAJ MC USA • Director, CME Physical Medicine and Rehabilitation Service, Department of Orthopedics and Rehabilitation, Walter Reed Army Medical Center, Washington, DC; Department of Neurology, Uniformed Services University of the Health Sciences, Bethesda, MD

GREGORY T. BALES, MD • Associate Professor, Section of Urology, Department of Surgery, University of Chicago Hospital, Chicago, IL

LESLIE BAUMAN, MD • Chief, Division of Cosmetic Dermatology, Department of Clinical Dermatology, University of Miami, Miller School of Medicine, Miami, FL

C. ROBERT BERNARDINO, MD, FACS • Assistant Professor, Section of Oculoplastics and Orbital Surgery, Department of Ophthalmology, Emory University School of Medicine, Atlanta, GA

ANDREW BLITZER, MD, DDS • Professor of Clinical Otolaryngology, Columbia University; Director, NY Center for Voice and Swallowing Disorders; Medical Director, NY Center for Clinical Research, New York, NY

REBECCA BROWN, MD • Resident, Department of Rehabilitation Medicine, Mount Sinai School of Medicine, New York, NY

AMIR COHEN, MD, MBA • Resident, Department of Ophthalmology, New York Medical College, New York, NY

GRANT COOPER, MD • Resident, Department of Physical Medicine and Rehabilitation, New York-Presbyterian Hospital, The University Hospital of Columbia and Cornell, New York, NY

FRANK FRIEDENBERG, MD • Associate Professor, Department of Medicine, Temple University Hospital, Philadelphia, PA

LOREN M. FISHMAN, MD, BPhil (OXON) • Assistant Clinical Professor, Department of Rehabilitation Medicine, Columbia College of Physicians and Surgeons, New York, NY

JOSEPH E. HERRERA, DO • Director of Sports Medicine, Interventional Spine and Sports Medicine Division, Department of Rehabilitation Medicine, Mount Sinai School of Medicine, New York, NY

SHAYAN IRANI, MD • Senior Fellow, Gastroenterology Section, Department of Medicine, Temple University School of Medicine, Philadelphia, PA

JOELY KAUFMAN, MD • Assistant Professor, Department of Dermatology, University of Miami, Miller School of Medicine, Miami, FL

DAVID KHORAMIAN, BA • New York Medical College, New York, NY

AVNIEL KLEIN, MD • Chief Resident, Department of Rehabilitation Medicine, Mount Sinai School of Medicine, New York, NY

DAVID LIN, MD • Associate Professor, Rehabilitation Medicine, Weil-Cornell University Hospital, New York, NY

ZINOVY MEYLER, DO • Resident, Department of Physical Medicine and Rehabilitation, New York-Presbyterian Hospital, The University Hospital of Columbia and Cornell, New York, NY

ISAAC M. NEUHAUS, MD • Assistant Professor, Department of Dermatology, University of California, San Francisco, San Francisco, CA

ALENA POLESIN, MD • Clinical Instructor, Department of Rehabilitation Medicine, Weill-Cornell Medical School, New York, NY

DAVID E. RAPP, MD • Resident, Section of Urology, Department of Surgery, University of Chicago Pritzker School of Medicine, Chicago, IL

STEVEN E. SAMPSON, MD • Chief Resident, Department of Rehabilitation Medicine, St. Vincent's Medical Center, New York, NY

JEROME S. SCHWARTZ, MD • Junior Attending, Department of Clinical Otolaryngology, St. Luke's-Roosevelt Hospital Center, New York Center for Voice and Swallowing Disorders, New York, NY

PHILLIP SONG, MD • Junior Attending, Department of Clinical Otolaryngology, St. Luke's-Roosevelt Hospital Center, New York Center for Voice and Swallowing Disorders, New York, NY

MARC SPIRN, MD • Resident, Department of Opthalmology, Emory University School of Medicine, Atlanta, GA

MICHAEL D. STUBBLEFIELD, MD • Assistant Attending, Rehabilitation Service, Memorial Sloan-Kettering Cancer Center; Rehabilitation Medicine, Weill Medical College of Cornell University, New York, NY

ALEX VISCO, MD • Attending, Physical Medicine and Rehabilitation, Private Practice, New York, NY

# History and Mechanism of Action

## Zinovy Meyler and Grant Cooper

### INTRODUCTION

Usage of botulinum toxin (BTX) for cosmetic treatment was approved by the Food and Drug Administration (FDA) only a few years ago and already Botox® has become a household name. Some people have substituted Tupperware® parties for Botox parties. Few, however, are aware of the fascinating history of Botox and its many therapeutic uses.

It was a bout of sausage poisoning that eventually led to the discovery of a protein we now know as BTX. During the Napoleonic Wars, the Duke of Württemberg in Stuttgart observed an epidemic of deaths resulting from food poisoning. Smoked sausages seemed to be the cause and the poison was referred to as the "sausage poison." In 1802, the government in Stuttgart issued a public notice and warning about the "harmful consumption of smoked blood-sausages." In 1811, the medical section of the Department of Internal Affairs of the Kingdom of Württemberg again discussed the problem of "sausage poisoning" and believed it was caused by prussic acid *(1)*.

### MEDICAL COMMUNITY GETS INVOLVED

Finally, the Medical Faculty at the University of Tübingen was asked for advice. The first answer came from Wilhelm Gottfried von Ploucqet (1744–1814), who disputed that prussic acid could be the toxic agent in sausages, suspecting a "zoonic, possibly organic poison"*(2)*. In a second statement, one of the prominent medical professors at the University of Tübingen, Johann Heinrich Ferdinand Autenrieth (1772–1835), asked the government to collect the reports of general practitioners and health officers on cases of food poisoning. After Autenrieth had studied these reports, he issued a list of symptoms of the so-called "sausage poisoning," such as gastrointestinal problems, double vision, and mydriasis, and added a comment in which he blamed the housewives for the poisoning because they did not boil the sausage long enough, trying to prevent the sausages from bursting *(1)*.

In 1815, a health officer in Herrenberg, J.G. Steinbuch (1770–1818), sent the case reports of seven intoxicated patients who had eaten the same meal (liver sausage and peas) to Professor Autenrieth. Three of the patients had died and the autopsies had been carried out by Steinbuch himself *(2)*.

Simultaneously with Steinbuch, Justinius Kerner, a poet and a medical officer in a small town in Germany also reported cases of lethal food poisoning. Autenrieth considered the two reports from Steinbuch and Kerner as accurate and important observations and decided to publish them

From: *Therapeutic Uses of Botulinum Toxin*
Edited by: G. Cooper © Humana Press Inc., Totowa, NJ

in 1817 in the Tübinger papers for natural sciences and pharmacology. Kerner observed more cases and published his first monograph in 1820 on sausage poisoning, entitled "New Observations on the Lethal Poisoning Occurring So Frequently in Württemberg Through the Consumption of Smoked Sausages." Kerner summarized the case histories of 76 patients and gave a complete clinical description of what neurologists now recognize as botulism *(2)*.

After he had moved to Weinsberg, Kerner intensified his activities in toxin research. In 1821, he started animal experiments as well as self-experimentation. Kerner had the objective to extract and isolate the unknown toxic substance from sausages that he called "sausage poison" or "fatty acid." In 1822, Kerner published the results of his work and his hypotheses on the sausage toxin in a second monograph: "Das Fettgift oder die Fettsäure und ihre Wirkungen auf den thierischen Organismus, ein Beytrag zur Untersuchung des in verdorbenen Würsten giftig wirkenden Stoffes" ("The fat poison or the fatty acid and its effects on the animal organism, a contribution to the examination of the substance which acts toxically in bad sausages") *(2)*. The monograph contained the clinical evaluation and summary of 155 case reports of patients with probable botulism, including postmortem studies. In addition, Kerner described his animal experiments in which he had administered BTX extracted from "sour" sausages to birds, cats, rabbits, frogs, flies, locusts, and snails. Kerner deduced from the clinical symptoms and his experimental observations that the toxin acted by an interruption of the signal transmission within the peripheral and the sympathetic and parasympathetic nervous systems, leaving the sensory signal transmission intact. He wrote: "The nerve conduction is brought by the toxin into a condition in which its influence on the chemical process of life is interrupted. The capacity of nerve conduction is interrupted by the toxin in the same way as in an electrical conductor by rust." In the eighth chapter of that monograph, he developed the idea of using the toxin for therapeutic purposes *(2)*.

Kerner performed various chemical reactions with the aqueous extracts from the sausages (e.g., with silver nitrate, mercuric chloride, and ferric chloride). When he had produced enough toxic extract from sausages, he mixed it with honey and fed it to mammals, birds, frogs, flies, locusts, and snails. The symptoms resulting from his cat experiments were particularly comparable with the symptoms of the intoxication Kerner had observed in humans: vomiting, intestinal spasms, mydriasis, ptosis, dysphagia, and finally, respiratory failure.

Finally, Kerner carried out experiments on himself, from which he found that the toxic sausage extracts in fact tasted sour and led to mild symptoms of beginning botulism *(2)*. For the prevention of sausage poisoning, Kerner suggested that sausages should be boiled long enough, stored under aerobic and dry conditions, and that bad parts should not be eaten.

In the final chapter of his 1822 monograph, Kerner discussed the possibility of using the sausage toxin as a remedy for a variety of diseases. Based on his previous experiences, he concluded that the toxin, applied in minimal doses, would lower or block the hyperactivity and hyperexcitability of the "sympathetic nervous system." The term *sympathetic nervous system*, as used during the Romantic period, encompassed nervous functions in general. "Sympathetic" overactivity then was thought to be the cause for many internal, neurological, and psychiatric diseases. Kerner considered other diseases associated with an overactive nervous system to be potential candidates for the toxin treatment: hypersecretion of body fluids, sweat, or mucus; ulcers from malignant diseases; skin alterations after burning; delusions; rabies; plague; consumption from lung tuberculosis; and yellow fever.

## DISCOVERY OF THE BACTERIUM

In 1895, Professor Emile Pierre van Ermengem of Ellezelles, Belgium identified the bacterium—and its toxin—that caused sausage poisoning and accordingly called it *Bacillus botulinus*, from the Latin *botulus* meaning sausage. A few years later, it was renamed *Clostridium botulinum*, hence the term *botulism* is now used to describe what was once known as sausage poisoning *(1)*.

BTX-A was first isolated in purified form as a stable acid precipitate in the early 1920s by Dr. Herman Sommer from California. This precipitate provided the basis of raw materials for future study *(3)*.

During World War II, Stanley Lovell, an American officer in the Office of Strategic Services, ordered the manufacture of gelatin capsules containing the toxin. The plan was for Chinese prostitutes to hide these capsules behind their ears and then slip them into the meals of high-level Japanese officials. In 1946, Dr. Edward Schantz, a young US army officer stationed at Fort Detrick, and other colleagues purified BTX in great quantities for use in government and educational institutes. In 1969, The United States declared that it would unilaterally destroy all their biological weapons stocks and in 1972 the Biological and Toxins Weapons Convention Treaty was signed by more than 100 countries. President Nixon ordered Fort Detrick to close all laboratories for biological agents offensive programs and Dr. Schantz went to the University of Wisconsin to continue his research *(4)*.

## BOTULINUM TOXIN STUDIED

The first major result of BTX studies occurred in the 1950s, when Dr. Vernon Brooks discovered that BTX type A (BTX-A), when injected into a hyperactive muscle, blocked the release of acetylcholine from motor nerve endings, thus inducing a temporary "paralysis" of the targeted muscle *(3)*. Dr. Brooks' breakthrough sparked new interest in BTX as a potentially significant therapeutic agent.

In the 1960s and 1970s, Dr. Alan B. Scott of the Smith-Kettlewell Eye Research Foundation tested BTX-A in monkeys to determine if the drug might be an effective therapy for strabismus, a type of "ophthalmic dystonia," in humans. Having heard about Dr. Schantz's research with BTX, Dr. Scott contacted Dr. Schantz at the University of Wisconsin to obtain product samples. Dr. Scott found that by injecting a small amount of BTX in the hyperactive ocular muscles in monkeys he was able to correct the strabismic condition. For the next 20 years, Dr. Schantz collaborated with Dr. Scott to develop BTX-A for human treatment.

In the late 1970s, Dr. Scott formed his own company, Oculinum, Inc., where he continued to study BTX-A. In 1978, Dr. Scott received permission from the FDA to test BTX-A in human volunteers *(3)*. The original batch of 150 mg was used for more than 250,000 injections in humans. For many years, this was the only batch approved by the FDA, which requires batch approval for biological drugs. It was not until 1997 that the FDA approved a new bulk toxin source for use in the manufacture of BTX-A *(4)*. The new product, today known as Botox, is comparable in clinical efficacy to the original Botox, but the higher specific potency reduces the amount of neurotoxin protein utilized, which in turn leads to a reduction in the production of antibodies. In 2000, the FDA approved Botox, manufactured by Allergan, Inc. (Irvine, CA), for the treatment of abnormal head positions and neck pain associated with cervical dystonia. At that time, the FDA also approved Myobloc® for the same indication.

Myobloc is the US trade name for BTX-B from Elan Pharmaceuticals (San Francisco, CA). Finally, in 2002 the FDA approved Botox, synthesized by Allergan, for cosmetic treatment of wrinkes at the brow line *(4)*.

## NORMAL NEUROMUSCULAR JUNCTION

The history of the discovery of BTX is indeed remarkable. What is even more remarkable is the way it produces its effect. Let us take a closer look at the action of BTX at the neuromuscular junction (NMJ) or as it is otherwise known, the myoneural junction.

First, a few words about the normal physiology of the NMJ. The NMJ is formed by the terminal branch of the motor neuron and the muscle fiber that it innervates. At this chemical synapse, the action potential causes release of the neurotransmitter (acetylcholine) from the presynaptic neuron. Acetylcholine then diffuses across the synaptic space and binds to the receptors on the postsynaptic neuron, causing a change in the electrical properties of that membrane, which ultimately results in the contraction of the muscle fiber.

Acetylcholine is stored in the synaptic vesicles that are released into the synaptic cleft by fusion with the presynaptic membrane, through the process of exocytosis. The fusion and exocytosis are a consequence of an influx of calcium ions through voltage-dependent channels that is triggered by a nerve action potential arriving at the terminal membrane. Let us take a closer look at the synaptic vesicle itself—the site of action of BTX.

Calcium-regulated exocytosis is a complicated process that involves the actions of proteins located on the vesicles in the cytosol and on the presynaptic membrane. Synapsin I links the synaptic vesicle to the cytoskeleton. Phosphorylation of synapsin I, which is a calcium-dependent process, leads to the release of the vesicle from the cytoskeleton, which is then transported into the active zone, where it fuses with the presynaptic membrane *(5)*. Synaptobrevin on the synaptic vesicle and syntaxin on the presynaptic membrane act as anchors that pull the membranes together. It is believed that synaptosome-associated protein-25, which is attached to the presynaptic membrane, binds two molecules of syntaxin, which forms a complex *(6)*. Synaptobrevin binds to this complex and displaces one of the syntaxin molecules from the complex, which brings the synaptic vesicle and the presynaptic membrane into the proximity that is necessary for fusion and exocytosis to take place *(5)*. As mentioned previously, the mechanism of exocytosis of synaptic vesicles is complex and not completely understood at this point; however, it has been demonstrated that a coordinated action of the above described proteins is necessary for the release of acetylcholine and subsequent contraction of the muscle fiber to occur. Therefore, anything interfering with the action of the proteins would cause a neuromuscular blocking effect, which is exactly where BTX comes in.

## BOTULINUM TOXIN MECHANISM OF ACTION

As previously mentioned, BTX is produced by *Clostridium botulinum*, a Gram-positive anaerobic bacterium. It is broken down into seven neurotoxins: types A, B, C1, C2, D, E, F, and G. The neurotoxin types are structurally similar, but serologically and antigenically distinct *(7)*. BTX effects in humans are mainly caused by types A, B, E, and rarely F. Types C and D affect animals only. Its molecule is synthesized as a single chain, which is then cleaved to form a two chain molecule with a disulfide bridge.

The light chain acts as a zinc endopeptidase with proteolytic activity at the N-terminal end. The heavy chain provides cholinergic specificity and binds the toxin to presynaptic

**Table 1**
**Botulinum Toxin Types, Target Sites, and Discoverers**

| Year | Discoverer | Type | Receptor | Clinical Use |
|------|------------|------|----------|--------------|
| 1897 | Wrmengem | B | Synaptobrevin | FDA Approved |
| 1904 | Landman | A | SNAP-25 | FDA Approved |
| 1922 | Bengston & Seldon | C | Syntaxin | Not FDA Approved |
| 1929 | Robinson | D | Synaptobrevin | Not FDA Approved |
| 1936 | Gunnison | E | SNAP-25 | Not FDA Approved |
| 1960 | Moller & Scheibel | F | Synaptobrevin | Not FDA Approved |
| 1970 | Gimenez & Ciccarelli | G | Synaptobrevin | Not FDA Approved |

receptors, in addition to promoting the light chain translocation across the endosomal membrane. The toxin produces its effect by cleaving the specific target proteins in the neuroexocytosis apparatus, thus impairing the docking and fusion of synaptic vesicles at the terminal presynaptic membrane.

BTX-A and BTX-E cleave synaptosome-associated protein-25. BTX-B, BTX-D, and BTX-F cleave synaptobrevin, and BTX-C cleaves syntaxin. Table 1 lists BTX types, receptors, year discovered, and discoverers *(3)*.

BTX, used therapeutically, gives a neuromuscular blocking effect as the basis of its effect. This effect is temporary. Currently, the exact mechanism of the recovery from the blocking effect is not well defined, but is thought to occur through proximal axonal sprouting and muscle re-innervation by formation of a new NMJ *(8)*. However, other researchers suggest that eventually, the original NMJ regenerates.

After more than 100 years of discoveries, tests, and more discoveries, BTX is nothing short of a phenomenon and a breakthrough that is being used in a growing variety of medical disciplines, for a growing number of medical conditions. It is doubtless that as our understanding of BTX grows, so too will our ability to use it with increasing efficacy for a growing number of patients.

## REFERENCES

1. Erbguth FJ. Historical notes on botulism, *Clostridium botulinum*, botulinum toxin, and the idea of the therapeutic use of the toxin. Mov Dis 2004;19:S2–S6.
2. Erbguth FJ, Naumann M. Historical aspects of botulinum toxin: Justinus Kerner (1786–1862) and the "sausage poison." Neurology 1999;53:1850.
3. Kedlaya D. Botulinum toxin: overview. Available from: http://www.emedicine.com/pmr/topic216. htm#section~author_information. Accessed Jan. 23, 2006.
4. Garland Science. Botulinum toxin: core materials. Available from: http://www.garlandscience.com/ textbooks/cbl/CoreMaterials/timeline.html. Accessed: Jan. 22, 2006.
5. Meriggioli MN, Howard JF Jr., Harper CM. Neuromuscular Junction Disorders, Diagnosis and Treatment. New York, NY: Marcel Dekker; 2003.
6. Blasi J, Chapman ER, Link E, et al. Botulinum neurotoxin A selectively cleaves the synaptic protein SNAP-25. Nature 1993;365:160–163.
7. Jankovic J, Brin MF. Botulinum toxin: historical perspective and potential new indications. Muscle Nerve Suppl 1997;6:S129–S145.
8. Brin MF. Botulinum toxin: chemistry, pharmacology, toxicity, and immunology. Muscle Nerve Suppl 1997;6:S146–S168.

## Elise Weiss and David Lin

## INTRODUCTION

Spasticity is a component of many neurological conditions, including multiple sclerosis (MS), cerebral palsy, spinal cord injury, stroke, and brain injury. First described in the 19th century, spasticity is a velocity-dependent increase in stretch reflex activity. Peter Nathan described it as "a condition in which stretch reflexes that are normally latent become obvious. The tendon reflexes have a lowered threshold to tap, the response of the tapped muscle is increased, and usually, muscles besides the tapped one respond; tonic stretch reflexes are affected in the same way" *(1)*. Although appearing straightforward, a search of current literature shows that there is disagreement over the exact definition of spasticity. Some authors include clonus, hyperactive tendon reflexes, and spasms, whereas others find these physical findings to be associated with spasticity but separate from what is a more restricted definition of velocity-associated increased muscle tone.

Decq recently suggested that spasticity is a "positive" sign of a more inclusive upper motor neuron syndrome. The "negative" signs include weakness and loss of dexterity *(1)*. The upper motor neuron syndrome is characterized by a generalized increase in spinal reflexes attributed to a hyperexcitable motor neuron pool. Decq further separated spasticity into categories of intrinsic tonic spasticity, intrinsic phasic spasticity, and extrinsic spasticity. Each of these categories is manifested as a different component of the overall clinical syndrome. Increased tonic spasticity equates to a generalized increase in tone, whereas intrinsic phasic spasticity results in tendon hyperreflexia and clonus. Extrinsic spasticity is seen as an exaggeration of spinal reflexes in response to what is usually a noxious stimulus.

## PATHOPHYSIOLOGY

The defining characteristic of spasticity is a muscle's excessive resistance to passive stretch. A complete explanation of the pathophysiology of spasticity does not exist but the exaggerated response of stretch reflexes is often used as a starting point to explain the clinical manifestations of this condition. At its most basic level, the stretch reflex is a monosynaptic reflex pathway originating in the muscle spindles positioned parallel to extrafusal muscle fibers *(2)*. Alterations in this pathway have been linked to spasiticty. Injury to the spinal cord, peripheral nerve, or cerebral cortex can alter the message that is ultimately delivered to a motor neuron.

From: *Therapeutic Uses of Botulinum Toxin*
Edited by: G. Cooper © Humana Press Inc., Totowa, NJ

Clinically, the stretch reflex causes a muscle that is stretched to respond by contracting. This response is owing in large part to the muscle spindle. The muscle spindle has its own motor efferent, the gamma neuron. The γ-efferents adjust the length of the muscle spindle by contracting or relaxing the intrafusal fibers. In this way, they maintain the spindle's comparative length relationship to the extrafusal fibers. Supraspinal control of γ-efferents is responsible for the inherent tone of muscle *(3)*.

It stands to reason that when a muscle stretches, everything within it stretches as well. If the intrafusal spindle fibers within the muscle are not altered by the γ-efferent in proportion to the stretch of the extrafusal fibers, then the spindle's receptor site will be altered *(4)*. In response, action potentials generate along the Ia afferent sensory endings. These impulses travel through the dorsal root of the spinal nerve trunk into the spinal cord where a monosynaptic connection occurs within the anterior horn of the gray matter. The motor neuron travels through the ventral root of the spinal nerve trunk to innervate the specific motor unit of the muscle in which the impulse originated. The Ia fiber also connects with an inhibitory interneuron that makes contact with the α-motor neurons of antagonistic muscles. The result is contraction of extrafusal fibers that comprise the agonist motor unit and inhibition of extrafusal fibers that comprise the antagonistic motor unit *(4)*. Action potentials from the receptor site cease when the extrafusal fibers surrounding the muscle spindle shorten the spindle length and remove the stimulus for Ia afferent impulses.

In this context, two pathological states working in conjunction or alone can favor an increased stretch reflex: a hyper-excitable efferent α-motor neuron or an increased excitatory Ia fiber in the spindle afferent. Either of these states can be attributed to increased primary excitation or decreased inhibition at either the spinal or the supraspinal level. With this in mind, spasticity is said to be cerebral or spinal in nature. Spasticity caused by spinal cord lesions is marked by a slow increase in excitation of flexors and extensors resulting in hyperactivity. Cerebral lesions often cause rapid excitation with antigravity muscles more commonly involved than other muscle groups *(5)*.

Using the stretch reflex model as outlined by Decq, the spasticity component of the upper motor neuron syndrome can be further defined. Tonic spasticity, or increased muscle tone, is thought to be the result of a combination of denervation hypersensitivity and changed muscle properties that result from an interrupted stretch reflex arc. Denervation leads to an initial downregulation of neuronal membrane receptors, followed by an upregulation, with enhanced sensitivity to neurotransmitters. Gradual changes in muscle properties also occur, such as fibrosis, atrophy of muscle fibers, decrease in the elastic properties, decrease in the number of sarcomeres, and accumulation of connective tissues. All of these changes alter the contractile properties of muscle, which likely contributes to increased passive tension of muscle to stretch *(6)*.

Intrinsic phasic spasticity includes symptoms such as tendon hyper-reflexia and clonus, and results from exaggeration of the phasic component of the stretch reflex. It is thought that the normal mechanism of presynaptic inhibition in the spinal cord is altered in patients with spasticity, creating an enhanced central excitatory state primed for exaggerated responses. Supraspinal influences adjust Ia afferent activity originating from the muscle spindle. It is thought that the interneuron responsible for this inhibition is less active in patients with spasticity, effectively making a patient's stretch reflex not subject to tonic presynaptic control. As a result, all afferent impulses are able to gain direct access to α-motor neurons allowing for hyperreflexia and clonus *(6)*.

In addition to the various intrinsic factors that contribute to symptoms of spasticity, involuntary muscle spasms can also occur in response to a perceived noxious stimuli originating extrinsic to the muscle. Flexion spasms are the most common form of extrinsic spasticity, triggered by afferent input from skin, muscle, subcutaneous tissues, and joints. These so-called flexor reflex afferents mediate the polysynaptic reflexes involved in the flexion withdrawal reflex *(6)*. Upon disruption of normal descending influences, the threshold for the flexor withdrawal reflex may become lowered, the response of the system may become raised, or both may occur together.

## RISK FACTORS

Overall, spasticity affects about 500,000 people in the United States and more than 12 million people throughout the world *(6)*. The number of people affected depends on the cause of the spasticity. It is present in many patients with cerebral palsy, traumatic brain injury, stroke, neurodegenerative diseases affecting the motor system, MS, and spinal cord injury. It is not influenced by age, race, or sex.

## HISTORY/CLINICAL EXAMINATION

Spasticity is characterized by muscle hypertonia and exaggerated tendon reflexes. Increased stretch reflex activity may be manifested as increased muscle tone, exaggerated tendon jerks, spread of phasic stretch reflexes in response to tendon hammer percussion, and repetitive stretch reflex discharges (clonus) generated by sustained stretch. It is often associated with weakness, slow building to maximal muscle power, and difficulty with voluntary muscle movement. These features can be attributed in large part to incoordination of synergistic muscle and failure to inhibit antagonistic muscles *(7)*. Despite the characteristic features of spasticity, it is quite diverse in its clinical manifestation secondary to differing etiologies, chronicity, and nervous system compensation.

A complete physical examination, including a thorough musculoskeletal and neurological evaluation is necessary when assessing a patient with spasticity. Strength, reflexes, and range of motion are all evaluated. The physician moves the patient's joints through achievable range of motion at various speeds. A spastic muscle may catch or snag midway. Patients must be examined very closely to determine which spastic muscles are detrimental to a patient's function. Many patients have a mixture of agonist and antagonist contraction, which may limit extremity motion. The patient may also have underlying muscle weakness. Treatment of spasticity in this case would be detrimental to a patient's overall function.

Chronic spasticity can lead to changes in muscle properties. Stiffness, atrophy, and fibrosis may impact limb movement and position. It is important to distinguish the level of impairment that is secondary to spasticity and the level of impairment that is secondary to pathological changes in the muscle itself. Electromyography (EMG) or nerve block may help in making this distinction *(5)*.

The original and modified Ashworth scales, physician rating scale (gait pattern and range of motion), and spasm frequency scale are widely used to measure exam findings. To use the Ashworth or physician rating scales, the clinician moves the patient's limb through a range of motion and scores the muscle tone for each limb. It is a subjective measure of spasticity. The Ashworth scale is rated 0 to 6 with 6 being severe spasticity. More often, the modified Ashworth scale is used. On this scale, 0 represents no increase in muscle tone while 4 represents increased tone in flexion or extension. The spasm scale requires the number of spasms in an hour to be counted. This is a more objective attempt to quantify spasticity. Zero represents no spasms while a maximum of 4 represents 10 or more spasms in the course of a day.

With rare exception, spasticity will impact a patient's function. Functional scales such as the functional independence measure or the Fugl-Meyer scale are widely used to capture the degree of disability and impairment. These are not direct scales of spasticity. Some believe the functional independence measure is insensitive to the functional changes in patients with spasticity. As such, the Fugl-Meyer scale, which uses a three-step approach to test function in the extremities is more widely used. A score of less than 50 out of 100 is consistent with severe motor impairment. Although not a specific test of spasticity, the Fugl-Meyer scale is a good measure of sensorimotor impairment.

## DIAGNOSTIC EVALUATION

EMG is a valuable tool in the assessment and treatment of spasticity. EMG recordings can determine which muscles are overactive or inappropriately contracting during a movement. Analysis of recruitment pattern can determine if the target muscle is paretic. A silent EMG may suggest contracture. The most frequently used technique is dynamic multichannel EMG. When matched with gait laboratory technology, electrical activity from multiple muscles can be obtained while the patient is moving. Gait analysis can be used alone to analyze the forces and angles of the joints while in motion. This can be quite useful in planning operations to treat spasticity *(1)*.

In general, objective measures of spasticity have been expensive and impractical in their application to a clinical environment. These research-oriented measurement tools include EMG-obtained H reflex and threshold angle torque measurements. The H reflex is essentially a measure of a monosynaptic reflex elicited by stimulating a nerve with an electric shock. It is often paired with the M response to quantify a patient's spasticity. The H/M ratio tends to be higher in those with spasticity. The threshold angle is defined as the joint angle at which torque, stretch reflex activity, and EMG activity begin to increase in an initially silent muscle. Although attempts have been made to use these measures in a clinical setting, they tend to be impractical and poorly correlate with clinical measures *(8)*.

## DIFFERENTIAL DIAGNOSIS

Spasticity is a symptom of many different conditions. Spinal cord injury, brain injury, tumor, stroke, MS, and cerebral palsy can all be associated with spasticity. It can co-exist with many other conditions that easily confuse the examiner. Spasticity should be carefully distinguished from rigidity, dystonia, athetoid, chorea, ballisms, and tremor. Rigidity is involuntary bidirectional resistance to movement that does not change with velocity. It should be present at rest, whereas spasticity is always velocity-dependent. Dystonia is involuntary sustained contractures that can result in abnormal positions. Athetoid movement is involuntary irregular writhing movements, whereas chorea is similar to athetoid but more abrupt, rapid, and irregular in nature. Ballism is involuntary movements of the limbs or body in which large flinging motions are made, whereas tremor is an involuntary rhythmic repetitive oscillation that is not self-sustaining. Spasticity may also be mistaken for seizure activity, but it is not followed by a postictal period and it tends to not be rhythmic.

As mentioned, the etiologies of spasticity are numerous. Some of the conditions are quite treatable and reversible. As such, an underlying cause for spasticity should always be sought.

Tethered spinal cord, central nervous system (CNS) tumor, nerve impingement, hydrocephalus, and intracranial bleeds can all result in spasticity. Symptoms can be eliminated with appropriate diagnosis and effective treatment of the underlying disorder.

It should also be noted that multiple factors can exacerbate the condition of an already spastic patient. Infection, pressure sores, noxious stimuli, deep venous thrombosis, bladder distention, bowel impaction, cold weather, fatigue, seizures, and malpositioning can all increase muscle tone and account for a patient presenting with increased symptoms. These conditions should always be ruled out when a patient presents with a change from baseline spasticity. This is particularly relevant in the spinal cord injury population, in which a change in spasm frequency may be the only sign of a more insidious process.

## TREATMENT APPROACH

When treating spasticity, a team approach is most appropriate. The team may include a physiatrist, physical therapist, occupational therapist, neurologist and/or orthopedic surgeon, and neurosurgeon. Typical goals of treatment include pain reduction, improved mobility, increased range of motion, avoidance or reversal of contracture, improvement in positioning, and proper fitting of bracing devices.

In meeting these goals, the advantages of increased tone must be considered. Spasticity can substitute for strength with direct improvements in walking, transfers, and assuming an upright posture. The intrinsic increase in muscle tone may also serve to reduce the risk of osteoporosis and decrease the risk of deep venous thrombosis and edema.

Despite the advantages of spasticity, it is obvious that there is quite a bit of morbidity associated with the condition. Tension on the bones while minimizing osteoporosis may lead to orthopedic deformity, such as hip dislocation, scoliosis, and contracture. This may make mobility and activities of daily living more difficult. It may also result in skin breakdown as additional pressure is added to areas not accustomed to mechanical stress. Pain is often associated with spasticity and should always be a consideration in formulating a treatment plan for patients.

With the above considerations in mind, patient function and quality of life is the ultimate measure of treatment success. As a result, the treatment plan varies from patient to patient and no distinct all-inclusive algorithm exists. Perhaps the only universal recommendation is that all patients participate in regular range-of-motion exercises, which may serve to prevent contractures, desensitize nociceptors, and reduce abnormal motor neuron activity *(1)*. Beyond this recommendation, the first step in evaluating a patient with spasticity is to determine if function is negatively impacted or deformity exists. If neither of these situations pertain to the patient, then no further treatment may be necessary.

If a patient is limited by spasticity, then a number of treatment strategies can be attempted. A treatment plan is formulated in conjunction with the patient and/or caregiver to meet agreed functional goals. Although an increase in mobility or dexterity is the desire of many, at times the ease of care-giving is the primary objective. Either of these functional goals can be further defined by what musculoskeletal alteration must be achieved. Depending on the limitation, tone reduction, improved range of motion, or altered joint position may be the goal of treatment. Each of these goals may require a different treatment strategy.

Chronicity, symptom distribution, and severity of spasticity will all influence the method by which musculoskeletal goals are achieved. A management plan may include less invasive treatments, such as physical and occupational therapy, splinting, bracing, and oral medications, or more invasive treatments, such as botulinum toxin (BTX) or phenol injections, intrathecal baclofen, or surgery. Additionally, treatment may be aimed locally as with Botox® injections or systemically as with intrathecal baclofen or oral medication.

Spasticity can develop after a variety of injuries to the upper motor neuron but its development is neither universal nor immediate nor permanent. Spasticity may improve as neurological recovery occurs; if a patient had a recent injury and symptoms are rapidly improving, no treatment may be necessary. If treatment is undertaken it will likely be conservative and aimed at aiding rehabilitation efforts during neurological recovery. Mild spasticity may initially be treated with splinting, orthotics, range-of-motion exercises, and oral medication. Severe spasticity is less likely to respond to these conservative measures and is more likely to entail long-term management strategies. Ultimately, surgery may be required because patients with chronic and severely spasticity are predisposed to the development of contractures.

The distribution of spasticity will guide whether treatment is aimed globally or at a more focal location. A patient with diffuse spasticity may benefit from intrathecal baclofen or oral medication, whereas a patient with more local symptoms may benefit from phenol or Botox injections. A patient with a local but fixed contracture may require surgery to release the joint. Similarly, the origin of injury must be considered. Spasticity of spinal cord origin tends to respond better to oral baclofen than that of CNS origin.

As stated previously, physical therapy is a mainstay of treatment. It is the most preferred intervention for children. Programs aim to improve range of motion and mobility, increase coordination and strength, improve self-care, and reduce muscle tone. Motivation of the patient is paramount to the success of any therapy program and results tend to vary with the physical therapist's skill and experience.

Stretching forms the central basis of physical therapy. It helps to maintain full range of motion of the joint and prevents contracture. Underlying spasticity, there may be muscle weakness. As such, strengthening exercises are aimed at restoring the proper level of strength to the affected limb. Orthoses, serial casting, and braces allow for more functional joint positions to be obtained and maintained. Proper limb positioning can improve comfort and reduce spasticity.

Modalities are of some use in the treatment of spasticity. Heat and cold packs are typically used to provide temporary relief of pain and have been shown to reduce tone. Electrical stimulation can stimulate a weak muscle to oppose the activity of a stronger spastic muscle. This may reduce spasticity and deformity even if for a limited amount of time. Biofeedback is yet another method that is increasingly employed. It uses an electrical monitor to create a sound that corresponds with muscle relaxation. With this auditory stimulus, some patients are able to voluntarily reduce muscle tone.

Although physical therapy can be quite effective, oral medications are often used to reduce symptoms in patients suffering from spasticity. Rizzo et al. found that the use of oral medication was proportional to the severity of spasticity. Analysis of 17,501 patients with MS showed that 78% of patients who were severely affected with spasticity used at least one drug, whereas 46% used at least two *(7)*. Baclofen was the most common agent, followed by gabapentin, tizanidine, and diazepam. Although very effective, at high doses these medications cause adverse effects such as sedation and mood changes that may limit their utility. These effects are particularly relevant in children, in whom schooling and learning are easily impaired by these additional obstacles. Systemic toxicities such as liver damage may also result.

Baclofen is a γ-aminobutyric acid (GABA) agonist with its primary site of action in the spinal cord, where it binds to the GABA-B receptor, thereby reducing excitatory neurotransmitters.

Baclofen is particularly effective in reducing spasm frequency and clonus. The oral dose ranges from 10 to 80 mg per day in divided amounts. Tolerance and withdrawal are both risks with this medication. Rapid cessation of the medication can result in seizures, hallucinations, and increased spasticity. Adverse effects include sedation, ataxia, dizziness, nausea, weakness, and fatigue. These effects tend to increase in frequency with dose *(9)*.

Intrathecal infusion of baclofen reduces the adverse effects of this medication. Rizzo et al. also found in the analysis of patients with MS that intrathecal baclofen provided better relief of spasticity, leg stiffness, pain, and spasms. These effects are likely because the drug is concentrated at the level of the spinal cord rather than the brain. Complications of intrathecal baclofen are usually related to mechanical failures of the pump or catheter. This intervention is particularly effective in children *(9)*.

Benzodiazepines also function in modulating the GABA system. Diazepam and clonzepam work at the level of the brain stem and the spinal cord. They increase GABA and GABA-A receptor complex affinity. In doing so, presynaptic inhibition prevails and monosynaptic and polysnaptic reflexes are reduced. While treating hyperreflexia and spasms, these medications also have an anxyolitc effect that can be beneficial. Diazepam has a long half-life of up to 80 hours, whereas clonazepam's half-life extends only to 28 hours. Both drugs should be started at low doses and gradually increased to minimize sedation. Adverse side effects include memory impairment, weakness, incoordination, confusion, depression, and hypotension. Tolerance, dependence, and withdrawal can all occur *(10)*.

Unlike baclofen and benzodiazepines, dantrolene does not act at the level of the CNS. Instead, it acts directly on the muscle decreasing release of calcium from the sarcoplasm reticulum and subsequent muscle contraction. It is most useful for spasticity of supraspinal origin such as cerebral palsy or traumatic brain injury and is less likely to cause adverse cognitive effects. Its half-life is 6 to 9 hours. Adverse effects include generalized weakness that can extend to the respiratory muscles, sedation, weakness, and diarrhea. Liver function should be carefully monitored. It should not be used with tizanidine because of the heaptotoxicity that is associated with both medications.

Numerous studies have shown that tizanidine is an effective option for those suffering from spasticity. It is a central $\alpha$2-noradrenergic agonist and it likely inhibits the H reflex. It may also favor inhibitory rather than excitatory neurotransmitters. Tizanidine is often combined with baclofen or benzodiazepines so that both can be used at lower dosages. In doing so, therapeutic benefits are maximized while adverse effects are reduced. With its extensive hepatic metabolism, tizanidine has a short half-life. As such, timing of use is of paramount importance and liver function should be monitored. Dry mouth, somnolence, orthostasis, and dizziness are common adverse side effects. Clonidine is a medication of the same class but carries a greater risk of orthostasis. As such, its use is less tolerated than tizanidine *(6)*.

Other medications have shown to be useful in select patients but have gained less widespread use. Gabapentin is a GABA analog that modulates enzymes that metabolize glutamate. Lamotrigine blocks sodium channels and reduces the release of glutamate. Cannabinoid compounds have been shown to reduce spasms in select patients. Any of these medications may prove beneficial where others have failed.

The surgical treatment of spasticity has targeted the brain, spinal cord, peripheral nerves, and muscle. Stereotactic brain surgery and cerebellar pacemakers have met with little success. By far the most promising surgical option is selective dorsal rhizotomy for lower extremity spasticity. This procedure involves cutting specific nerve roots between the L2 and S1 or

S2 levels. These fibers enter the posterior spinal cord and carry sensory information from the muscle to the spinal cord. They are targeted in an attempt to restore physiological balance to the alpha motor neuron system. It is thought that brain or spinal cord damage prevents adequate inhibitory signals from dampening the incoming sensory excitatory signals. Selective dorsal rhizotomy is thought to counter this pathology by reducing incoming sensory excitatory signals by 25 to 50%. The best candidate is a person with good strength and balance without contractures in the lower limbs. Many show improvements in range of motion immediately after surgery. Pain, altered sensation, sleep disturbance, bowel and bladder dysfunction, and fatigue may persist after surgery *(11)*.

Musculoskeletal surgery remains an important procedure for the treatment of spasticity. These surgeries are used frequently and aim to lengthen or release muscles and tendons. The majority of these operations are performed on children aged 4 to 8 years to relieve contractures. The most common site for contracture release is the Achilles tendon. The tendon of the contractured muscle is cut and the joint is positioned at a more physiological angle after which a cast is applied. Regrowth of the tendon to this new length occurs over the following weeks. Another procedure often employed is a tendon transfer, in which the attachment point of a spastic muscle is moved so that the muscle is no longer pulling the joint into a deformed position. The split anterior tibial tendon transfer procedure originated by Garrett is one such surgery, which is performed alone or with Achilles release may allow a patient with equinovarus to effectively use an orthotic to ambulate. Osteotomy is also used to correct deformity. In this procedure, a small wedge is removed from a bone to allow it to be repositioned or reshaped. A cast is applied to allow healing. This is used most often to correct hip displacements. A less commonly used procedure is arthrodesis, which involves fusing together bones so that the spastic muscle has a limited opportunity to pull the joint into abnormal position *(11)*.

Many clinicians use a variety of treatments to achieve the overall goal of increased function. Sometimes more local treatments are indicated. Injections of phenol, alcohol, lidocaine, and BTX are appropriate in select patients. Treatment with BTX type A (BTX-A) is particularly useful in patients with focal spasms.

### BTX Injection

Food-borne botulism was recognized as a threat in the 10th century by Emperor Leo VI of Byzantium, but it was not until 1820 that the first clinical description of botulism was documented. The German physician Kerner observed not only flaccid paralysis, but also the associated absence of autonomic secretions, including saliva, tears, sweat, and ear wax. Incredibly, he foresaw the use of BTX in the treatment of muscle tone disorders. It was not until 1989 that Botox therapy was approved by the United States Food and Drug Administration for the treatment of strabismus, blepharospasm, and hemifacial spasm in patients older than 12 years. The use of BTX to treat spasticity in adults and children remains off-label at the time of this chapter's completion *(1)*.

BTX inhibits acetylcholine release at the neuromuscular junction by preventing neurotransmitter-filled vesicles from reaching the presynaptic membrane. Initially, the toxin is internalized via receptor-mediated endocytosis. Once internalized, the light chain, a zinc-dependent protease, begins to exert its effect on its substrate, the synaptosome-associated protein 25 protein of the SNARE docking complex. Cleavage of this complex prevents neurotransmitter exocytosis and results in neuromuscular blockade. The effect of the toxin is seen as early as hours and can last as long as 3 to 4 months. Over this time, muscle function is gradually restored. This is believed to be owing at least in part to regeneration and sprouting of nerve terminals.

BTX injections have several advantages over conventional drug and surgical therapy in the management of spasticity. Permanent destruction of tissue does not occur and systemic effects are rare. In addition, graded degrees of therapeutic effect can be achieved by altering the dosage. Although BTX, with its self limiting effect, may require repeated office visits, it also allows for an overly vigorous response to therapy to be short-lived.

It should be noted that BTX injection is almost never used in isolation but rather it is part of a comprehensive treatment strategy. At the very least, it is complimented by physical and occupational therapy, including bracing when appropriate, to maximize functional gains. At times it is combined with phenol or alcohol neurolysis. With this combination, BTX injection can remain below maximum dosage. This may prove important when there are numerous muscle targets or a patient proves extremely sensitive to its effects. Added benefits of the use of phenol or alcohol include its inexpensive long-term effects.

Clinical trials support the efficacy of BTX injection in the treatment of spasticity associated with a variety of conditions, including MS, stroke, brain injury, neurodegenerative disease, cerebral palsy, and spinal cord injury. Simpson et al. reviewed 18 open-label or double-blind placebo-controlled trials. All showed that BTX injection was effective in the reduction of focal spasticity. No adverse effects were reported and improvements were documented in tone, range of motion, hygiene, gait, and positioning *(7)*.

A series of studies have disputed the efficacy of BTX in treating spasticity. It is thought that these findings have often been owing to poorly designed studies or inadequate measures of disability. For instance, Lagalla et al. found that disability scores were unchanged when stroke patients with upper extremity spasticity were injected with BTX. This did not consider the fact that the patients were newly able to perform self-care activities despite the lack of change in disability scores. It is important to consider areas of importance to study subjects as opposed to global assessment scores *(12)*.

One of the most frequently sited clinical trials supporting the use of BTX for spasticity was performed by Brashear et al. and appeared in the *New England Journal of Medicine* in 2002 *(13)*. In this study, 126 subjects with flexor tone in the wrist and fingers following stroke were identified. When BTX was injected into these spastic muscles, functional disability was reduced as compared with placebo. This study stressed the importance of identifying spasticity that was disabling rather than just symptomatic.

These results have been replicated in patients suffering from other primary conditions. MS is said to be a good disease model to study treatment of spasticity because clinical scales are well developed and validated. Snow et al. performed a double-blind placebo-controlled study of BTX use in patients with MS *(14)*. BTX injections provided significant improvement in spastic contraction of the thigh adductor muscles. This is of particular importance because contracture in this pattern significantly influences sitting, self-care, positioning, and urethral catheterization. Similar results were reproduced by Hyman et al. *(15)*.

It is apparent from clinical trials that choosing an appropriate patient is necessary when considering BTX injections. As with any other treatment strategy, the goals of the intervention must be carefully reviewed with the patient and caregiver. Controlled tone reduction may be practical but it is not enough to validate BTX treatments. The justification of treatment will depend on the ability of the procedure to assist in meeting functional goals. For instance, patients with spasticity tend to have limited underlying voluntary motor control. Spasticity reduction in a patient with poor motor control is unlikely to improve mobility; however, a patient with the treatment goals of improved positioning, self-care, personal hygiene, or comfort may be a more appropriate candidate.

Patterns of spasticity in the upper extremity that have proven particularly responsive to BTX injection include an adducted and internally rotated shoulder, flexed elbow, pronated forearm, flexed wrist, thumb-in-palm, and clenched fist *(16)*. In the lower extremity, BTX injections are most useful in the flexed hip, flexed knee, adducted thighs, extended knee, equinovarus foot, and striatal toe *(16)*.

BTX dosing is individualized to the patient and dependent on target muscle. Usually, one or two joints with their associated muscles are targeted per session. Conservative doses should be used when treating patients with swallowing dysfunction. Adverse effects tend to be minimal but certain conditions require caution. These include patients who have been hypersensitive in the past, those using aminoglycoside antibiotics, those with neuromuscular disease, and women who are pregnant or potentially lactating *(8)*.

The form of BTX most typically used for spasticity in the United States, and the form of BTX used in our clinics, is BTX-A (Botox, Allergan, Inc., Irvine, CA). Dysport®, Linurase™, and Chinese toxin are other formulations of BTX-A not available in the United States. BTX-B (Myobloc®, Solstice Neurosciences, Inc., South San Francisco, CA) is another formulation of BTX available in the United States. This chapter discusses the dosages of BTX-A (Botox) because this is the form of choice discussed most widely in the literature and also the form used for spasticity in our institution. Dosage adjustments need to be made with other formulations.

Botox is supplied in 100 U vials and can be diluted to various concentrations. It is reconstituted with normal saline. Determination of dilution takes into account muscle size and the desired level of effect. For most muscles of average size, a concentration of 1–10 U/0.1 mL is appropriate with a volume of 1.0 mL per site. In very tiny muscles, a smaller volume with higher concentration may be desirable: 10–20 U/0.1 mL with an injected volume of 0.1–0.2 mL per site. Generally it is better to use lower concentrations in multiple sites rather than greater concentrations in one site. The total maximum body dose per visit is usually 400–600 U. This is well below the lethal dose ($LD_{50}$) of Botox at 3000 U *(8)*.

Some practitioners look to past clinical trials to further guide their dosing decision. Injection of 400 U Botox into thigh adductors resulted in significant improvement in spasticity and hygiene versus placebo. Injection of 4.0 U/kg Botox into the medial and lateral gastrocnemius of one or both legs resulted in improved gait pattern and ankle position in patients with cerebral palsy. Seventy-five to 300 U Botox into the elbow and wrist flexors resulted in improvement in patients suffering from a stroke. In general, physicians tend to combine recommendations, clinical data, past patient response, and personal experience when determining appropriate Botox dosage *(2)*.

Once an appropriate dose has been determined, Botox is injected using a 23- to 27-gauge needle. Larger and superficial muscles are identified by palpation, while small or deep muscle groups can be identified by EMG. When using EMG, the objective is to record motor unit potentials that are in close proximity to the needle tip. After palpating for proper anatomy, a reference lead is appropriately placed and a hollow Teflon® EMG needle is inserted into the target muscle. Active maneuvers of the muscle can confirm proper needle placement within the desired muscle. Proximity of the needle to a contracting fascicle can be demonstrated by bi- or triphasic motor unit potentials with a "crisp" sound *(17)*. Further, electrical stimulation can be used to confirm injection placement because the motor point can be accurately localized with a cannulated monopolar needle cathode.

Follow-up appointments are usually scheduled at 3- to 6-month intervals. At that time, the effect of prior doses can be assessed and used to further guide treatment decisions. This timeframe coincides with the return of muscle function and therefore spasticity. Another reason for this dosing schedule is that at intervals less than 3 months, patients are predisposed to the formation of antibodies.

Most people injected with Botox show continued responsiveness, but others do not respond initially or fail to respond with repeated injections. Antibody resistance should be suspected in such cases. The existence of antibodies is suggested by a lack of a beneficial effect following injection. Resistance has been reported in 3 to 10% of patients (5). Less frequent low-dose injections are less likely to result in antibody formation. As such, the smallest amount of Botox necessary to achieve a therapeutic effect should be used. If resistance should develop, some studies suggest that other serotypes of BTX such as Myobloc might provide some benefit. This is an area that needs elucidation from further research.

## CONCLUSION

The etiologies and pathophysiological mechanisms of spasticity are varied and affect a wide array of patients. Although Botox has relatively few approved indications, its use has expanded over the past decade to include the treatment of spasticity, which has proven to be of great benefit in patients with disabling focal muscle overactivity. Appropriate patients must be chosen and functional goals must be clearly outlined and discussed with the patient and caregiver. Once defined, Botox may become part of an overall treatment protocol aimed at maximizing patient function. As further research provides a stronger scientific foundation, the use of BTX injection to treat spasticity as well as numerous other medical conditions will gain wider acceptance.

## REFERENCES

1. Jankovic J, Brin MF. Botulinum toxin: historical perspective and potential new indications. In: Mayer NY, Simpson DM, eds. Spasticity: Etiology, Evaluation, Management and the Role of Botulinum Toxin. New York: WE MOVE; 2005.
2. Jabbari B, Polo KB, Ford G, Grazko MA. Effectiveness of botulinum toxin A in patients with spasticity. Mov Disord 1995;10:379.
3. Koman LA, Mooney IF, Smith BP, Goodman A, Mulvaney T. Management of spasticity in cerebral palsy with botulinum-A toxin: report of a preliminary, randomized, double-blind trial. J Pediatr Orthop 1994;14:299–303.
4. Simpson D. Editorial. Treatment of spasticity with botulinum toxin. Muscle Nerve 2000;23: 447–449.
5. Gormley M, O'Brien C. A clinical overview of treatment decisions in the management of spasticity. In: Mayer NY, Simpson DM, eds. Spasticity: Etiology, Evaluation, Management and the Role of Botulinum Toxin. New York: WE MOVE; 2005.
6. Brin M, Aoki R. Botulinum Toxin Type A: Pharmacology. In Mayer NY, Simpson DM, eds. Spasticity: Etiology, Evaluation, Management and the role of Botulinum Toxin. New York: WE MOVE; 2005.
7. Simpson DM. Clinical Trials of botulinum toxin in the treatment of spasticity. In Mayer NH, Simpson DM, eds. Spasticity: Etiology, Evaluation, Management and the Role of Botulinum Toxin. New York: WE MOVE; 2002, pp. 125–130.
8. Shaari CM, Sanders I. Quantifying how location and dose of botulinum toxin injections affect muscle paralysis. Muscle Nerve 1993;16:964–969.

 9. Van Hemert JCJ. A double-blind comparison of baclofen and placebo in patients with spasticity of cerebral origin. In: Feldman RG, Young RR, Koella WP, eds. Spasticity: Disordered Motor Control. Chicago: Year Book Medical Publishers; 1980, pp. 41–56.

10. Verrier M, MacLeod S, Ashby P. The effect of diazepam on presynaptic inhibition in patients with complete and incomplete spinal cord lesions. Can J Neurol Sci 1975;2:179–184.

11. Bakheit AM. Management of muscle spasticity. Crit Rev Phys Rehabil Med 1996;8:235–252.

12. Lagalla G, Danni M, Reiter F, et al. Post-stroke spasticity management with repeated botulinum toxin injections in the upper limb. Am J Phys Med Rehabil 2000;79:377–384.

13. Brashear A, Gordon MF, Elovic E, et al. Intramuscular injection of botulinum toxin for the treatment of wrist and finger spasticity after stroke. N Engl J Med 2002;347:395–417.

14. Snow BJ, Tsui JK, Bhatt MH, Varelas M, Hashimoto SA, Calne DB. Treatment of spasticity with botulinum toxin: a double blind study. Ann Neurol 1990;28:512–515.

15. Hyman N, Barnes M, Bhakta B, et al. Botulinum toxin (Dysport®) treatment of hip adductor spasticity in multiple sclerosis: a prospective, randomised, double blind, placebo controlled, dose ranging study. J Neurol Neurosurg Psychiatry 2000;68:707–712.

16. Fehlings D. An evaluation of botulinum-A toxin injections to improve upper extremity function in children with hemiplegic cerebral palsy. J Pediatr 2000;137:331–337.

17. O'Brien C. Injection techniques for botulinum toxin using elecromyography and electrical stimulation. In: Mayer NY, Simpson DM, eds. Spasticity: Etiology, Evaluation, Management and the Role of Botulinum Toxin. New York: WE MOVE; 2005.

# 3

# Radiation Fibrosis Syndrome
## *Trismus, Trigeminal Neuralgia, and Cervical Dystonia*

## Michael D. Stubblefield

## INTRODUCTION

Cancer has recently surpassed heart disease as the number one killer of Americans younger than 85 *(1)*. Although prostate and breast cancers are the most common, lung cancer continues as the top killer among cancers because of its relatively poor prognosis *(2)*. Improved survival across most cancer types is the result of progress in cancer prevention, early detection, and better treatment *(3)*.

Although the mortality associated with cancer is relatively easy to characterize, the morbidity often is not. The morbidity associated with cancer is generally related to cancer type and location. The central and peripheral nervous system, for instance, can be involved directly, in spinal cord compression from epidural metastases or leptomeningeal disease, or indirectly from paraneoplastic phenomenon *(4)*. Cancer-related morbidity results not only from the direct and indirect effects of disease, but as importantly, from its treatment *(5)*. Such treatments include surgery, chemotherapy, and radiation therapy, which often result in neuropathic or muscle pain, muscle spasm, spasticity, loss of sensation, or weakness *(6)*. Radiation-induced toxicity is a major cause of long-term disability following cancer treatment. Approximately 50% of cancer patients will receive radiation therapy at some point during the course of their disease and it may play a critical role in 25% of cancer cures.

Botulinum toxin (BTX) injection has emerged as both a primary and adjunctive treatment for musculoskeletal pain, muscle spasms, spasticity, migraines, neuropathic pain, and a variety of other disorders *(7)*. The successful use of BTX in such diverse clinical settings coupled with better understanding of its novel mechanism of action in pain relief has encouraged translation of its use to the cancer setting *(8)*. This chapter discusses the use of BTX injections in the treatment of focal neuropathic pain and painful muscle spasms associated with radiation fibrosis. A variety of other cancer-related disorders will also likely benefit from the use of BTX and will require the application of similar principles and techniques.

## PATHOPHYSIOLOGY

Radiation therapy uses high-energy radiation to kill proliferating tumor cells with relative sparing of the surrounding normal cells, which are typically less active. Two main types of radiation are external beam radiation and internal radiation, also known as brachytherapy. A variety of new dose-sculpting techniques for delivering radiation have been developed.

From: *Therapeutic Uses of Botulinum Toxin*
Edited by: G. Cooper © Humana Press Inc., Totowa, NJ

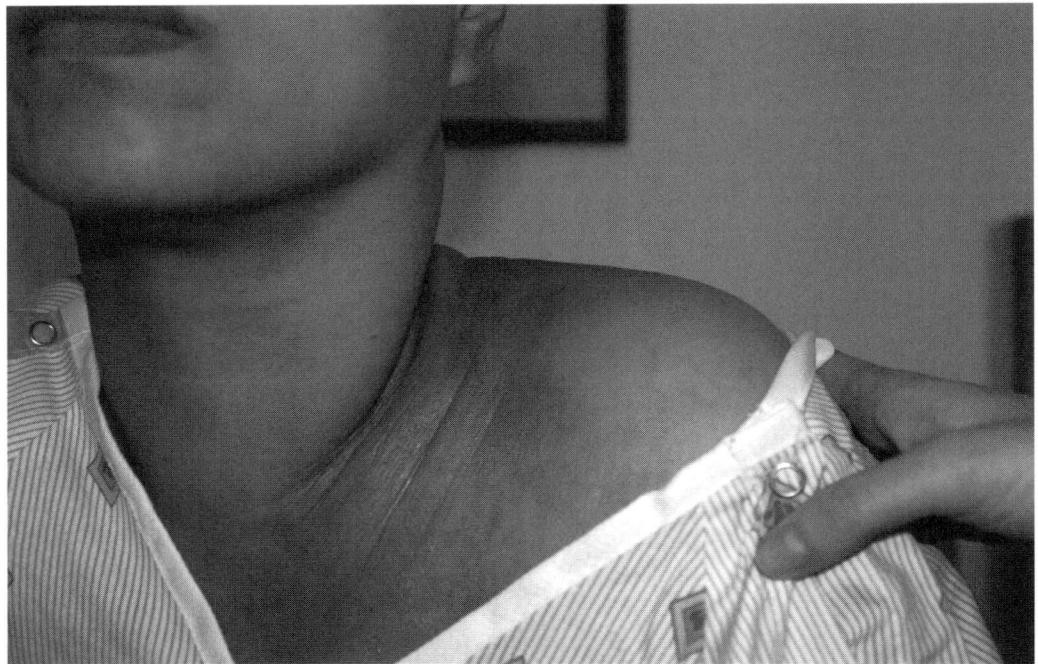

**Fig. 1.** Radiation fibrosis syndrome following radiation to the chest wall for a breast cancer recurrence. Note the dermal erythema and the contracture of the skin and underlying soft tissues.

These include intensity-modulated radiotherapy and image-guided radiotherapy, which allowed the radiation to be conformed to the size and shape of the tumor thereby delivering higher doses of radiation to the tumor while decreasing the radiation exposure to surrounding tissues with a high degree of accuracy *(9)*. Radiation can be used either for intent to cure or palliatively with the intention of prolonging life or function or decreasing pain *(10,11)*. Radiation is often used adjuvantly with surgery or chemotherapy to maximize its potential benefit *(12,13)*.

The primary effect of radiation on tissues is the induction of apoptosis or mitotic cell death from free radical-mediated DNA damage. A variety of other secondary effects occur that are mediated by cytokines, chemokines, and growth factors. These secondary effects include activation of the coagulation system, inflammation, epithelial regeneration, and tissue remodeling that is mediated by a number of interacting molecular signals that include cytokines, chemokines, and growth factors. Radiation causes endothelial cell apoptosis, increased endothelial permeability, expression of chemokines, and expression of adhesion molecules with the subsequent loss of vascular thrombo-resistance. The loss of vascular thrombo-resistance is a result of decreased fibrinolysis, increased expression of tissue factor and von Willebrand factor, and decreased expression of prostacyclin and thrombomodulin. The increased expression of tissue factors and increased local thrombin formation occurs intravascularly and in the perivascular areas and extracellular matrix because of the increased vascular permeability. The accumulation of thrombin in the intravascular and extravascular compartments causes the progressive fibrotic sclerosis of the tissues that characterizes radiation fibrosis *(14)*.

Radiation fibrosis can damage any tissue type, including skin, muscle, ligament, tendon, nerve, viscera, and even bone (refs. *15–17*; Figs. 1 and 2). The effects of radiation can be acute

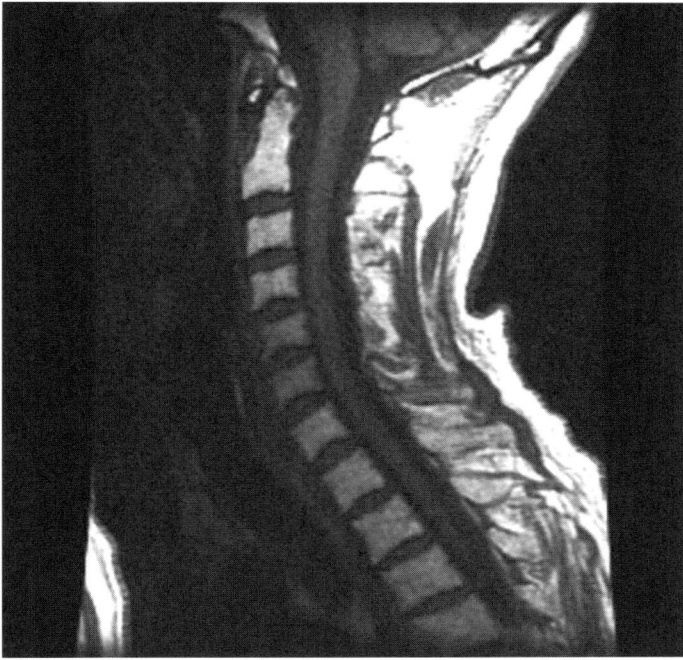

**Fig. 2.** Late effects of XRT on bone as seen on a T1-weighted magnetic resonance imaging scan. Note the increased signal in the C1 through C4 vertebral bodies. The signal change results from radiation damage to the normal marrow, which is replaced with fat, which in turn has a higher signal.

(occurring during or immediately after treatment), early-delayed (occurring up to 3 months after completion of treatment), or late-delayed (occurring more than 3 months following completion of treatment; ref. *18*). Radiation fibrosis is an example of a late complication of radiation therapy, which may manifest years after treatment, progress rapidly or insidiously, and is not reversible *(19,20)*.

The term *radiation fibrosis syndrome* (RFS) describes the clinical manifestations that result from the progressive fibrotic sclerosis that follows radiation treatment. RFS can result locally from treatment of any tumor or malignancy with radiation on any part of the body *(21)*. Some radiation fields are quite extensive, as in the mantle field radiation used to treat Hodgkin's disease that involves all lymph nodes in the neck, chest, axilla, and at times the upper abdomen (Fig. 3). Such broad radiation fields can result in wide-spread sequelae of RFS *(22)*. The radiation field can be focal, as when treating isolated vertebral metastases, an extremity sarcoma, a local breast cancer recurrence in the chest wall, or a head and neck neoplasm *(23,24)*. Patients radiated for head and neck cancers are very likely to develop RFS because of the high doses of radiation often needed for tumor control and the close proximity of many vital tissues.

Patients with head and neck cancer typify the RFS and are often likely to benefit from treatment with BTX. Disorders attributable to the RFS in this population include radiation-induced trigeminal neuralgia, dermal sclerosis, cervical dystonia, trismus, and migraines. The spinal cord and peripheral nervous system can be affected *(25)*. Radiculopathy, plexopathy, and neuropathy are very common and likely contribute to neck pain and spasms.

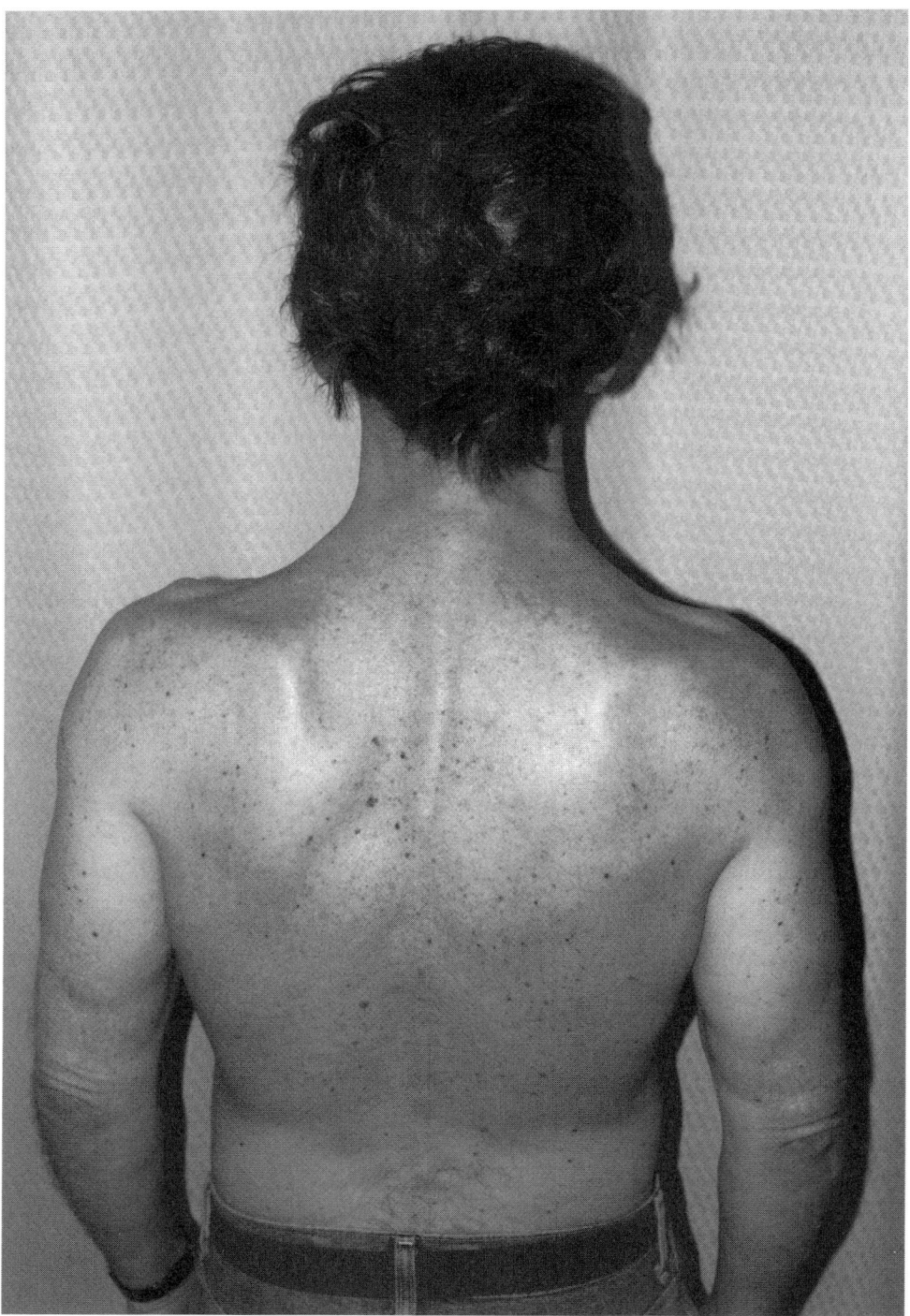

**Fig. 3.** Radiation fibrosis syndrome 20 years following mantle field radiation treatment for Hodgkin's disease. Note the marked atrophy in the cervical and thoracic paraspinal, bilateral supraspinatus, infraspinatus, and rhomboid muscles. The deltoids and triceps are preserved. Electromyography demonstrated cervical radiculoplexopathy and myopathic changes in the radiation field.

Such peripheral nervous system disfunction can result from ischemia resulting from fibrosis and stenosis of the vaso vasorum, from external compressive fibrosis of the skin and soft tissues, or both *(26,27)*.

Muscle cramps are thought to arise from spontaneous discharges of the motor nerve sending volleys of activity to and across the neuromuscular junction *(28)*. Ectopic activity in the spinal accessory nerve may be causally related to the spasms of the sternocleidomastoid muscle and trapezius that often characterize cervical dystonia. The spinal accessory nerve is involved in the radiation field of many head and neck cancers because it receives a large contribution of fibers from upper cervical nerve roots and the cervical plexus *(29)*. Similarly, radiation damage to the cervical nerve roots can cause focal cervical paraspinal muscle spasms, pain, as well as weakness of the rotator cuff (C5 and C6) and other extremity muscles *(30)*. Brachial plexus damage can be profound with resultant weakness and pain. The upper plexus may be more prone to damage because its superior location puts it within the field of many head and neck radiation ports and because the pyramidal shape of the chest provides less protective tissue around the upper plexus *(31)*. As with C5 or C6 cervical radiculopathy, damage to the upper brachial plexus can weaken the rotator cuff muscles, biceps, and deltoid. Weakness of the rotator cuff with subsequent perturbation of normal shoulder motion is causally related to the development of rotator cuff tendonitis and adhesive capsulitis in this population *(32)*. It is difficult to distinguish an upper trunk brachial plexopathy from an upper cervical radiculopathy both clinically and electrophysiologically in most instances because they are generally seen together in RFS.

Progressive fibrosis in muscle fibers within the radiation field can cause a focal myopathy that is associated with nemaline rods *(16)*. Myopathic muscles are weak relative to normal muscle and prone to spasm and pain. Cervical myopathy, cervical radiculopathy, and brachial plexopathy are commonly seen together often with devastating effects. Progressive damage to the cervical paraspinal muscles and nerves can lead to severe head drop as a potentially devastating complication of the RFS (Fig. 4).

Our understanding of the mechanism of action of BTX in pain and spasm has continued to progress. Our understanding of BTX's role in the inhibition of muscle spasms and spasticity is well developed and discussed in Chapter 2. The mechanism by which BTX treats pain, particularly neuropathic pain, is less clear. Early studies demonstrated that BTX can inhibit the release of substance P from cultured rat dorsal root ganglion cells and regulate calcitonin gene-related peptide secretion from cultured rat trigeminal nerve cells *(33,34)*. These findings initially led to speculation that BTX injected peripherally would somehow be transported centrally to inhibit the release of pain neurotransmitters in the central nervous system. This speculation has not been supported experimentally because intact BTX cannot be demonstrated centrally following peripheral injection. Other evidence suggests that the anti-nociceptive effects of BTX are in fact peripheral and related to a dose-dependent decrease in the release of glutamate and most likely other pain neurotransmitters (substance P and calcitonin gene-related peptide) at the site of peripheral inflammation *(35)*. A BTX-induced block of peripheral pain neurotransmitter release would inhibit nociceptor sensitization and thus pain. Indirect central effects likely result from the secondary inhibition of central sensitization that occurs as a result of hyperexcitability in the peripheral nervous system *(36)*. The mechanism of inhibition of release of the peripheral neurotransmitters is most likely, as at the neuromuscular junction, related to the cleavage of synaptosome-associated protein-25 and the resultant inhibition of vesicle release *(37)*.

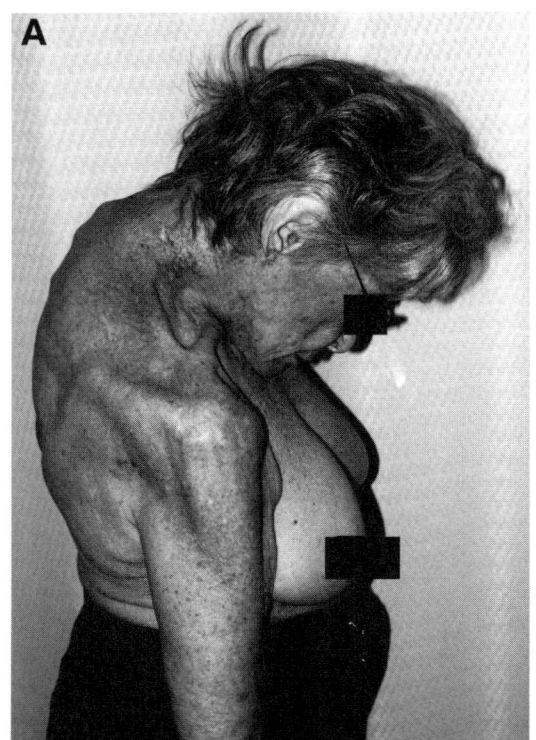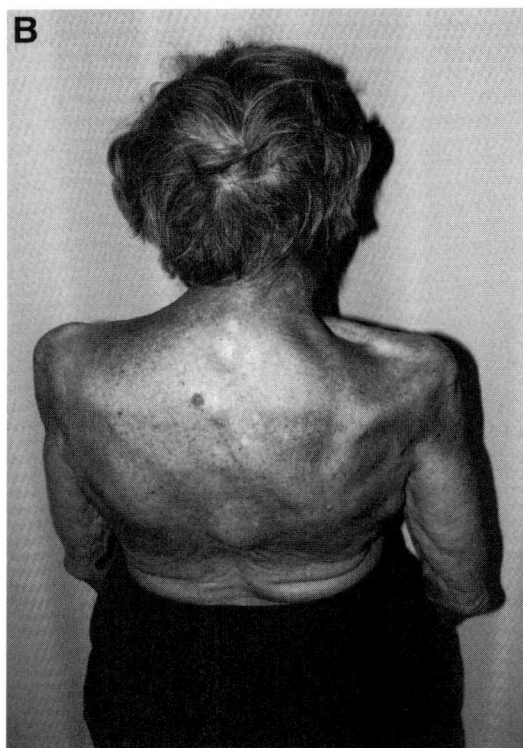

**Fig. 4.** Radiation fibrosis syndrome in a woman 5 years after radiation of a nasopharyngeal carcinoma. Note the dropped head from severe cervical paraspinal weakness as well as the marked atrophy of the rotator cuff muscles. Electromyography demonstrated cervical radiculoplexopathy involving predominately the upper cervical nerve roots and plexus as well as myopathic muscles in the radiation field.

## RISK FACTORS

The clinical manifestations of RFS depend largely on the distribution and amount or radiation given. For instance, patients radiated for a nasopharyngioma may have relatively circumscribed symptoms compared with a patient who has received mantle field radiation. Although confined to a small area, the manifestations of head and neck radiation for nasopharyngioma are often worse than those of the mantle field radiation given for Hodgkin's disease because of the high doses of radiation used and the proximity of vital structures within the field. As previously noted, radiation to any part of the body can have severe consequences with marked tissue damage to skin, nerve, muscle, bone, viscera, and other tissues. The manifestations of RFS that result depend on the structures involved in the radiation field, the dose and type of radiation given, and importantly, factors intrinsic to the patient, such as pre-existing medical conditions *(38)*.

The effects of radiation are cumulative and patients radiated more than once at the same location for recurrent disease can be expected to develop worse radiation fibrosis. Similarly, patients given higher-than normal doses of radiation are more likely to develop complications of the radiation. It is likely that certain patients are more prone to the effects of radiation based on a variety of genetic, environmental, and other as yet uncharacterized factors *(39)*. The presence of pre-existing disorders, such as cervical radiculopathy, neuropathy (from chemo-therapy, paraneoplastic effects, diabetes), and arthritis can predispose patients to or hasten the development of pain and functional disorders when combined with the effects of radiation. Recurrent or progressive tumors can severely affect nerves, bone, joint, muscle, and other tis-sues. Unfortunately, recurrence and progression of disease is common in cancer and represents a major diagnostic and therapeutic obstacle that cannot always be overcome.

## HISTORY

The diagnosis of RFS is not always straightforward. Symptoms should be referable to and anatomically consistent with a history of prior radiation therapy. A complete history should include all pre-existing medical conditions including musculoskeletal and neurological con-ditions, such as rotator cuff tendonitis, cervical radiculopathy, neuropathy, and so on. The importance of pre-existing or developing musculoskeletal and neurological conditions should not be discounted because these can impact greatly the development of symptoms in the set-ting of radiation.

A complete oncological history should be detailed from diagnosis to present. All oncological therapies given, such as surgeries, chemotherapy, and radiotherapy, should be documented and include the specifics of type, dosing, duration, and location where appropriate. The time course of the development of symptoms should be carefully documented because they may give clues to comorbid disorders that are contributing to symptoms and dysfunction and may be of prognostic importance.

Symptoms of radiation fibrosis can develop during radiation or years later. More rapidly progressive symptoms may indicate a worse prognosis in some instances but may also suggest a superimposed disorder that is not directly related, such as an acute cervical radiculopathy from a disk herniation that might change the treatment strategy.

The specific radiation-induced muscular disorders that are likely to be amenable to BTX injections include focal muscle spasms, such as trismus, cervical dystonia, paraspinal muscle spams, and extremity muscle spasms *(40,41)*. Focal disorders of neuropathic pain, such as trigeminal neuralgia, post-mastectomy syndrome, and migraines are also potentially respon-sive to BTX injections *(8,42)*. Widespread spasms and pain are not usually treatable with BTX because the amount of tissue that would need to be covered generally is too great.

The details of the patient's pain, tightness, spasm, and the language used to describe symp-toms are important. Discomfort that is intermittent and rare is not as likely to respond to BTX injections as symptoms that are more frequent. Patients often describe constant or frequent muscle spasms in or outside the radiation field. Symptoms may be nonspecific but are often described as "tight," "pulling," or "cramping." Neuropathic terms such as "burning," "stabbing," "searing," and so on may be used to describe the pain associated with nerve injury. The prac-titioner should make every effort to differentiate symptoms associated with muscle spasms from those associated with neuropathic pain because this difference will determine whether BTX injections will be given intramuscularly, intradermally, or both.

The patient's description of symptoms should be anatomically related to the radiation field either directly (within the radiation field) or indirectly (within the myotomal or dermatomal distribution of nerves involved by the radiation field). If the patient's symptoms are not anatom-ically congruent, other diagnostic possibilities other than RFS should be strongly considered.

Spasms can be associated with fixed contractures and loss of both active and passive range of motion as symptoms progress. Contractures can occur in the jaw, neck, extremities, or any joint involved in the radiation field (Fig. 5). In general, fixed contractures cannot be treated

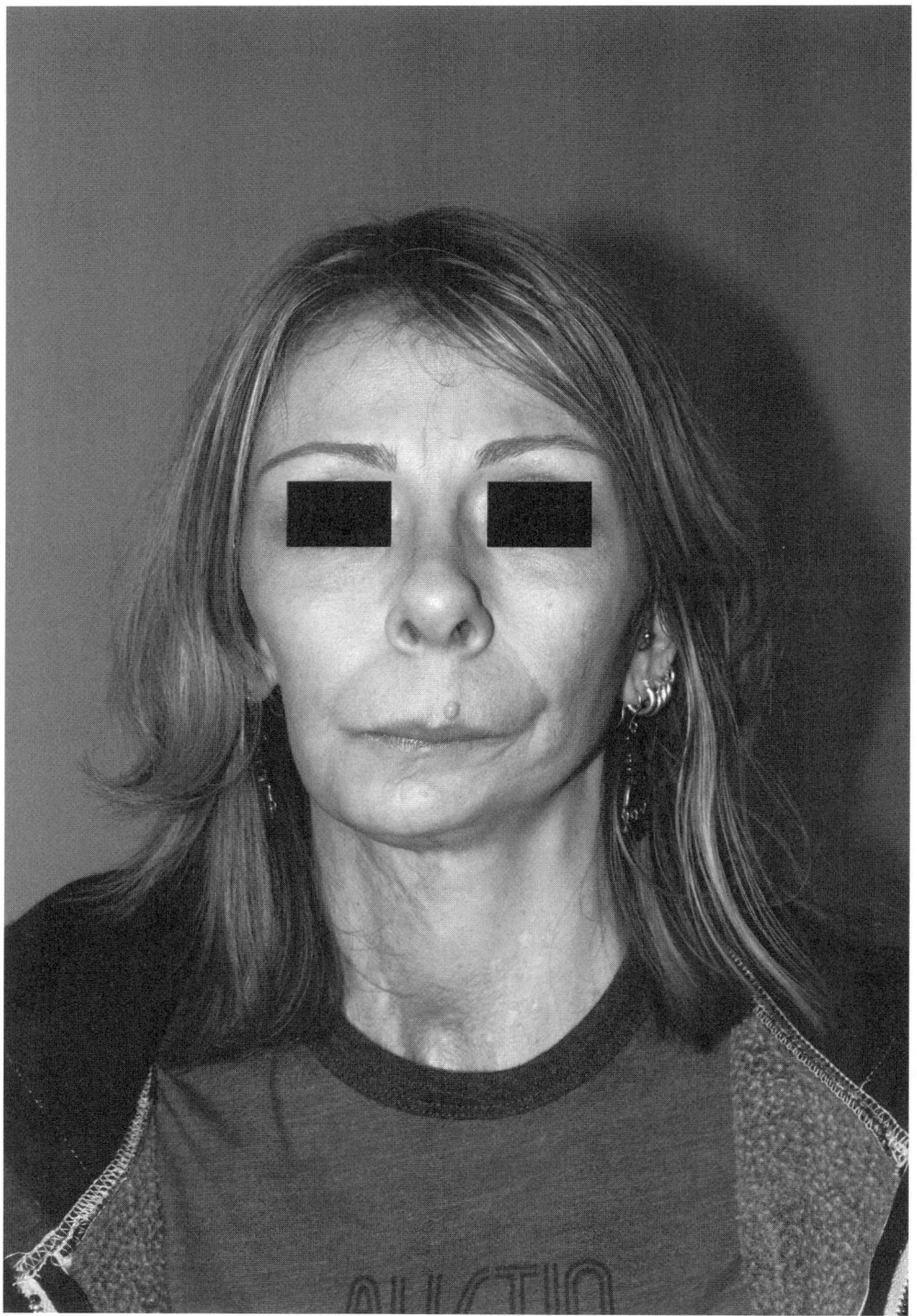

**Fig. 5.** Jaw contracture in a woman treated for adenoid cystic carcinoma of the soft pallet with resection, reconstruction, and radiation. Note that the jaw is pulled to the right. The patient suffers from radiation-induced trismus, cervical dystonia, and right V2 and V3 trigeminal neuralgia.

by BTX injection alone. The use of BTX in patients with contractures complicated by muscle spams, however, often facilitates therapy and range-of-motion exercises intended to reduce the contractures by alleviating pain and in some cases selectively weakening the contracting muscles *(43)*.

## CLINICAL EXAMINATION

In general, BTX only works where it is injected. It is therefore extremely important that the targeting of injections be precise. For intramuscular injections, the decision on which muscles to inject should be based on both the history and physical examination. Patients can usually describe which muscles or muscle groups produce pain and spasm. Although muscle spasms cannot always be appreciated on physical examination, tenderness in muscles usually can. Muscle tenderness can help guide a "follow the pain" strategy for BTX injections.

In patients with head and neck cancer and RFS, tenderness is most often appreciated in the upper cervical paraspinal muscles at the base of the skull, including the splenius capitis and longissimus, the mid and lower cervical paraspinal muscles, the mid trapezius, and the sternocleidomastoids. The masseters are often described to spasm historically in patients with trismus but do not always exhibit tenderness to palpation. In RFS of the extremities, muscles distal to the site of radiation, the gastroc-soleus complex for instance, are often described to spasm historically and can be painful and spasmodic on physical examination.

Great caution should be used in determining which muscles are likely to benefit from BTX injections. As a general rule, only muscles that are relatively strong should be subject to injection unless there is a compelling reason to do otherwise. This is particularly true in patients who have received radiation to the neck because one of the most common complications of BTX injections is worsening neck weakness and swallowing. An overdose of BTX in these situations can precipitate a neck drop or dysphagia that may persist for weeks until the effects of the toxin wear off. In the extremities, the focal weakness caused by BTX injections may be a welcome effect that facilitates functional bracing, improves gate, improves upper extremity function, and so on.

In disorders of focal neuropathic pain, such as radiation-induced trigeminal neuralgia, physical examination should focus on determining the areas most affected by positive neuropathic phenomenon such as paresthesias, dysesthesias, hyperpathia, and allodynia. Identification of the location and extent of such findings will guide the injection of BTX. Failure to adequately identify all affected skin may result in underdosing of toxin or in a penumbra effect, wherein areas of treated skin are surrounded by painful untreated skin. Often, the initial BTX treatment results in a penumbra effect that is corrected on subsequent treatments by escalation of dose and skin coverage.

## DIAGNOSTIC EVALUATION

Patients are often referred for BTX injections in the setting of worsening signs and symptoms, such as pain, spasms, and weakness. Although progressive cancer and superimposed benign musculoskeletal or neuromuscular disorders are not generally a contraindication to the use of BTX, their identification is imperative to its safe and effective use. BTX injections can be used palliatively and can be particularly effective when pain and spasms are directly related to progressive tumor. The use of BTX in benign pathology is discussed elsewhere in this text.

The choice of imaging for evaluation for metastatic, recurrent, or progressive disease depends on the type of cancer and its location. Magnetic resonance imaging (MRI) is the test of choice for evaluating the spine, soft tissues of the head, and joints such as the shoulder. The addition of gadolinium contrast is needed when a brain metastases, intramedullary spinal tumor, or leptomeningeal disease are diagnostic possibilities. Gadolinium is also required when a post-operative or previously irradiated site is being evaluated to facilitate differentiation of tumor from a background of scar or fibrotic tissue. A computed tomography (CT) scan with contrast is usually the test of choice to evaluate the viscera of the chest, abdomen, and pelvis for metastatic or progressive disease. CT may also be used when MRI is contraindicated (pacemaker, aneurism clips, breast tissue expanders). A CT myelogram is indicated when metallic hardware, such as from previous spinal instrumentation, causes excessive artifact that precludes adequate visualization of the spinal canal. Bone scan is useful for identification of most bony metastases but does not generally provide adequate anatomical information because the soft tissues are not visualized. X-rays are useful when evaluating spinal stabilization hardware or joint replacement prostheses for loosening or failure.

BTX is often injected in close proximity to tumor or surgical hardware. Injection into tumor or directly adjacent to hardware may increase the risk of bleeding and infection and is unlikely to be as beneficial as injection into contractile tissue. Available imaging should be reviewed and new imaging obtained so that the practitioner can be sure of the exact location of tumor, previous surgery, and hardware.

Electrodiagnostic evaluation is useful to identify, localize, confirm, and differentiate radiculopathy, plexopathy, neuropathy, or myopathy in patients with RFS. Needle electromyography (EMG) can confirm muscle denervation and may identify myokymia, fasciculations, and muscle spasm. Needle EMG localizaton is often useful to confirm injection into contractile tissue and not scar or tumor and to localize the motor end plate zone.

Laboratory evaluation of platelets is particularly important in patients with cancer because disease and treatment, including chemotherapy and radiotherapy, can be myelosuppressive. The patient's coagulation status should be assessed because liver dysfunction and treatment of and prophylaxis for thromboembolism are common in the cancer population.

## DIFFERENTIAL DIAGNOSIS

A major factor in the successful use of BTX injections in muscular spasm is the correct assessment the muscles involved. This determination is made predominately by history and physical examination with potential contributions from electrodiagnostic testing and imaging in select cases. Often, the decision on the muscular targets chosen for injection will change over time based on the patient's response to past injections and the progression of their underlying pathology.

In neuropathic pain, BTX is injected subdermally into the skin affected. Multiple small (usually 0.1 cc) injections are used at regular intervals until all affected skin is covered. Clinical assessment should emphasize the patient's historical account of pain location and physical examination should identify dysesthetic and allodynic areas of skin. Causes of focal pain that are nociceptive and not neuropathic in etiology, such as infection, bone infarct, and oral caries, should be excluded because the treatment of these conditions may be more successful with modalities other than BTX injection.

Aside from bleeding and infection, the major potential complication of BTX injection is focal muscular weakness, which can be as benign as a droopy eyelid or as serious as major dysphagia requiring the placement of a feeding tube. Neck drop is particularly common in the head and neck cancer population because the target muscles are often weak. In general, BTX should only be used in relatively strong muscles. Overzealous use of BTX injections in weakened muscles, such as the trapezius or cervical paraspinal muscles for pain or spasm, can make the symptoms worse by forcing compensation from muscle fibers not affected by the injection. Great care should be used when clinical weakness is found and starting doses of BTX should be small.

Patients should be continually re-assessed for worsening of both benign and malignant pathology because these pathologies may significantly alter if, where, and how BTX injections are used. A patient with worsening upper cervical metastases, for instance, may develop instability pain that requires surgical cervical stabilization and may be worsened by BTX injections. Progression of radiation fibrosis with worsening paraspinal muscle strength can facilitate the development of neck drop from BTX injections in a patient who had previously benefited from them.

## TREATMENT APPROACH

Once it has been determined that a patient's symptoms of focal muscle spasm or focal neuropathic pain are a complication of RFS, initial management should start conservatively and progress to more interventional therapies, such as BTX injection, based on the patient's response to therapy. A few common clinical scenarios will be detailed. All dosing is for BTX type A (BTX-A; Botox®, Allergan, Inc., Irvine, CA), which is used preferentially in cancer patients because of its efficacy, duration of action, predictable spread within tissues, and minimal systemic absorption.

Radiation-induced trigeminal neuralgia is a common complication of radiation to the head and neck for nasopharyngioma and other neoplasms. Extensive surgical resections are often used with radiation and may significantly contribute to damage of one or more branches of the trigeminal nerve. The symptoms of trigeminal neuralgia may be in any trigeminal nerve distribution, with V2 and V3 being the most common. The anterior neck is also commonly affected because of damage to the cervical plexus. Symptoms are generally ipsilateral to the side of the tumor but can be bilateral.

Initial treatment of radiation-induced trigeminal neuralgia is similar to that for idiopathic or traumatic etiologies of trigeminal neuralgia. Conservative therapy such as skin desensitization and transcutaneous electrical nerve stimulation may be of limited benefit. "Nerve stabilizing" medications can be useful. Pregabalin is generally our preferred initial medication, particularly in the cancer population, because of its efficacy, rapid onset of action, lack of drug–drug interactions, and favorable side effect profile (44). Doses higher than 600 mg per day may be used if there is incremental efficacy without a significant increase in adverse events, such as somnolence or peripheral edema. Other nerve-stabilizing medications, such as oxcarbazepine, carbamazepine, and phenytoin, can be considered as alternatives but are prone to more serious adverse events. The addition of medications with differing mechanisms of action is often beneficial but may run the risk of potentiating additive side effects (such as somnolence) and drug–drug interactions (45). Tricyclic antidepressants (amitriptyline, nortriptyline), serotonin-norepinephrine re-uptake inhibitors (duloxetine, venlafaxine), and narcotics (methadone, oxycodone) may improve efficacy when combined with drugs that have differing mechanisms of action such as pregabalin (46).

If conservative and pharmacological therapies have not resulted in adequate pain reduction in radiation-induced trigeminal neuralgia, then the addition of BTX injections should be

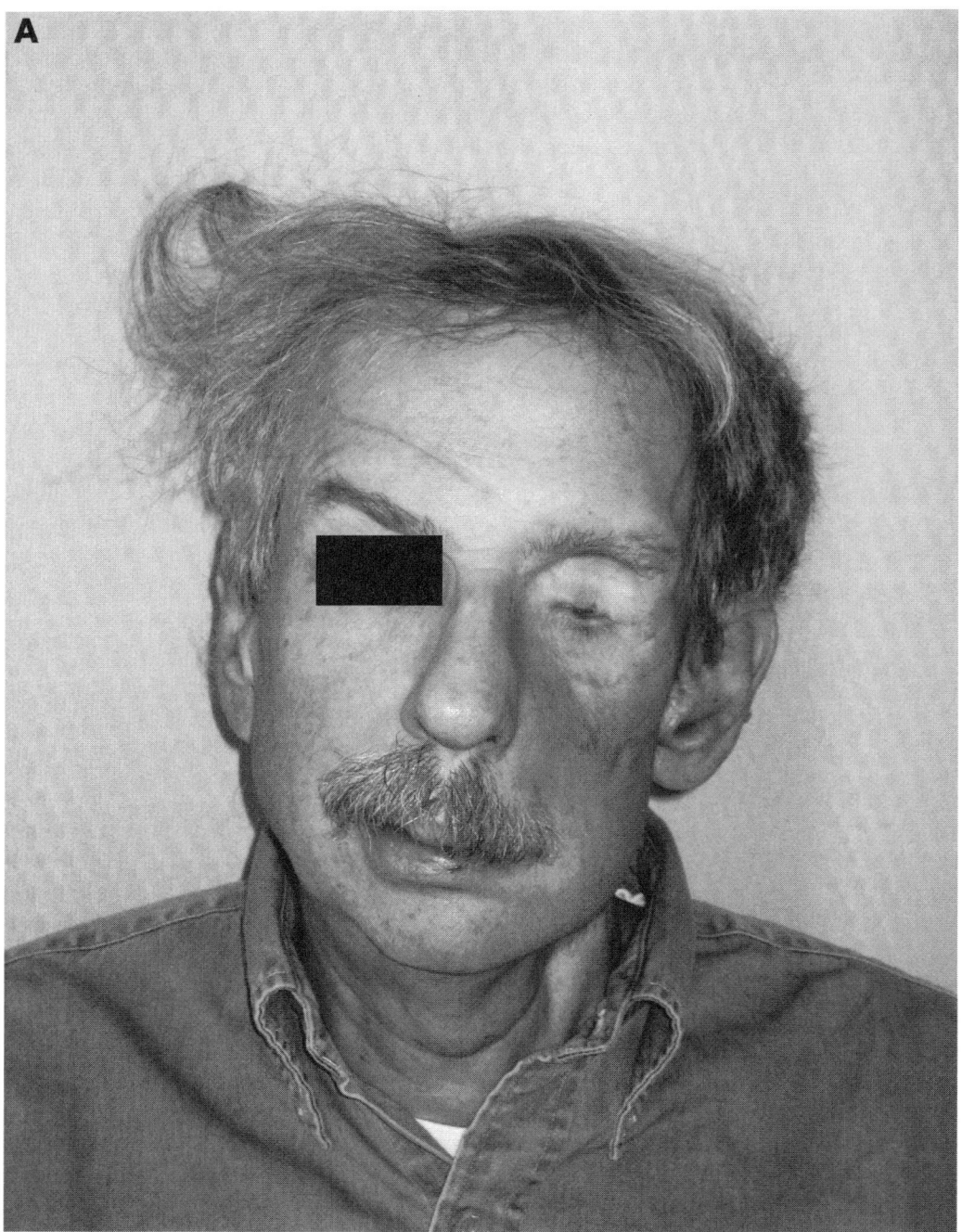

**Fig. 6.**

considered. Treatments with even partial efficacy should not be withdrawn until adequate efficacy with the BTX injections has been achieved. It may take several treatments until the location and dosing of the injections is optimized. In most patients, multimodal treatment is generally required to achieve satisfactory pain control.

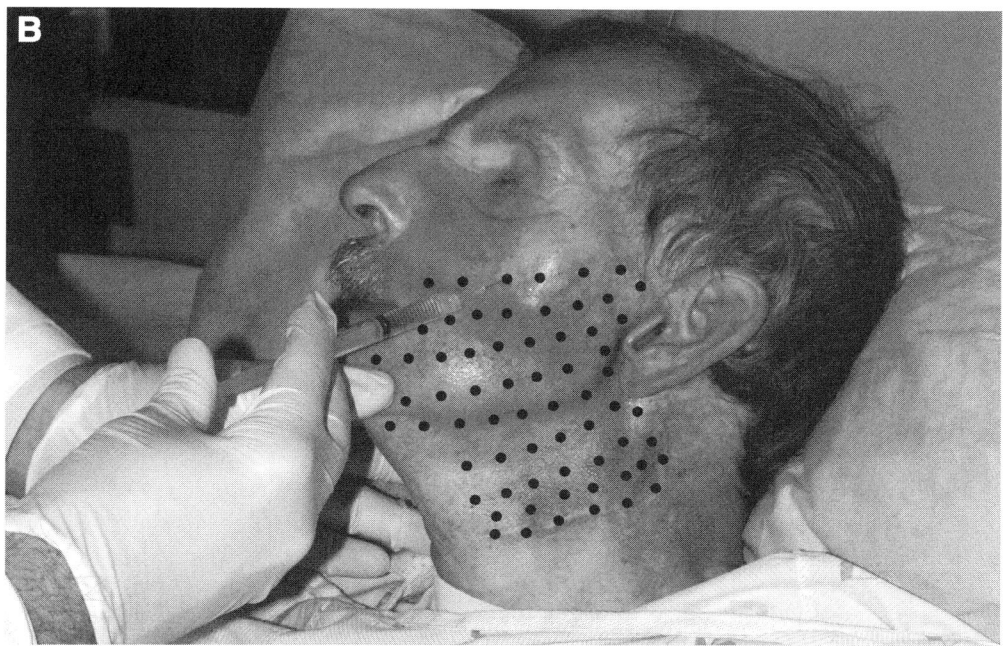

**Fig. 6.** *(Continued)* Radiation-induced trigeminal neuralgia resulting from surgical and radiation treatment of a left maxillary sinus squamous cell carcinoma. Note the extensive surgical resection of the left face including eye enucleation. The patient suffers from severe trigeminal neuralgia in a partial V2, V3, and anterior cervical distribution. Two hundred units of botulinum toxin into 5 cc of normal saline produces a concentration of 5 U/0.1 cc. Injections of approximately 0.1 cc are spaced about 1.5 cm apart (illustrated by black dots) should spread to cover all affected skin.

BTX injections will be performed intradermally or subdermally over the areas of skin affected as determined by the patient's historical account and the physician's physical exam. BTX-A is delivered in 100 U vials that are stored frozen and must be reconstituted with normal saline. The concentration of BTX can be varied at the physician's discretion based on how much saline is used to reconstitute the toxin. In general, 2.5 cc of normal saline injected into a 100-U vial is used to produce a concentration of 5 U per 0.1 cc.

The anticipated amount of spread of BTX-A is approximately 1 cm from the site of injection (2 cm diameter) from 5 U in 0.1 cc in normal skin. Spread is probably significantly lower in patients affected by radiation fibrosis because of the abnormal accumulation of protein. Injections should be spaced about 1.5 cm apart so that the spread from each injection overlaps the next and all affected skin is covered (Fig. 6). It is not necessary to cover all radiation-damaged skin, only the skin that the patient reports is painful or physical examination determines to be dysesthetic or allodynic.

The usual starting dose of BTX needed to treat radiation-induced trigeminal neuralgia is about 100 U. More BTX should be used if the area of skin to be injected is extensive. The skin should be clean and sterilized with alcohol. Patients should be encouraged to not wear makeup to the office visit. A 30-gage needle is generally used and syringe size ranges from 1 to 10 cc based on physician preference. Smaller syringes allow for more precise volume delivery and should be used by beginning practitioners. With practice, the volume of solution injection into the patient can be accurately determined by the size of the bleb raised under the skin.

**Table 1**
**Disorders of Focal Neuropathic Pain Associated With RFS**

| Disorder | BTX-A dose range (units) |
|---|---|
| Intercostal neuralgia | 50–300 |
| Migraine | 50–200 |
| Occipital neuralgia | 50–300 |
| Post-mastectomy syndrome | 50–300 |
| Stump pain | 100–300 |
| Thoracic radiculopathy | 50–300 |
| Trigeminal neuralgia | 50–300 |

RFS, radiation fibrosis syndrome; BTX-A, botulinum toxin type A.

It is common for initial BTX injections to only provide a partial benefit, generally resulting from either failure to overlap the spread from injections, too low a concentration of BTX in each aliquot delivered, or a penumbra effect. The penumbra effect occurs when the most severely affected skin is adequately treated but the surrounding, less affected areas are not. In such cases the injection procedure should be modified to include more of the surrounding skin. Closer spacing of BTX injections should be used if spread is insufficient. A more concentrated BTX solution should be considered if the injections are properly spaced and all affected skin is covered, but the patient still has inadequate efficacy.

The effect of BTX injections in radiation-induced trigeminal neuralgia should take approximately 2 to 3 days to begin and are maximal at about 10 days. EMLA cream can be used pre-procedure and ice post-procedure to alleviate discomfort. The area injected can be gently washed but makeup should not be applied for several hours to decrease the chance of it entering or irritating the skin. Normal activities can be resumed following injection without limitation.

The major potential complication of BTX injections for radiation-induced trigeminal neuralgia is infection. Weakening of the orbicularis oris or orbicularis oculi may cause or worsen drooling and ptosis respectively. Injection over the anterior neck can cause dysphagia or dysarthria. Wrinkles on the face may be reduced. This is often considered a cosmetic benefit in patients whose face has been deformed by the radiation and scaring of treatment but is not pleasing to all patients. Weakness caused by BTX injections is not permanent and should resolve spontaneously in approximately 6 weeks.

It should be noted that the techniques used for radiation-induced trigeminal neuralgia are likely widely applicable to any focal neuropathic pain disorders associated with radiation (Table 1).

Radiation-induced trismus is a complication of RFS and may co-exist with radiation-induced trigeminal neuralgia. Ectopic activity in trigeminal nerve motor fibers resulting from radiation fibrosis results in spasm and pain, particularly in the masseter. Unchecked, persistent spasms of the masseter can contribute to fixed contracture and ultimately inability to open the jaw. Patients with severe trismus and jaw contracture may have difficulty speaking and may not be able to ingest food or liquid orally.

Antispasmodic medications may offer some relief from spasms. Nerve stabilizers such as pregabalin and analgesics such as oxycodone have some efficacy in relief of pain. A trial of medications should be used initially to relieve pain and spasms. Often more than one medication with differing mechanisms of action is required. Evaluation and treatment by physical, occupational, or speech therapy is extremely important and should be ordered early in the course of disease. Therapy should emphasize maintenance of jaw excursion to prevent progression to fixed contracture. Treatment of fixed jaw contractures required progressive static or dynamic stretching using such devices as tongue depressors or the Therabite® system *(41,47)*.

BTX injections may alleviate the spasm and pain associated with radiation-induced trismus but will not directly treat jaw contracture. The masseter is most often targeted but injection into the temporalis muscle may also be useful in some instances. Although the medial and lateral pterygoid muscles may be involved in radiation-induced trismus, their location behind the ramus of the maxilla makes their injection difficult. It should be noted that the masseter is commonly subject to resection depending on tumor type, extent, and location. The presence or absence of a masseter (palpable on the ramus of the jaw with volitional jaw clinching) may not always be obvious on physical examination because of scar and deformity. When the anatomy is uncertain, surgical records and imaging (MRI) should be reviewed before initiating BTX injections for trismus to be sure of the presence and location of critical structures. Injection can be either unilateral or bilateral depending on the patient's anatomy and symptoms.

EMG guidance is very useful to confirm needle placement within the masseter, which is often atrophic and fibrotic. Marked spontaneous activity including fibrillation potentials, positive sharp waves, myokymia, and fasciculation potentials are usually seen. A hollow monopolar needle (such as the Ambu® Neuroline Inoject) is used. Needle size varies but a 30-mm, 28-gage needle is usually sufficient to achieve adequate muscle purchase in most patients.

Because of the size of the masseter, no more than 0.5 to 1 cc of volume is typically injected. The volume injected should be divided into two to three muscle sites, preferably in and around the motor endplate zone. The concentration of BTX varies to accommodate the total number of units the clinician intends to inject. For instance, if 50 U in 0.5 cc are to be injected, then 1 cc of saline should be used to dilute a 100-U vial of BTX-A. The dose used varies from 25 total units per masseter at the conservative end to as high as 200 or more units per masseter as needed by the patient's response to past injections. The site of injection should be sterilized with alcohol. Titration of dose should occur at approximately 6-week intervals unless symptoms are so severe as to warrant rapid dose escalation on repeat injections every several days.

The technique and doses used for injection of the temporalis is similar but EMG guidance is not generally needed. A 30-gage needle should be used to inject at least four separate sites within the temporalis.

The major potential complications of injection for radiation-induced trismus include infection and bleeding. Dysphagia and dysarthria are uncommon at lower doses of BTX but become more likely as doses are increased.

Radiation-induced cervical dystonia can result not only from the treatment of head and neck cancers, but from treatment of any tumor treated with radiation that involves occiput, cervical spine, or upper thoracic spine *(48)*. This includes metastatic disease from any cancer type, sarcomas, lymphomas such as Hodgkin's disease, thyroid cancer, and so on.

Idiopathic cervical dystonia is broadly defined as a movement disorder characterized by involuntary contractions of the head and shoulders, which may be twisted into aberrant positions including torticollis, laterocollis, retrocollis, and anterocollis *(49)*. In radiation-induced

**Table 2**
**Disorders of Focal Muscle Spasm Associated With RFS**

| Disorder | Muscle | BTX-A dose range (units) |
|----------|--------|--------------------------|
| Trismus | Masseter | 25–200 |
| Cervical dystonia | Cervical paraspinals | 25–200 |
| | Levator scapulae | 25–50 |
| | Longissimus | 25–100 |
| | Scalene complex | 10–50 |
| | Splenius capitis | 50–100 |
| | Sternocleidomastoid | 10–50 |
| | Trapezius | 25–100 |

RFS, radiation fibrosis syndrome; BTX-A, botulinum toxin type A.

cervical dystonia, radiation fibrosis likely contributes to ectopic activity in the distribution of the spinal accessory nerve and cervical nerve roots, which may be asymmetric and cause aberrant positioning of the head and neck. More often, symptoms are at least partially bilateral. As radiation fibrosis progresses, posturing of the head and neck becomes less pronounced and fixed contractures develop. Most patients complain of neck tightness that progresses slowly and insidiously and is almost always accompanied by pain. Inability to position the head because of progressive fibrosis can affect swallowing, phonation, and activities of daily living, such as driving and work-related tasks.

As in radiation-induced trismus, the natural history of radiation-induced cervical dystonia is one of progression. Aggressive physical therapy with emphasis on a life-long home exercise program designed to maintain head and neck range of motion is critical. It is generally easier to prevent a contracture than to treat one. Medications may be useful in treating the symptoms of radiation-induced cervical dystonia but cannot substitute for range-of-motion exercises. Medications of possible benefit are similar to those discussed in the treatment of trismus and include muscle relaxants, such as baclofen, nerve stabilizers such as pregabalin, and analgesics.

BTX injections can be extremely effective in treating the pain and spasms associated with radiation-induced cervical dystonia (Fig. 6). As in other disorders, BTX injections will not directly treat fixed contractures but may facilitate the progression of range of motion through physical therapy. Techniques used in the treatment of radiation-induced cervical dystonia are very similar to those used to idiopathic cervical dystonia. Clinical evaluation with particular emphasis on the patient's historical account of symptoms and physical examination are instrumental in choosing targets and dosing for therapy. As with other inductions for BTX injection, technique is often modified on subsequent injection visits to maximize efficacy.

The dose, volume, and concentration of BTX injected for radiation-induced cervical dystonia varies widely (Table 2). The most frequently injected muscles are the cervical paraspinal muscles, sternocleidomastoid, and trapezius. A "follow the pain" tactic wherein the point of maximal muscle tenderness is injected is often effective when muscles demonstrate tenderness to palpation. In muscles that are symptomatic from spasm more than pain, injection into the motor endplate zone is indicated. More than one injection point may be necessary in long or broad muscles, such as the sternocleidomastoid, to ensure maximal efficacy. Choice of needle is determined by the muscle to be injected. EMG guidance may be used when the

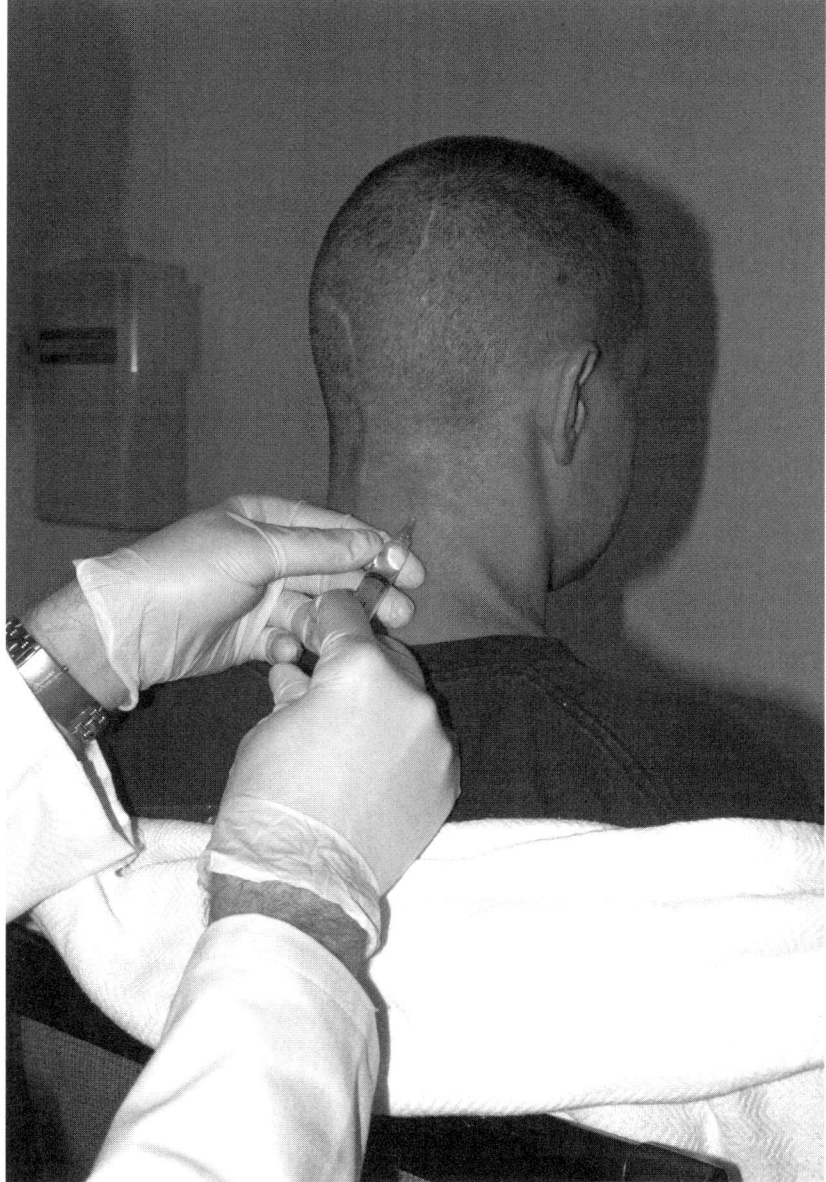

**Fig. 7.** Injection of the mid cervical paraspinal muscles for painful radiation-induced cervical dystonia. The patient has adenocarcinoma of unknown primary metastatic to the upper cervical spine previously treated with external beam radiation. The surgical scar is from resection of a meningioma several years earlier. The lower cervical paraspinal muscles and trapezius will be injected bilaterally. The patient's spine is imaged by magnetic resonance imaging every 3 months or sooner as indicated and the imaging is reviewed before every procedure to ensure there is no significant progression of disease including paraspinal mass. Initial injections were electromyography (EMG)-guided to ensure position within contractile tissue. More comfortable non-EMG-guided injections were started once familiarity with this individual patient's anatomy was gained. A total of 200 U of botulinum toxin type A is used approximately every 6 weeks in conjunction with a nerve stabilizer (pregabalin) and narcotic (oxycodone).

4

anatomy is not easily palpable, when injecting near tumor or surgical scar, or when injecting around spinal stabilization hardware to ensure the needle is in contractile tissue. In most instances, a 25-gage needle 1- to 1.5-in. long is sufficient. Injections are usually repeated every 6 weeks.

Potential major complications include bleeding and infection, especially if injections are near spinal stabilization hardware or tumor. Neck drop can occur when injecting weak spinal muscles. Precipitation or worsening of dysphagia is particularly problematic because patients with RFS that involves the neck often have pre-existing difficulty. Overtreatment with BTX can result in aspiration or the need for a feeding tube.

## CONCLUSION

RFS is a common complication of cancer treatment. Although the natural history of radiation fibrosis is one of invariable progression, the associated symptoms and dysfunction can, in most instances, be alleviated with multimodal therapy. BTX is a novel treatment modality with tremendous promise in alleviating the focal muscular spasms and neuropathic pain associated with RFS. Although little research on the role of BTX in the cancer setting is currently available, translation of research in disorders with similar pathophysiology is promising and clearly indicates the need for investigation of BTX's role in alleviating the pain and dysfunction associated with cancer and its treatment.

## REFERENCES

1. Jemal A, Siegel R, Ward E, et al. Cancer statistics, 2006. CA Cancer J Clin 2006;56:106–130.
2. Kuzniar T, Masters GA, Ray DW. Screening for lung cancer—a review. Med Sci Monit 2004;10:RA21–30.
3. Stewart SL, King JB, Thompson TD, Friedman C, Wingo PA. Cancer mortality surveillance—United States, 1990–2000. MMWR Surveill Summ 2004;53:1–108.
4. Patchell RA, Posner JB. Neurologic complications of systemic cancer. Neurol Clin 1985;3:729–749.
5. Plotkin SR, Wen PY. Neurologic complications of cancer therapy. Neurol Clin 2003;21:279–318.
6. Falah M, Schiff D, Burns TM. Neuromuscular complications of cancer diagnosis and treatment. J Support Oncol 2005;3:271–282.
7. Royal MA. The use of botulinum toxins in the management of pain and headache. Phys Med Rehabil Clin N Am 2003;14:805–820.
8. Okereke LI, Stubblefield MD, Custodio CM. Botulinum toxin type A for radiation-induced trismus and facial pain: a case report. Arch Phys Med Rehabil 2004;85:E37.
9. Chou WW, Puri DR, Lee NY. Intensity-modulated radiation therapy for head and neck cancer. Expert Rev Anticancer Ther 2005;5:515–521.
10. Saarto T, Janes R, Tenhunen, Kouri M. Palliate radiotherapy in the treatment of skeletal metastases. Eur J Pain 2002;6:323–330.
11. Chow E, Wu J, Loblaw A, Perez CA. Radiotherapeutic approaches to metastatic disease. World J Urol 2003;21:229–242.
12. O'Meara WP, Lee N. Advances in nasopharyngeal carcinoma. Curr Opin Oncol 2005;17:225–230.
13. Tannock IF. Combined modality treatment with radiotherapy and chemotherapy. Radiother Oncol 1989;16:83–101.
14. Hauer-Jensen M, Fink LM, Wang J. Radiation injury and the protein C pathway. Crit Care Med 2004;32:S325–S330.
15. Libshitz HI, DuBrow RA, Loyer EM, Charnsangavej C. Radiation change in normal organs: an overview of body imaging. Eur. Radiol 1996;6:786–795.

16. Portlock CS, Boland P, Hays AP, Antonescu CR, Rosenblum MK. Nemaline myopathy: a possible late complication of Hodgkin's disease therapy. Hum Pathol 2003;34:816–818.
17. Johansson S, Svensson H, Larsson L, Denekamp J. Brachial plexopathy after postoperative radiotherapy of breast cancer patients: a long-term follow-up. Acta Oncologica 2000;39:373–382.
18. New P. Radiation injury to the nervous system. Curr Opin Neurol 2001;14:725–734.
19. Johansson S, Svensson H, Denekamp J. Dose response and the latency for radiation-induced fibrosis, edema, and neuropathy in breast cancer patients. Int J Radiation Oncology Biol Phys 2002;52:1207–1219.
20. Johansson S, Svensson H, Denekamp J. Timescale of evolution of late radiation injury after posoperative radiotherapy of breast cancer patients. Int J Radiation Oncol Biol Phys 2000; 48:745–750.
21. Stone HB, Coleman CN, Anscher MS, McBride WH. Effects of radiation on normal tissue: consequences and mechanisms. Lancet Oncol 2004;4:529–536.
22. Lund MD, Kongerud J, Boe J, et al. [Late complications after treatment of Hodgkin's disease] [Article in Norwegian]. Tidsskr Nor Laegeforen 1999;10:933–937.
23. Falkmer U, Järhult J, Wersäll P, Cavallin-Ståhl. A systematic overview of radiation therapy effects in skeletal metastases. Acta Oncologica 2003;42:620–633.
24. Paulino AC. Late effects of radiotherapy for pediatric extremity sarcomas. Int J Radiation Oncology Biol Phys 2004;60:265–274.
25. Cross NE, Glantz MJ. Neurologic complications of radiation therapy. Neurol Clin N Am 2003;21:249–77.
26. Gillette EL, Mahler PA, Powers BE, Gillette SM, Vujaskovic Z. Late radiation injury to muscle and peripheral nerves. Int J Radiation Oncology Biol Phys 1995;31:1309–1318.
27. Greenfield MM, Stark GM. Post-irradiation neuropathy. AJR Am J Roentgenol 1948;60: 617–622.
28. Miller TM, Layzer RB. Muscle cramps. Muscle Nerve 2005;32:431–442.
29. Karuman PN, Soo KC. Motor innervation of the trapezius muscle: a histochemical study. 1996; 18:254–258.
30. Stubblefield MD, Custodio CM. Upper-extremity pain disorders in breast cancer. Arch Phys Med Rehabil 2006;87:S96–S99.
31. Jaeckle KA. Neurological manifestations of neoplastic and radiation-induced plexopathies. Semin in Neurol 2004;24:385–393.
32. Tytherleigh-Strong G, Hirahara A, Miniaci A. Rotator cuff disease. Curr Opin Rheumatol 2001;13:135–145.
33. Welch MJ, Purkiss JR, Foster KA. Sensitivity of embryonic rat dorsal root ganglia neurons to clostridium botulinum neurotoxins. Toxicon 2000;38:245–258.
34. Durham PL, Cady R, Cady RK. Regulation of calcitonin gene-related peptide secretion from trigeminal nerve cells by botulinum toxin type A: implications for migraine therapy. Headache 2004;44:35–42.
35. Cui M, Li Z, You S, Khanijou S, Aoki KR. Mechanisms of the anti-nociceptive effect of subcutaneous Botox®: inhibition of peripheral and central nociceptive processing. Naunyn Schmiedebergs Arch Pharmacol 2002;365:R17.
36. Aoki KR. Review of a proposed mechanism for the antinociceptive action of botulinum toxin type A. Neurotoxicology 2005;26:785–793.
37. Cui M, Khanijou S, Rubino J, Aoki KR. Subcutaneous administration of botulinum toxin A reduces formalin-induced pain. Pain 2004;107:125–133.
38. Zackrisson B, Mercke C, Strander H, Wennerberg J, Cavallin-Ståhl E. A systematic overview of radiation therapy effects in head and neck cancer. Acta Oncologica 2003;42:443–461.
39. Jung H, Beck-Bornholdt H, Svoboda V, Alberti W, Herrmann T. Quantification of late complications after radiation therapy. Radiother Oncol 2001;61:233–246.
40. Lou JS, Pleninger P, Kurlan R. Botulinu toxin A is effective in treating trismus associated with postradiation myokymia and muscle spasm. Mov Disord 1995;10:680–681.

41. Dijkstra PU, Kalk WWI, Roodenburg JLN. Trismus in head and neck oncology: a systematic review. Oral Oncol 2004;40:879–889.
42. Piovesan EJ, Teive HG, Kowacs PA, Della Coletta MV, Werneck LC, Silberstein SD. An open study of botulinum-A toxin treatment of trigeminal neuralgia. Neurology 2005;65:1306–1308.
43. O'Brien CF. Treatment of spasticity with botulinum toxin. Clin J Pain 2002;18:S182–S190.
44. Shneker BF, McAuley JW. Pregabalin: a new neuromodulator with broad therapeutic indications. Ann Pharmacother 2005;39:2029–2037.
45. Fine PG, Miaskowski C, Paice JA. Meeting the challenges in cancer pain management. J Support Oncol 2004;2:5–22.
46. Finnerup NB, Otto M, McQuay HJ, Jensen TS, Sindrup SH. Algorithm for neuropathic pain treatment: an evidence based proposal. Pain 2005;118:289–305.
47. Cohen EG, Deschler DG, Walsh K, Hayden RE. Early use of a mechanical stretching device to improve mandibular mobility after composite resection: a pilot study. Arch Phys Med Rehabil 2005;86:1416–1419.
48. Astudillo L, Hollington L, Game X, et al. Cervical dystonia mimicking dropped-head syndrome after radiotherapy for laryngeal carcinoma. Clin Neurol Neurosurg 2003;106:41–43.
49. Costa J, Espirito-Santo C, Borges A, et al. Botulinum toxin type A therapy for cervical dystonia. Cochrane Database Syst Rev 2005;25:CD003633.

# Low Back Pain

**Rebecca Brown, Avniel Klein, Alex Visco, and Joseph E. Herrera**

## INTRODUCTION

Low back pain (LBP) is the most common musculoskeletal complaint in the general population. It is one of the major reasons patients seek medical evaluation *(1)*, second only to upper respiratory illness *(2,3)*. Approximately 50 to 90% of the adult population will suffer from pain related to their back during their lifetime *(4,5)*. Each year, 15 to 45% of adults suffer LBP, and 1 out of 20 people present to the hospital with a new episode of back pain.

A review of worker's compensation cases cites LBP as the most common injury reported. Two percent of the workforce submits disability claims each year for LBP, as a result, back pain has a vast effect on workforce in terms of disability and lost productivity. It is currently the most common cause of disability in workers 45 years of age and younger *(6)*.

In one recent comparative literature study exploring demographic information and its association with back pain, the following predictive variables for duration of sick leave were found:

1. Predictors for a longer duration of sick leave: specific LBP, higher disability levels, older age, female gender, heavier work, receiving higher compensation, more social dysfunction, and more social isolation.
2. Variables with no influence on duration of sick leave because of LBP: a history of LBP, job satisfaction, educational level, marital status, number of dependants, smoking, working longer than 8-hour shifts, occupation, and size of industry or company *(7)*.

About 2 to 7% of patients with acute LBP will go on to become chronic. In the United States, cost estimates of LBP have exceeded $50 billion when considering both health care costs and costs resulting form disability payments and work loss *(8)*. It is also known that the majority of these costs are associated with a small number of LBP sufferers—that is, those having prolonged disability *(9)*. The percentage of patients with acute LBP that go on to a chronic state ranges from 2 to 34%.

## RISK FACTORS

The risk factors associated with LBP range from external causes, such as occupation and athletic activities, to intrinsic risk factors such as physiological and psychological composition of each individual patient. The following are the common risk factors associated with LBP.

### Occupational Factors

Heavy labor and jobs that require lifting and bending have been cited as being the chief cause of pain by more than 60% of patients with LBP *(10)*. Physical risk factors at work

From: *Therapeutic Uses of Botulinum Toxin*
Edited by: G. Cooper © Humana Press Inc., Totowa, NJ

include heavy manual work, lifting and carrying, whole body vibration, frequent bending and twisting, and static work postures.

## Patient-Related Factors

### Age

LBP is most common between the ages of 35 and 55 years, with the incidence gradually increasing over this period. According to statistics acquired from the Workman's Compensation database, the most common cause for disability in those under the age of 45 is LBP. The incidence for LBP increases as the population ages, but the complaints of those over the age of 60 is related to the degenerative process affecting the low back as opposed to occupational causes.

### Gender

When comparing genders, LBP is more prevalent in males between the ages of 35 and 45. This finding may be attributed to the fact that more males are involved in jobs that require manual heavy labor.

### Physical Fitness and Smoking

Risk factors for disc herniation, which may or may not be associated with axial LBP, include smoking, weight-bearing sports (e.g., weight lifting, hammer throw, etc.), and certain work activities, such as repeated lifting. Driving motor vehicles is also associated with increased risk *(11)*.

## Anthropomorphic Factors

There is a higher risk of LBP in very obese people. It has been postulated that the combination of weak abdominals and increased anterior load leads to stress on the posterior elements of the lumbar spine.

## Psychosocial Factors

The psychological and social aspect of LBP is one that is challenging and complex. The psychological component alone may cause the perpetuation of symptoms and may play a major role in those with chronic LBP. Psychosocial risk factors at work include perceived high pressure on time and workload, low job control, job dissatisfaction, monotonous work, and low support from co-workers and management *(12)*.

## ETIOLOGY OF BACK PAIN

LBP is a complex ailment with multiple etiologies that range from primary spinal causes to referred sources. Primary spinal back pain originates from the spinal structures, such as the vertebral bodies, discs, nerve roots, muscles, and tendons. Secondary spinal sources for LBP include infection, systemic disease, metabolic, and neoplastic causes. Lastly, referred pain may stem from viscerogenic or vascular causes.

## Primary Spinal Causes of LBP

### Spinal Osteoarthritis (Spondylosis and Degenerative Joint Disease)

Spinal osteoarthritis occurs with aging and overuse. It usually includes findings consistent with spondylosis and facet joint degeneration. Spondylosis is the formation of osteophytes or bony overgrowth of the vertebral body. Osteophytes are usually located on the anterior and lateral aspects of the vertebral body endplates. Although these findings show evidence of osteoarthritic changes, they may also be found in asymptomatic patients.

Osteoarthritis of the facet joints is another cause of localized back pain. Distortion of the normal anatomy or function of the facet joint disrupts the normal biomechanics of the joint, causing subsequent hyaline cartilage damage and periarticular hypertrophy, which can be secondary to degenerative disc disease or a primary process. If bony changes are significant, it may cause nerve root compression and patients may present with symptoms consistent with lumbar radiculopathy.

Morning pain and stiffness is a common symptom of this disease. Pain is often described as intermittent and can present with painful radiation to the buttock or posterior thigh. Pain is increased by activity, especially with extension and twisting motions of the spine, and relieved by rest. Patients demonstrate decreased range of motion and localized back pain. Radiographic findings frequently include spondylosis and facet joint hypertrophy.

*Lumbar Spondylolisthesis*

Spondylolisthesis is the displacement of one vertebral body on another resulting from different etiologies. One of the more common causes includes lumbar spondylolysis, which is a bony fracture of the pars interarticularis. Often the defect in the pars will be quiescent until some inciting event triggers the onset of pain. These patients present with localized back pain with or without radiation. Pain-provoking positions include extension and rotation of the lumbar spine.

Lumbar spondylolysis is only one of the causes of spondylolisthesis. There are several different classifications of spondylolisthesis that include the following *(13)*:

1. Dysplastic: congenital dysplasia in the superior sacral facet or inferior L5 facet allows L5 vertebral body subluxation on S1.
2. Isthmic: defects of the pars interarticularis.
   a. Lytic type also known as spondylolysis are stress fractures of the pars interarticularis.
   b. Elongated but intact pars results from microfractures that fill with bone over a long period of time.
3. Degenerative: results from degenerative changes at the disc and facet joints.
4. Traumatic: results from fracture of posterior elements other than pars (facet joints, lamina, pedicles).
5. Pathological: secondary to pathological changes in posterior elements secondary to malignancy, bone disease or infection.

*Degenerative Disc Disease*

The spine is made up of vertebral bodies and intervertebral discs. The disc is located between the bony vertebrae and acts as the shock absorber of the spine. The disc is composed of a tough outer annulus surrounding a soft center called the nucleus pulposus. In the normal course of aging, the annulus becomes more friable and is subject to cracking and fissuring called annular tears. The annulus is highly innervated and these tears can be painful. Typically, patients will present with localized back pain with occasional radiation to paravertebral musculature, buttocks, groin, and proximal thighs. Common complaints include back pain with bending or twisting movements.

If the annulus is significantly torn, and in the setting of continual axial loading, the softer nucleus pulposis can be forced to herniate through the torn annulus, which can occur posteriorly (most common), laterally, or anteriorly. When the herniated nucleus pulposis occurs in a posterior direction, it can cause nerve root impingement. This causes pain in the distribution of the nerve root and, if compression is significant enough, motor dysfunction. Midline disc protrusions can cause localized back pain and, if large enough, can cause radiculopathies or canal stenosis leading to cauda equina syndrome.

## Spinal Stenosis

Spinal stenosis occurs when the canal through which the spinal nerves pass becomes narrowed secondary to degenerative disc disease in the front of the canal and facet arthropathy in the back of the canal. This compression affects the nerve roots by limiting the blood supply and decreasing venous drainage. Symptoms then occur with increased activity when the nerve has higher metabolic demands and is unable to get the oxygen and nutrients that it needs.

Activities that flex the spine, such as sitting and walking slightly bent forward (such as in walking up a hill), increase the diameter of the spinal canal and alleviate some of the symptoms. Activities that involve extension of the spine, such as lying supine or prone, decrease the canal diameter exacerbating symptoms. Patients will often complain of pain in the legs while walking that is relieved by sitting.

## Coccyx Pain (Coccygodynia, Coccydynia)

The coccyx is the most inferior portion of the spine, most commonly called the tail bone. Pain originating from this area usually has an unknown etiology but has been associated with a sudden fall and childbirth. Patients present with tenderness over the coccyx and pain while sitting.

## Sacroiliac Pain

The sacroiliac (SI) joint connects the spine to the pelvis and is a common source of LBP. Pain evolving from the SI joint (SIJ) may be resulting from arthritic and/or inflammatory changes. The diagnosis can be confirmed by injecting the SIJ with a short-acting analgesic under fluoroscopic guidance.

## Traumatic Causes

### FRACTURES OR DISLOCATIONS

Fractures generally occur in the young, very active population and in the elderly. Women tend to get fractures earlier than men secondary to the added effect of bone weakness caused by osteoporosis. Compression fractures can occur spontaneously in patients with osteoporosis, multiple myeloma, metastatic cancer, and hyperparathyroidism. Compression fractures usually result from compressive flexion trauma, although spontaneous fracture can occur in patients with underlying pathology. The upper lumbar spine or the middle to lower thoracic spine is most commonly affected and pain is localized and is perceived immediately after the fracture occurs.

## Musculoligamentous/Myofascial

### ACUTE OR CHRONIC SPRAINS OR STRAINS OF LUMBAR, LUMBOSACRAL OR SI MUSCLE OR LIGAMENTS/MECHANICAL LBP

This is defined as nondiscogenic back pain that is exacerbated by physical activity and relieved by rest. It does not usually point to a particular cause, but is often caused by an amalgamation of stress and strain to tendons, muscles, and ligaments of the back. The pain often worsens throughout the day as daily activities add to stress on the back. Deconditioning and decompensation also can cause a mechanical back pain that is secondary to obesity, and weak abdominal and back muscles also known as the core stabilizers.

A sprain is a stretching or a tearing injury to a ligament. A strain is an injury to either a muscle or a tendon. Depending on the severity of the injury, a strain may be a simple over-stretch of the muscle or tendon or it can result in a partial or complete tear.

MYOFASCIAL PAIN SYNDROME AND TRIGGER POINTS

Myofascial pain syndrome (MPS) is a common cause of musculoskeletal pain. MPS is characterized by the development of trigger points that are locally tender when active and refer pain through specific patterns to other areas of the body. A trigger point or sensitive, painful area in the muscle or the junction of the muscle and fascia (hence, myofascial pain) develops as a result of any number of underlying causes. Trigger points are usually described as a taut band of ropey thick muscle tissue. When a trigger point is palpated, it causes referred pain. If there is no referral pain pattern, the area is termed a tender point.

The following factors can cause trigger and/or tender points:

1. Sudden trauma to musculoskeletal tissues (muscles, ligaments, tendons, bursae).
2. Injury to intervertebral discs.
3. Injury to the facet joints, ligaments, or other deep structures in the back.
4. Generalized fatigue (fibromyalgia is a perpetuating factor of MPS, perhaps chronic fatigue syndrome may produce trigger points as well).
5. Repetitive motions, excessive exercise, muscle strain resulting from overactivity.
6. Systemic conditions (e.g., gall bladder inflammation, heart attack, appendicitis, stomach irritation).
7. Lack of activity (e.g., a broken arm in a sling).
8. Nutritional deficiencies.
9. Hormonal changes (e.g., trigger point development during premenstrual syndrome or menopause).
10. Nervous tension or stress.
11. Chilling of areas of the body (e.g., sitting under an air conditioning duct, sleeping in front of an air conditioner).

The fascia is a tough connective tissue that spreads throughout the body in a three-dimensional web from head to foot without interruption. The fascia surrounds every muscle, bone, nerve, blood vessel and organ of the body, all the way down to the cellular level. Therefore, malfunction of the fascial system because of trauma, posture, or inflammation can create a binding down of the fascia, resulting in abnormal pressure on nerves, muscles, bones, or organs.

This binding can create pain or malfunction throughout the body, sometimes with side effects and seemingly unrelated symptoms. It is thought that an extremely high percentage of people suffering with pain and/or lack of motion may have myofascial problems, but most go undiagnosed, as the importance of fascia is just now being recognized. Many of the standard tests, such as X-rays, myelograms, computed axial tomography scans, electromyography, and so on, do not show the fascia.

Occasionally, trigger points produce autonomic nervous system changes such as flushing of the skin, hypersensitivity of areas of the skin, sweating in areas, or even "goose bumps." The trigger points cause localized pain, although trigger points can involve the whole body.

The characteristic electrical activity of myofascial trigger points most likely originates at dysfunctional endplates of extrafusal muscle fibers. This dysfunction appears to play a key role in the pathophysiology of trigger points *(14)*.

FIBROMYALGIA

Fibromyalgia is a pain syndrome that is defined as widespread pain of at least 3 months' duration both above and below the waist and on both right and left sides of the body, along with axial pain. Patients must have at least 11 of 18 tender points as designated by the American College of Rheumatology. Other associated symptoms and syndromes include disturbances in sleep, fatigue, swelling, tension-type headaches, and irritable bowel syndrome. Patients may also have a history of psychological disturbance, depression, and anxiety/panic disorder.

### Secondary Causes of LBP

*Inflammatory Causes*

SPONDYLOARTHROPATHIES (ANKYLOSING SPONDYLITIS)

Ankylosing spondylitis is a chronic inflammatory seronegative rheumatic spondyloarthropathy that affects skeletal and extraskeletal tissues. It is one of a group of rheumatic disorders. The spinal column, SIJs, and peripheral joints are commonly affected. Males are approximately three times more likely to get ankylosing spondylitis than females with a prevalence of about 1 in 1000 in the white population.

*Infectious Causes*

PYOGENIC VERTEBRAL SPONDYLITIS

*Intervertebral Disc Infection (Discitis) and Infectious Vertebral Osteomyelitis.* Discitis and infectious vertebral osteomyelitis can occur postoperatively as well as via lymphatic or hemotagenous seeding from a distant site of infection. It is more common in immunocompromised patients. Sources for infection include pneumonia, urinary tract infections, and cutaneous and dental infections. Pyogenic vertebral spondylitis is associated with spinal epidural abscesses, which can cause cauda equina syndrome and are a surgical emergency. Onset is often acute, with associated fever, malaise, and back pain in the setting of a concomitant infection or after spine surgery, discography, or spinal interventional procedures.

*Metabolic*

OSTEOPOROSIS/OSTEOPENIA

Osteoporosis is the most prevalent metabolic bone disease in the United States. It consists of a group of bone disorders in which there is reduced bone mass per unit volume as compared with normal bone. There is an increase in bone porosity and a decrease in bone density that results in more fragile bone structure. This fragile bone has an increased likelihood of fracture leading to pain.

PAGET'S DISEASE OF BONE

Paget's disease of bone is a common disease that is characterized by focal increase in osteoblastic activity in bone. It can present in a single bone or in many bones. Lesions in the vertebral bones or in the pelvis can cause focal pain.

*Neoplastic Causes*

Spinal: benign or malignant bony or soft tissue tumors/metastasis of spine.

Neoplasms of the spine are typically metastatic lesions from distant primary tumors. The cancers that most typically metastasize to spine are lung, prostate, breast, kidney, thyroid, multiple myeloma, malignant melanoma, and malignant lymphomas. Night and resting pain are often associated with neoplastic and infectious space-occupying lesions of the spine. All patients should be questioned on history of cancer as well as recent weight loss, pain that wakes the patient up from sleep, and fevers.

### Referred Causes for Back Pain

*Non-Spine-Related Causes of Back Pain*

Although the structures of the spine are the major cause of back pain, it is important to know the structures that can refer pain to the back. These structures include but are not limited to the following:

1. Viscerogenic:
    a. Upper genitourinary disorders.
    b. Retroperitoneal disorders (often neoplastic).
2. Vascular:
    a. Abdominal aortic aneurysm or dissection.
    b. Renal artery thrombosis or dissection.
    c. Stagnation of venous blood.

## DIAGNOSTIC APPROACH

As described previously, numerous pain generators—acting singly or in combination—may be responsible for a complaint of back pain. Furthermore, back pain may be the presenting complaint in a wide variety of pathologies, not only those intrinsic to the back. Proper diagnosis is therefore crucial, yet can be quite challenging. The goal of the diagnostic approach when confronting back pain is twofold. Obviously, one goal is to identify the relevant pain generator so that appropriate treatment can be initiated. Equally important, however, is to rule out the "red flags" that can present as back pain, but that may in fact be manifestations of more serious medical conditions. Causes of back pain can range from acute to chronic, focal to systemic, and can involve virtually any of the body's systems including neurological, cardiovascular, renal, musculoskeletal, and psychiatric. For these reasons, a thorough, focused history and physical examination are crucial first steps in the diagnostic approach to back pain.

### History

The history is necessarily the first step in the diagnostic approach, because the information obtained in this step guides subsequent actions. An appropriate history narrows the differential, focuses the physical exam, and directs one's choice of laboratory work and imaging. Because back pain can be the result of a variety of diverse etiologies, the history for back pain is a superset of the general medical history. In other words, the history should obtain information relating to past medical/surgical history, social/occupational setting, allergies, medications taken, and a complete review of systems.

The general medical history helps to place patients' complaints in the proper context. For example, diagnoses such as spondylosis, spinal stenosis, compression fractures, or malignancy are more likely in older individuals. Other pathologies, including acute disc herniation and ankylosing spondylitis, may be found more prominently in younger patients. Medical conditions or prior surgeries can play a significant role in pain-generating processes and so must be considered in the differential. Similarly, back pain can be related to one's vocational or avocational practices, so a social history that explores work, leisure activities, drug use, and smoking is needed.

The patient's medication list is another valuable source of information. Naturally, one cannot prescribe new medications without knowing whether the patient has drug allergies or is taking potentially interacting medicines. Moreover, patients have been known to omit crucial aspects of their history, and one may, for example, not determine that the patient has diabetes until noticing that the patient is on oral hypoglycemics.

The review of systems can elicit specific and useful information, and is an important place to check for "red flags." A history of unintentional weight loss and pain that is worse at night may signal malignancy. Changes in bowel or bladder function may indicate cauda equina syndrome. Complaints of chronic night sweats and chills may be a sign of an infectious cause.

In addition, there are elements of the history more specific to back pain, which are discussed in the following Subheadings.

*Duration*

"How long have you had your pain? Has the pain been present for days, weeks, months, years?" Knowing the duration allows one to immediately begin to narrow the differential in terms of acute versus chronic etiologies.

*Onset*

"How did the pain start? Did the pain start suddenly, or gradually?" Try to determine whether there were any unusual events that the patient can associate with the onset of symptoms. Did the pain begin while lifting? While bending? After surgery? Perhaps there was no inciting event, but the pain has been getting progressively worse for several months. Any of these descriptions can help to order the differential possibilities.

*Pattern*

Along with onset, it is important to identify the pattern of pain. Typically, benign musculoskeletal back pain is intermittent, worsening with activity and going away with rest. Chronic back pain may develop a constant component, with activity-related exacerbations. One should take note of pain that is constant and unremitting or that is intermittent but unpredictable or spasmodic. Establish the pattern of pain with relation to the patient's day. Does the pain get worse toward the end of the day, or is it present upon awakening? Also determine the pattern of pain in terms of the longer time course. Has the pain remained at the same level, has it worsened over time, or was the pain initially more severe, but has lessened?

*Alleviating/Exacerbating Factors*

The pattern of pain is often related to the factors that make the pain better or worse. Knowing these factors is useful as one attempts to localize the pain generator, and helps focus the physical exam. As mentioned previously, back pain is often activity-dependent, and improved with rest. Generally, however, patients can provide more specific information. Is the pain worse when walking, standing, or sitting? Is the pain relieved when lying down or when sitting? Pain resulting from sacroiliitis is often noticed when sitting and standing for prolonged periods and during sit-to-stand maneuvers. Ask whether the pain is better when bending forward or when leaning back? For some patients, pain from spinal stenosis is improved when sitting or bending forward. Classically, one may find these patients using a shopping cart to lean on as they walk. On the other hand, some patients with discogenic pain may find leaning back more comfortable. These patients may state that their pain is worse with Valsalva maneuvers or coughing or sneezing. Certain complaints may be a clue that the pain is not intrinsic to the back. For example, if the pain is worse when taking a deep breath, it may indicate respiratory or pulmonary pathology. Back pain that is particularly worse after meals may be cholecystitis or pancreatitis.

## Quality

Back pain can be variously described. The subjective nature of pain makes such descriptors of questionable value, but certain words can be helpful when trying to differentiate neuropathic from nociceptive pain. Specifically, neuropathic pain is often described as electrical in quality, burning, tingling, or shooting. It may be described as toothache-like, and may be associated with numbness. It is not typically described as dull or throbbing.

## Location/Radiation

Back pain that radiates to the legs is the hallmark of neurogenic pain. However, some types of nociceptive pain can also present with a radiating type of picture, and the diagnosis is not always obvious. SI pain, in particular, can cause pain in a similar distribution as that produced by irritation of sacral nerve roots. This type of nonspecific finding is not uncommon when confronting back pain, and for this reason, the other elements of the history as well as physical exam findings need to all be taken together to arrive at the most likely diagnosis.

A pain map can be a useful way to elicit information regarding quality, location, and radiation of pain. When looking at patients' pain maps one may see common patterns emerging. Localized, unilateral, paraspinal, non-radiating pain is typical of musculoskeletal strain. Pain from a herniated nucleus pulposus is commonly seen as a band of pain combined with pain in a scleratome radiation pattern. Pain from spinal stenosis is often symmetric presenting in the lower back and radiating to both legs.

## Quantification

The most commonly used clinical tool for quantifying a patient's pain is the numeric rating scale (NRS). The NRS is an eleven-step (0–10) scale. Patients are ask to rate their pain from 0 to 10, with the instructions that 0 represents no pain at all, and 10 represents the worst pain the patient can imagine. It is important to instruct the patient appropriately as to the endpoints of the scale, as many patients incorrectly assume that a 10 represents the worst pain they have experienced.

Because pain is subjective, the pain scale is most useful to assess the patient's pain over time. In this way the practitioner can determine whether various interventions are effective. Because pain varies with time and activity, it does not suffice to simply ask the patient to rate their pain. Rather, one should try to determine the range of pain the patient is currently experiencing. For example, one may ask a series of three questions. "On a scale from 0 to 10, please rate the worst pain you have felt in the past 7 days." Then, "Please rate the best your pain has been in the past 7 days." Finally, "Please rate how your pain is right now." Ideally, pain should be assessed with a pain rating at each office visit. In addition, after any intervention, whether therapeutic or diagnostic, a pain diary should be sent home with the patient.

## Physical Exam

The physical exam for back pain should be part of a focused general physical examination. Vital signs must be taken and the patient should be assessed systematically from head to foot. Begin with the patient's general habitus—is he or she obese? Excess weight puts additional strain on the musculoskeletal system and is associated with increased risk for diabetes and cardiovascular disease, all of which may be relevant to the diagnosis of back pain. On the other extreme, is the patient cachectic, which may prompt the need to consider malignancy or HIV in the differential. Does the patient appear comfortable or in acute distress? Assess the patient's respiration—is he or she breathing comfortably or is there dyspnea or wheezing? Take the patient's pulse to evaluate its rate and rhythm. Inspect and palpate the abdomen, keeping in mind that intra-abdominal pathology may present as back pain. Examine the legs. Are the pulses palpable? Are there stigmata of peripheral vascular disease? Ruling out vascular claudication simplifies the diagnosis of neurogenic claudication.

The systematic general physical examination helps to avoid missing red flags. Once this is done, one's attention can be turned to the musculoskeletal exam that is at the heart of the exam for back pain.

*Inspection*

The process of inspection begins before the patient has even entered the exam room. Observe how the patient is sitting. Observe how the patient rises from the chair. Observe the patient's gait as he or she walks to the exam room. Gait can be formally assessed later in the exam, but often one can appreciate subtle findings that may disappear when the patient knows he or she is being watched. The main goal of this step is to identify asymmetries or postural problems that may play a role in the patient's pathology. Normally, shoulders should be level, as should the pelvis. The spine should be midline and the paravertebral muscles should appear symmetric around the midline. One would expect some degree of lordosis in the lumbar spine. Absence of this may be indicative of paravertebral muscle spasm.

In addition, be alert for subcutaneous masses, skin markings, or tufts of hair, as these findings can result from pathologies such as neurofibromatosis or spina bifida. Surgical scars or evidence of trauma may bring to light information that was missed in the initial history.

*Palpation*

Gently palpate the skin and musculature of the back. At this point, one may discover neuropathic findings of hyperesthesia or allodynia. One may note areas of localized warmth that can signal an infectious or inflammatory process. While palpating the musculature, feel for spasm of the paravertebral muscles, which may be symmetrical or unilateral. When unilateral, paravertebral muscle spasm can cause a listing to that side. Muscle spasm may be the result of acute injury of the muscle itself, but more often, when muscle spasm persists, it is the result of guarding because of an underlying pathology.

Next, palpate the bony structures. Stand behind the patient, placing one's hands on the iliac crests. Bring the thumbs to the midline at the level of the iliac crests. The L4/L5 interspace is at this level, and can be used as a reference point to identify the other vertebrae. While palpating the iliac crests, assess again for symmetry, making sure the pelvis is level. Palpate along the spinous processes in the midline. Note deviations from midline, or deviations in the anterior/posterior plane, felt as a discrete step-off. This step-off is the hallmark of spondylolisthesis, which is a subluxation of one vertebra relative to its neighbor. This is most commonly seen at L5/S1, but is also relatively common at L4/L5.

Once the architecture of the back is assessed, one should palpate the structures of the back again, using firmer pressure to identify areas of tenderness. Apply firm (but not undue) pressure to the musculature of the back. Tender areas may be related to muscle in spasm, trigger points, tender points, or fibromyalgia. Palpate again along the midline, both on the spinous processes as well as the interspinous ligaments. Tenderness during this portion of the exam helps to localize the area of the pain generator, although it will not specifiy the etiological source. Attention should be paid to the SIJs because these are a common source of lower back or buttock pain. The SIJs can be located by placing one's hands along the patient's iliac crests, and letting one's thumbs rest at the SIJs located just inferior and medial to the posterior superior iliac spines (often marked by skin dimples).

When eliciting pain as part of the physical exam, either while palpating or with the provocative tests described in the following sections, it is very important to ask, "Is this your pain?" It is easy to elicit incidental pain and to then assume that one has correctly located the relevant pain generator. Rather, one must be certain that the pain elicited on exam is the pain for which the patient sought medical assistance.

*Range of Motion*

The examination for back pain includes an assessment of the range of motion in the spine and extremities. Limited range of motion in the spine is not itself specific to any particular disease entity, and can be found in any setting of back pain. Taken in context of the rest of the diagnostic data, the degree and areas of limitation can aid in localizing pathology as well as identifying functional deficits that need to be addressed as part of the therapeutic goal.

Motion in the cervical spine and upper extremities should be briefly evaluated as well. With the patient seated, one can begin by testing flexion, extension, rotation, and lateral flexion of the cervical spine. Watch for asymmetries in motion and evidence of pain. Then have the patient abduct both arms from his or her sides outward until they meet over the patient's head. One can ask the patient to return his or her arms to their sides and forward flex the arms until they are again meeting over the patient's head. External and internal rotation can be gauged by having the patient place his or her arms behind the head then behind the back, respectively.

Lumbar range of motion is tested with the patient standing. The basic movements to test for are flexion, extension, rotation, and lateral bending. The lumbar spine, aside from supporting the entire upper body, is the region responsible for the most of the motion of the back. Therefore, the lumbar spine is subject to a great deal of stress in everyday activity and is at higher risk for injury.

To test flexion, stand behind and to the side of the patient. The examiner should place his or her hand on the patient's lower back, spanning L4, L5, and S1 (i.e., with the top of the hand at the iliac crests). With appropriate flexion of the lumbar spine, the examiner should be able to appreciate a flattening of the lumbar lordosis, under the examiner's hand. Forward flexion of the back occurs both at the lumbar spine and at the hips. If the spine is hypomobile with respect to forward flexion, the normal lumbar lordosis will *not* reduce, indicating that the patient is mainly exhibiting hip flexion. Another useful test for identifying limitations in lumbar range of motion is Schober's test. A mark is made on the lumbar spine at the level of the posterior superior iliac spines. A second mark is made 10 cm superior. With normal lumbar range of motion, the two marks should become 2 to 3 cm farther apart.

Full range of motion for forward flexion allows the patient to touch the floor without bending the knees. This degree of flexibility is, more often than not, an ideal. For the average patient who can not touch the floor, gauge range of motion by the distance from the outstretched fingertips to the floor. Limited range of motion may be multifactorial. Hamstring tightness is very common and will result in increased finger-to-floor distance but without limitation in lumbar spine motion, and with a characteristic discomfort in the posterior thigh.

A positive Schober's test is characteristic of ankylosing spondylitis but may also be the result of any number of painful conditions causing guarding.

Lower extremity range of motion can then be tested in a straightforward manner by asking the patient to bend his or her knees to their chest, testing hip and knee flexion. Ankle dorsiflexion and plantar flexion are tested next. Limitations of lower extremity range of motion can lead to postural problems causing back pain or, conversely, limitations may be resulting from neurological compromise originating from back pathology.

After having the patient perform active range, the patient should be ranged passively. This is particularly important for areas in which the patient is lacking active range of motion, but the quality of motion should be evaluated even in patients with full range of motion. Various abnormalities can be found when examining range of motion. A patient may have increased resistance to moving through the range. This can be because of structural limitation from tight musculature, or in the extreme, contractures. This is a progressive problem resulting from some initial relative immobility, and which inevitably worsens if not corrected. Increased resistance can also result from increased motor tone, which is a sign of upper motor neuron damage, and will be found in association with brisk and pathological reflexes on neurological examination. Spasticity is a form of increased tone that is commonly mistaken for contracture, but can be distinguished by the fact that spasticity is velocity-dependent. Thus, a knee that is contracted into flexion by shortening of the hamstrings will not be brought into extension, regardless of the examiner's technique. A knee with a great deal of flexor tone or spasticity, however, should be extendable if the motion is done very slowly.

Also observed during range-of-motion exam is the quality of motion. Does the joint move smoothly on passive range, or can the examiner feel crepitations, characteristic of degenerative joints? Pain within the range of motion is abnormal, and the extent of pain-free range of motion should be noted.

*Neurological Exam*

Performance of a neurological exam helps to determine if there is a neuropathic component to the patient's complaint. The neurological exam must, of course, be taken in the context of the patient's complaints. Weakness, numbness, tingling, lancinating, and radiating pain all are indicators of neuropathic pain.

Manual muscle testing is most easily done as part of the range-of-motion testing during the physical examination. As the patient actively moves through the range of motion, ask him or her to stop and resist while the examiner applies an opposing force. It is important to determine if what appears to be weakness is true neurological weakness or simply an inability to resist secondary to pain. True weakness is felt simply as decreased resistance to opposing force. One may also note asymmetry in the speed or smoothness with which the patient moves through the range of motion. One may also notice asymmetrical patterns of atrophy. On the other hand, inability to resist because of pain often takes the form of "give-way" weakness. This is characterized by initial strong resistance followed by a sudden loss of resistance.

Manual muscle testing can help to determine the level of pathology of a radiculopathy. Weakness from radiculopathy is usually a late finding, and is indicative of a severe nerve compression. L2 and L3 innervate the iliopsoas and can be tested with resisted hip flexion. L2–L4 innervate the quadriceps and can be tested via knee extension. L4 is also tested in ankle dorsiflexion. L5 innervates extensor hallicus longus and so can be tested via extension of the great toe. S1 can be tested through plantarflexion of the ankle. The muscles supporting ankle dorsiflexion and plantarflexion can be very strong, and subtle weakness can be missed. One simple screen for this weakness is to have the patient take several steps on his or her heels (dorsiflexion) then on his or her toes (plantarflexion). Of course, balance or coordination issues can confound this test.

Muscle testing is complemented by examination of deep tendon reflexes. Patellar reflex is mainly an indicator of L4, ankle jerk reflex mainly reflects S1. Lower motor neuron pathology, such as that produced by radiculopathy, may cause decreased reflexes, whereas pathologically brisk reflexes indicate an upper motor neuron source. Person-to-person variability is considerable when it comes to reflex responses, and as such, asymmetry is the more crucial finding rather than absolute magnitude.

Sensory testing is the third component of the focused neurological exam for back pain. Herniated discs more typically cause a chemical radiculitis rather than a true compression radiculopathy, and altered sensation is therefore more common than frank weakness. Altered sensation may present as either hypo- or hypersensitivity, as well as hyperpathia or allodynia. It is important to delineate the distribution of the sensory changes to help localize the pathology. Scleratomal maps can be a great assistance, but again, one must realize that there is considerable variability, and the scleratome map is only a guide. As in the other components of the exam, asymmetries are often the signal to the pathology; however, some etiologies such as spinal stenosis classically cause bilateral symptoms, as differentiated from the more typical unilateral radiculopathy.

*Provocative Tests*

A great number of provocative tests have been described to aid in determining the proper diagnosis for back pain, which has led to the misconception that the reproduction of pain as a result of a particular provocative movement is diagnostic for a particular condition. This is not the case. On the contrary, provocative tests are essentially movements that put a greater than usual amount of stress on numerous aspects of the neural and musculoskeletal system. If there are active pain generators, they may be activated by the provocative tests. However, a given provocative test can activate a variety of pain generators. Thus, it is not merely the presence of pain that is significant during provocative testing, but rather the specific pattern of pain that is produced in the context of the rest of the examination.

For example, straight leg raising is often mentioned as being a test for a herniated lumbar disk. To perform the test, the patient should lie flat while the examiner holds the leg from underneath the heel and smoothly flexes the hip while keeping the knee extended. A straight leg raise is considered positive if pain is produced between 30 and 70° of hip flexion. However, straight leg raising can produce several different types of pain, reflecting different pathologies. Radicular pain, as from herniated intervertebral discs (although also possible from spondylosis) should result in reproduction of a neuropathic-type (e.g., tingly, deep, burning, electrical) pain with a characteristic scleratomal distribution. On the other hand, the straight leg raise may also be "positive" in cases of degenerative joint disease of the spine, paravertebral muscle, or SIJ arthropathy. In these cases, there may also be pain during the maneuver, but the pain should be localized to the pathological area rather than radiating to the leg.

Similarly, flexion, abduction, external rotation (FABER) test of the hip can be painful in several pathologies. FABER causing groin pain is typically indicative of hip pathology. FABER causing posterior buttock or lower back pain, is more likely the result of SI pain.

Another common maneuver that can be useful in isolating the cause of back pain is Kemp's maneuver. This test consists of passively leaning the patient back into lumbar extension while simultaneously rotating the spine in one direction or the other. This can be achieved by the examiner having one hand stabilizing the lower back while the other hand holds the patient's shoulder and pulls back. Non-radiating back pain associated with this "lean back and twist" is often found in association with facet joint (zygapophyseal) pathology. Characteristically, facet joint pain will also be provoked by palpation over the affected joint.

In all cases, provocative testing must be evaluated in the overall context of the history and physical examination. By the time provocative testing is done, the differential should be narrowed down to one of a few possibilities, in which case the result of a particular provocative maneuver can help to confirm one's suspicions. It bears repeating that any pain elicited during palpation or provocative testing must be "the patient's pain." It is not difficult to find painful areas on anyone in the course of a thorough examination. One must be careful not to subject the patient to unnecessary tests or interventions to define and eliminate pains that were only elicited incidentally.

## *Imaging*

Imaging studies may be done after the history and physical examination have significantly narrowed down the differential diagnosis. The main difficulty with the interpretation of imaging for back pain is that the findings are generally not specific. More to the point, finding abnormalities on imaging studies does not predict whether a patient's pain complaints are related to the imaging abnormalities. A 1994 study by Jensen et al. in the *New England Journal of Medicine* showed that 64% of *normal* adults had abnormalities found on magnetic resonance imaging (MRI) of the spine. They concluded that "the discovery by MRI of bulges or protrusions in people with low back pain may frequently be coincidental" *(15)*. Thus, an MRI cannot diagnose the etiology of back pain in most cases. An MRI done on a typical 60-year-old man may discover disc bulges, spondylosis, and neural foramen narrowing, but this does not give any indication whether the patients back pain is related to one or all of those findings.

Nevertheless, imaging does have its place in the diagnostic workup for back pain. Even after one is fairly sure of the patient's diagnosis, an imaging study can help to confirm the diagnosis or to give information about the severity of the pathology. Additionally, imaging may be needed to rule out red flags that may change the diagnostic or therapeutic plan. Some practitioners do not automatically proceed to imaging if the diagnosis seems clear, the patient is otherwise healthy, and the treatment plan is noninvasive. In these cases, it may be justifiable to proceed with treatment and image the patient only if the conservative treatment fails, particularly to help rule out other etiologies such as malignancy. Many practitioners will insist on imaging before any invasive interventions to rule out structural abnormalities or pathologies that may interfere with treatment or require additional planning or testing.

The type of imaging needed is guided by the information one is looking to obtain. To evaluate vertebral alignment, stability, and screen out fractures, a plain film is a sensible first step. Flexion/extension films are requested to evaluate dynamic stability. Oblique views are needed to adequately evaluate facet joints and to diagnose spondylolisthesis (a fracture of the pars interarticularis). A computed tomography (CT) scan is a more expensive and time-consuming modality, but provides excellent axial views of bony structures and information about surrounding soft tissue. Sagittal reconstructions can be generated, but the quality will be no better than the underlying axial films from which they are calculated. CT scans also subject the patient to radiation, as do plain films. MRI is more expensive and time-consuming still, but provides the best images for the purpose of evaluating soft tissues, including intervertebral discs and nerve tissue. The lengthiness of the scan and the relatively tight confines of the scanner may preclude some patients from undergoing MRI. Additionally, a careful history must be obtained to ensure that the patient does not have any embedded or implanted metal that may be incompatible with a safe MRI scan.

## Treatment

The treatment of LBP ranges from conservative noninvasive options to surgical intervention. The presentation and severity of each case dictates the type of treatment needed. The initial step for the majority of back pain sufferers usually involves medication and physical therapy. Most people find benefit from a well structured physical therapy program that teaches specific stretching and strengthening exercises to improve biomechanics. Over-the-counter medications such as nonsteroidal anti-inflammatories and acetaminophen can provide some relief. Prescribed medications, such as prednisone, muscle relaxants, and narcotic pain relievers, can also ease the pain.

When medication and physical therapy are not sufficient, fluoroscopically guided injections, such as epidurals, joint blocks, and radiofrequency ablation, may be necessary. The most commonly used intervention is the epidural injection in which cortisone is placed directly on the affected nerve root. If all the injections, medications, and physical therapy fail, surgery is an option. Surgical procedures such as discectomies, laminectomies, fusion, and disc replacement may be required.

When conventional treatment is not sufficient, more patients have been looking to alternative treatment such as yoga, hypnotism, acupuncture, herbals, and prolotherapy. One promising alternative is the use of botulinum toxin (BTX) for back pain.

### BTX and LBP

In recent years, BTX type A (BTX-A; Botox®) has found a place in the treatment algorithm for certain types of LBP. The success of BTX in the treatment of disorders such as spasticity, cervical dystonia, blepharospasm, and cervicogenic headaches has guided researchers and clinicians in extending its range of therapeutic uses. It has now been recognized that its primary power as a paralytic agent can translate into analgesic benefits for LBP sufferers. As more is learned about how BTX works, its role in the treatment of back pain, and pain in general, may continue to grow.

### Why Botox for LBP?

BTX-A is a *Clostridium*-derived neurotoxin that acts to prevent the release of acetylcholine from the presynaptic nerve terminal at the neuromuscular junction. This results in a flaccid paralysis owing to chemical denervation. This pharmacological property of BTX is thought to be primarily responsible for its therapeutic effects; it is the basis for which it has been tried for the treatment of certain types of LBP. New research, however, has pointed to other potential mechanisms by which BTX may induce analgesia. The latest theories consider a cascade of potential in vivo events that contribute to the overall therapeutic effect, beginning with the direct effect of muscle paralysis.

Muscle paralysis may help reduce LBP because it causes a reduction in local muscle spasm and tone associated with certain conditions. Prolonged muscle contraction, spasms, and increased tone have been thought to decrease local blood supply while increasing the oxygen demand of muscle tissue. The resultant ischemic muscle triggers the release of pain-related chemicals, including bradykinins, serotonin, potassium, prostaglandin E, and neuropeptides such as substance P *(16)*. This triggers a "pain cascade" that may increase both the number of nociceptors in the affected region and the sensitivity of existing nociceptors. This can contribute to the developing chronicity of pain. BTX can theoretically break this cycle by paralyzing the affected muscles.

This theorized analgesic effect of BTX has application to musculoskeletal disorders, in which increased muscle spasm and tone is a contributing factor. However, it has been reported in multiple studies that the analgesic effects of BTX can outlast or even precede a clinically noted reduction in muscle spasm *(16,17)*. These observations have led researchers to postulate that BTX may reduce pain through other mechanisms as well. Among these are the effects of BTX on autonomic function, central nervous system neuroplasticity, and non-acetylcholine neurons.

BTX has traditionally been thought to affect only striated muscle; however, many preganglionic motor neurons in the autonomic nervous system are cholinergic and can also be directly impacted by BTX. The interaction of BTX with the autonomic nervous system is complex, but there are several mechanisms by which this interaction may modify the perception of pain. Neurogenic inflammation, for instance, has been associated with MPS and may be influenced by the autonomic nervous system. Mediated primarily by substance P and nitrous oxide, it is a complex process that consists of an inflammatory response followed by an alteration in the permeability of the peripheral vasculature. Local edema, erythema, and pain result. It is theorized that BTX may block early events in the cascade and prevent deleterious changes in regional blood flow patterns *(16)*.

Central nervous system neuroplasticity is a process by which prolonged exposure to painful stimuli can result in the anatomical modification of the neurological elements of pain recognition and perception. Essentially, peripheral pain such as that caused by local inflammation can trigger a "feedback" mechanism to the central nervous system that results in increased sensitization to painful stimuli and a prolonged pain response. Most theories of this biological mechanism involve anatomic changes in the excitatory and/or inhibitory sensory pathways in the spinal cord and, possibly, the cerebral cortex. The effect of BTX on peripheral sensory pathways discussed previously may have beneficial effects on the anatomic reorganization of higher pain pathways. In this way, analgesic effects can theoretically outlast the direct paralytic effects of the toxin *(16)*.

BTX may also directly affect the release and function of non-acetylcholine neurotransmitters; this is the least understood potential effect of BTX. Several in vitro studies have shown that BTX can exert direct effects on important compounds involved in pain pathways, such as glutamate, vasopressin, and substance P *(16,18)*. Further study is required in this area and is ongoing.

*General Overview of Treatment Approaches*

With respect to LBP, BTX-A has been used most frequently and with the greatest success when selectively injected into the lumbosacral paravertebral musculature. Although somewhat controversial, many clinicians associate paravertebral muscle spasm with a variety of common pathologies that cause LBP. These include, but are not limited to, radiculopathy, facet joint pathology, spinal osteoarthritis, degenerative disc disease, MPSs, acute and chronic sprains, and inflammatory disorders. There is currently little information on the use of BTX-B for LBP.

Spinal pathologies are generally complex and the pain associated with them is often multifactorial. For instance, a compressed spinal nerve root can cause symptoms consistent with a lumbosacral radiculopathy. Affected patients may complain of burning radiating pain down one leg. They may also complain of stiffness and spasm in the lower back. BTX may ultimately be useful in treating paravertebral muscle spasm by mechanisms discussed earlier. Other treatment options must be explored to treat the nerve compression itself. In this respect, BTX can be considered part of a multifaceted treatment plan, a pharmacotherapy that addresses part of the symptom complex.

For local spasm of unknown or unclear etiology or for isolated trigger points in the lower back region secondary to MPSs or muscle microtrauma, BTX injections may be sufficient as stand-alone therapy. In these cases, expense may be a limiting factor and BTX would be considered after other less costly therapies are trialed, including physical therapy, dry needling, and or local injection with anesthetic and/or steroid medications.

However, as its mechanisms of action become clearer, earlier and more liberal use of BTX may be indicated. Its potential effects on the autonomic nervous system, for instance, may have new implications for the treatment of MPS where autonomic dysfunction has been described. In these cases, early treatment with BTX may justifiably supercede traditional treatment.

*Current Research*

Research on BTX and its role in the treatment of LBP is limited. There are few randomized, placebo-controlled studies that have clinical applications; much of what is published is in the form of case reports or preliminary studies with very small sample sizes. Several of the larger studies are reviewed here.

Foster et al. studied the use of BTX-A injections in the lumbar paravertebral muscles versus placebo (saline) in 31 subjects with chronic LBP in a randomized, double-blind study. The inclusion criteria included LBP of 6 months or longer duration and pain laterality (either unilateral or bilateral if one side was more painful than the other). Patients were excluded if they had a systemic inflammatory disorder, acute pathology observed on MRI of the spine, a recent injection of elements of the lumbosacral spine with anesthetic and/or corticosteroid, or evidence of secondary gain. Subjects were examined and assessed for the presence or absence of increased paravertebral muscle tone, back tenderness, and focal trigger points. Most patients had no clear cause for their back pain. Several had a remote history of back trauma. Others had a history of disc disease, including three with remote discectomies. Chronic degenerative changes of the spine were seen on MRI of the spine in several older patients *(19)*.

BTX-A was prepared by reconstituting freeze-dried toxin with 0.9% saline to 100 U/mL concentration. This was drawn into a 1-mL syringe with a 27-gage needle. Injections of Botox or placebo were given at five lumbar or lumbosacral paravertebral muscle sites, 40 U per injection, unilaterally *(19)*.

Pain intensity was measured using the visual analog scale (VAS) at baseline and 3 and 8 weeks after injection. Function was measured using the Oswestry low back pain questionnaire at baseline and 8 weeks after injection. For the VAS, significant improvement was considered a 50% improvement over the pretreatment value. For the Oswestry LBP questionnaire, a two-grade improvement was defined as significant. At 3 weeks, some degree of pain relief was reported in 86% of patients in the Botox group and 31% in the placebo group. The pain relief (VAS) was significant in 73.3% of the Botox group and 25% of the placebo group. At 8 weeks, significant pain relief continued in 60% of the Botox group and 12.5% of the saline group. Functional improvement was demonstrated in 66.7% of the Botox group and 18.8% of the placebo group at 8 weeks. No patient in the Botox group worsened from baseline and injections were well tolerated with no side effects. Six-month follow-up revealed no further analgesia.

De Andres et al. investigated the use of BTX-A intramuscular injections for the treatment of MPS in an open-label prospective clinical trial. Inclusion criteria after a diagnosis of refractory MPS included the presence of muscle spasm in the form of a taut band with a zone of tenderness, pain on stretching, existence of trigger points with associated referred pain, and failure of conservative therapy to relieve pain. Exclusion criteria included neurological deficits involving the painful area, history of disc or bone disease with associated radiculopathy, motor neuron disease, or disorders affecting the neuromuscular junction. A number of different affected muscles were treated. A total of 90 subjects were included. Of these, a total of 17 subjects received injections into the quadratus lumborum, which was identified as a muscle responsible for LBP in certain subjects with MPS. All received physical therapy and were continued on their medications, if any, throughout the study *(20)*.

Freeze-dried BTX-A was reconstituted in 0.9% normal saline to a concentration of 10 U/mL. The dosage used for the quadratus lumborum muscle was 50 U, delivered once with a 3.5-in. spinal needle using fluoroscopic guidance. Pain levels were measured using the VAS at baseline, 15, 30, and 90 days post-injection. Functional questionnaires (Lattinen) and a psychological impairment assessment tool were also utilized.

The results revealed an improvement in the mean VAS score for all subjects at 15, 30, and 90 days posttreatment, but significant at 15 and 30 days only. Functional improvement was significant post-treatment. No significant improvement was noted for the psychological assessment. Unfortunately, statistics are in the aggregate and results for individual muscles are not available *(20)*.

Studies of the effectiveness of BTX-B in the treatment of LBP are limited. A poster presentation of an open-label prospective study by Opida examined the use of BTX-B for chronic LBP. A total of 35 subjects with LBP and/or spasms and reduced range of motion of the spine for 6 months or longer were included. Subjects with radicular symptoms were excluded. A total of 10,000 U BTX-B was injected into the lumbosacral paravertebral muscles at four levels in equal doses. Of the subjects, 66% reported improved pain and range of motion at 4 and 12 weeks posttreatment, although pain relief was most significant at 4 weeks *(21)*.

*When to Consider BTX for LBP*

Research and clinical experience has shown that BTX may be used safely to treat pain secondary to spasm and increased tone in the musculature of the lower back. It may also be used to effectively treat local "trigger points" in deep or superficial muscles of the lower back. As discussed earlier, spasm and increased tone may occur secondary to a number of different spinal pathologies or local disorders or muscle. Trigger points, meanwhile, are traditionally associated with MPSs, and can be associated with both superficial and deep muscles.

Most clinical uses of BTX have focused on patients suffering from chronic LBP, usually defined as LBP for more than 6 months. Because BTX is a relatively new treatment for pain and is relatively costly, established treatments are usually attempted first. Furthermore, most back pain is self-limiting and can be expected to improve after a period of several months, obviating the need for expensive or experimental treatments. However, as more is learned about BTX and its potential for analgesia, earlier use may be justified.

Once any potential malignant, systemic, or otherwise emergent causes for LBP are ruled out, treatment is conservative at first and should involve a multidisciplinary approach, including physical therapy and oral medications as needed. Trigger points may be "dry needled" or injected with local anesthetics during this time. If there is no satisfactory improvement after a 4 to 6 week trial, interventional spinal procedures may be indicated if a spinal pathology is suspected. Afterward, if spasm and local tenderness in the lower back continue to be significant, regardless of the primary pathology, BTX can play a role as part of the continuing treatment plan.

*How to Use BTX-A*

BTX-A (Botox) is supplied in single-use vials containing 100 U each. It is in the form of a vacuum-dried solid that must be reconstituted with preservative-free 0.9% sodium chloride sterile saline. The proper amount of dilutant should be drawn into an appropriate syringe and slowly injected into the vial of Botox. If the vacuum does not draw the dilutant in to the vial, the vial should be discarded. The solution should then be gently mixed and administered no longer that 4 hours after reconstitution, during which time it should be refrigerated at 2 to 8°C. The reconstituted Botox should be clear, colorless, and free of particulate matter. The solution should then be drawn up into an appropriately sized sterile syringe. Any air bubbles should be expelled *(22)*.

A history should be taken before injection, including patient allergies, medications, and a past medical history specifically inquiring as to coagulation disorders. Patients on Coumadin® therapy or with signs of infection at the injection site should not be injected. Injection landmarks should be identified and marked before injection. For the lumbosacral paravertebral muscles, tender areas should be manually palpated 2 cm lateral to the spinous processes. Given the proximity of the paravertebral muscles to sensitive structures, such as the spinal roots and nerves, EMG guidance is recommended. Up to eight bilateral spinal levels (four per side) may be injected at one time. No more than 200 U total should be injected, divided equally among the injection sites. The Botox should be diluted to a concentration of 100 U/mL and drawn into a suitably sized syringe. A 25- or 27-gage sterile needle may be used effectively. Once the injection sites are identified, proper sterile preparation of the area should be performed. The patient should in prone or side-lying position and should be as relaxed as possible. The needle should be carefully inserted lateral to the spinous processes and angled slightly laterally. If the patient experiences any neuropathic-type pain, the needle should be withdrawn. Once proper placement is obtained, the syringe should be aspirated slightly to exclude placement in a blood vessel. If there is no aspirate, the BTX may be slowly injected. Up to 40 U per site is appropriate. This approach may be used for both spasm and/or local trigger points found within the lumbosacral paravertebral muscles.

Deeper muscles such as the quadratus lumborum should be injected using fluoroscopic or CT guidance and should be attempted only by experienced clinicians. A detailed discussion of these techniques is beyond the scope of this chapter. With respect to dosing, however, a one-time injection of 50 U BTX-A is appropriate.

It has generally been reported that pain relief may last up to a period of 3 to 4 months post-treatment. The effect may wane over this time. Repeat injections may be performed, but the cumulative dose of Botox treatment in a 30-day period should not exceed 200 U. With repeated exposure, the formation of neutralizing antibodies to BTX-A may occur, which may reduce its effectiveness in these individuals *(22)*.

*Other Concerns*

BTX causes paralysis of muscle. Excessive weakness after administration is therefore a potential side effect when treating LBP. Several authors and clinicians have expressed concern over the risk of possible impairment of ambulation secondary to weakening of the paravertebral muscles. This side effect was not a factor in the study performed by Foster et al. *(19)*. In another study, patients with truncal dystonia were treated with BTX-A injections to the paravertebral muscles at doses ranging from 150 to 500 U per session. No cases of impaired ambulation were reported among the study subjects *(23)*.

## CONCLUSION

Studies have shown that BTX-A is a useful option for patients with LBP. This treatment seems most helpful in those with MPS and lumbar paraspinal spasm. Its proposed efficacy stems from reducing muscle tone, decreasing the amount of inflammatory factors such as substance P, and affecting neurotransmitter release. Although the current research is promising, further clinical trials are needed. Clinicians should also be aware of the potential generalized side effects, drug interactions, and contraindications of treatment with BTX before they incorporate it into their practice.

## REFERENCES

1. Benn RT, Wood PHN. Pain in the back: an attempt to estimate the size of the problem. Rheumatol Rehabil 1975;14:121–128.
2. Andersson GBJ. Epidemiologic features of chronic low-back pain. Lancet 1999;354:581–585.
3. Hart LG, Deyo RA, Cherkin DC. Physician office visits for low back pain: frequency, clinical evaluation, and treatment patterns from a U.S. national survey. Spine 1995;20:11–19.
4. Keller GC. Low back pain: Where does it come from and how do we treat it? Jacksonville Medicine. 1999;April:143–149.
5. Andersson GBJ. The epidemiology of spinal disorders. In: Frymoyer JW, ed. The Adult Spine: Principles and Practice. 2nd ed. New York: Raven Press, 1997, pp. 93–141.
6. Shelerud R. Epidemiology of occupational low back pain. Occup Med 1998;13:1–22.
7. Steenstra IA, Verbeek JH, Heymans MW, Bongers PM. Prognostic factors for duration of sick leave in patients sick listed with acute low back pain: a systematic review of the literature. Occup Environ Med 2005;62:851–860.
8. Frymoyer JW, Cats-Baril WL. An overview of the incidences and costs of low back pain. Orthop Clin North Am 1991;22:263–271.
9. Loisel P, Lemaire J, Poitras S, et al. Cost-benefit and cost-effectiveness analysis of a disability prevention model for back pain management: a six year follow up study. Occup Environ Med 2002;59:807–815.
10. Pope MH. Risk indicators in low back pain. Ann Med 1989;21:387.
11. Kelsey JL, Githens P, O'Connor T, et al. Acute prolapsed lumbar intervertebral disc: an epidemiologic study with special reference to driving automobiles and cigarette smoking. Spine 1984;9: 608–613.
12. Devereux JJ, Buckle PW, Vlachonikolis IG. Interactions between physical and psychosocial risk factors at work increase the risk of back disorders: an epidemiological approach. Occup Environ Med 1999;56:343–353.

13. Mokri B, Sinaki M. Painful disorders of the spine and back pain syndromes. In: Sinaki M, ed. Basic Clinical Rehabilitation Medicine. 2nd ed. St Louis: Mosby-Year Book, 1993, pp. 489–502.
14. Bendtsen L, Jensen R, Olesen J. Qualitatively altered nociception in chronic myofascial pain. Pain 1996;65:259–264.
15. Jensen MC, Brant-Zawadzki MN, Obuchowski N, Modic MT, Malkasian D, Ross JS. Magnetic resonance imaging of the lumbar spine in people without back pain. N Engl J Med 1994;331:69–73.
16. Arezzo J. Possible mechanisms for the effects of botulinum toxin on pain. Clin J Pain 2002; 18:S125–S132.
17. Freund B. Temporal relationship of muscle weakness and pain reduction in subjects treated with botulinum toxin A. J Pain 2003;4:159–165.
18. Mense S. Neurobiological basis for the use of botulinum toxin in pain therapy. J Neurol 2004; 251:I1–I7.
19. Foster L. Botulinum toxin A and chronic low back pain: a randomized, double-blind study. Neurology 2001;56:1290–1293.
20. De Andres J, Cerda-Olmedo G, Valia JC, Monsalve V, Lopez-Alarcon, Minguez A. Use of botulinum toxin in the treatment of chronic myofascial pain. Clin J Pain 2003;19:269–275.
21. Opida CL. Open-label study of Myobloc/Neurobloc (botulinum toxin type B) in the treatment of patients with chronic low back pain. Poster 202 presented at International Conference 2002: Basic and Therapeutic Aspect of Botulinum and Tetanus Toxins. June 2002, Hanover, Germany.
22. Allergan, Inc. Botox® package insert. Irvine, CA.
23. Comella CL, Shannon K, Jaglin J. Extensor truncal dystonia. Successful treatment with botulinum toxin injections. Mov Disord 1998;13:552–555.

# 5

# Piriformis Syndrome

## Loren M. Fishman, Alena Polesin, and Steven Sampson

### INTRODUCTION

Piriformis syndrome (PS) is the reversible compression of the sciatic nerve by the piriformis muscle. It may cause deep and severe pain in the buttock, hip, and sciatica, with radiation into the thigh, leg, foot, and toes. Like carpal tunnel or pronator syndromes, it may cause damage to the peripheral nerve through excessive pressure *(1)*. In PS, piriformis muscular tension presses the sciatic nerve anteriorly and inferiorly against the sharp tendinous edges of other muscles, such as the gemellus superior and obturator internus *(2,3)*. The painful condition that results may become chronic and debilitating.

### HISTORY OF PS

The syndrome was actually known in 15th century Florence, when hospitals were filled with cases of sciatica, a term used by Hippocratres, Galen, and Dioscorides (ischiatica). *Ischiatica* originally meant haunches or hip and gave its name to the ischial tuberosity *(4)*, the approximate anatomical location of the pain's origin and its imagined cause in that era. Sacroiliac arthritis and tuberculosis of the iliopsoas muscles were the proposed pathogenetic mechanisms.

After the work of Mixter and Barr in 1932 *(5)*, people began to accept spinal and intramedullary pathology as the chief causes of sciatica. Effective surgical techniques combined with improvements in anesthesiology and antibiotics made surgery for spinal conditions much more practical. Imaging studies advanced from tomograms through computed tomography (CT) scans to ever more sophisticated magnetic resonance imaging (MRI), rendering diagnosis within the reach of any internist or specialist.

It is this foraminal or intramedullary condition that comes to every clinician's mind when he or she is presented with a patient suffering from sciatica. A group of leading physicians and epidemiologists have defined sciatica as "…symptoms and findings considered to be secondary to herniations of a lumbar disc" *(6)*. However, sciatica is a symptom, not a diagnosis. It describes pain and feelings in the distribution of a peripheral nerve. It stands to reason that pain along the course of the sciatic nerve would at times be caused by pathological involvement of the nerve itself, and that rational diagnosis and treatment would then focus on the site of the pathology.

From: *Therapeutic Uses of Botulinum Toxin*
Edited by: G. Cooper © Humana Press Inc., Totowa, NJ

## EPIDEMIOLOGY

Because an estimated 80 million Americans suffer from low back pain and sciatica annually, any sizeable percentage of that group suffering from PS would be significant. One reason the syndrome is underdiagnosed is that MRI, myelogram, CT, and other imaging studies are very unlikely to turn up real evidence of PS *(7–9)*. Rather, it is a functional syndrome, in which only certain positions and pressures will bring out the pain, paresthesias, and weakness that come with it. Therefore, traditional structural imaging studies are of minimal value *(10–14)*.

In February 2005, a group at the University of California, Los Angeles shimmed an otherwise standard MRI device for the pelvis and used software to subtract the fat-suppression signals from the full image, leaving only the fat-covered nerve to highlight the neuroanatomy from the cauda equina through the lumbosacral plexus and the buttock *(15)*. Examining 229 patients that either had remained undiagnosed or had undergone unsuccessful lumbar spinal surgeries, they identified 161 patients (67.8%) with PS. These patients had suffered an average of 4.2 years, and had averaged more than eight visits with clinicians in that time. The group concluded:

> The true incidence of piriformis syndrome is not clear at this time. Lacking agreement even on the existence of the diagnosis and on how to establish the diagnosis if it does exist, epidemiological work has been scarce; however, there is a reasonable inference to be made from the fact that of 1.5 million patients with sciatica severe enough to require MR imaging, only 200,000 prove to have a treatable herniated disc. One interpretation of the results obtained in our study population is that piriforms syndrome may be as common as herniated discs in the cause of sciatica. [...] The low rate of referral and frequent failure to recognize the diagnosis, however, should not be mistaken for evidence of a low incidence in the population (15).

In 1983, without the aid of MRI or electromyography (EMG), it was estimated that 6% of all patients presenting to a back pain service at the Mayo Clinic had PS *(16)*. Records from 1976 to 1979 in Olmstead County, where the Mayo Clinic is located, found the diagnosis of PS was made 11 times out of 4416 cases, or 0.25% *(17)*. The same county had 54 of 4349 piriformis diagnoses in 2001, a fivefold increase to 1.24%, but still another fivefold short of the naïve diagnostic incidence seen at Mayo. In 2002, Walter Reed Hospital had 54 of 9161 piriformis diagnoses or 1.58% *(17)*.

This tendency, as well as general underemphasis on anatomical and functional matters in contemporary American medical education, suggests that the syndrome is probably significantly underdiagnosed. In many quarters, it is even considered a "diagnosis of exclusion," although there is good evidence that the diagnosis may co-exist with herniated disc, spinal stenosis, and sacroiliac derangement *(17,18)*. This tendency has led to a large but unquantifiable group of patients receiving an ever-increasing number of painful and pointless surgical and nonsurgical procedures based on limited inquiries and faulty diagnosis.

Given 80 million yearly complaints of sciatica, even the Mayo Clinic's 6% of all back pain estimated made more than 25 years ago would suggest that there are 4.8 million cases of PS annually. Considering the years from onset to diagnosis, that leaves an eight-digit reservoir of patients with PS.

Two groups are primarily affected: active individuals (such as athletes, health club users, joggers, and performers) and people in vocations that require prolonged sitting (such as financial workers, lawyers, psychotherapists, secretaries and vehicular drivers). The most common cause is overactivity, followed by occupational factors, trauma, improper lifting, and back strain. There are many other initiating events, including misplaced gluteal injections and lipomas.

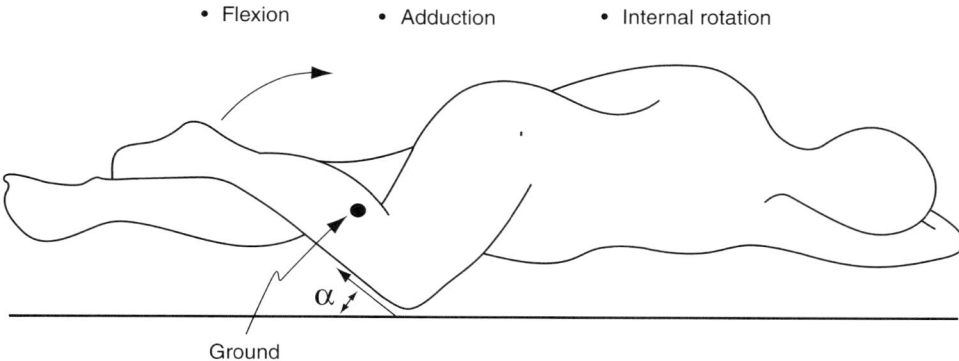

Pace sign: Abduction weak
Solheim sign: Adduction painful

• Flexion      • Adduction      • Internal rotation

α

Ground

**Fig. 1.** The most reliable signs are weakness in resisted abduction of the flexed thigh (Pace) and buttock pain with passive adduction of the flexed thigh (Solheim). This is the flexion adduction and internal rotation test (FAIR-test) position as well. The solid angle α is the independent variable; H-reflex delay is the dependent variable.

## DIAGNOSIS

On physical examination, there is generally tenderness in the buttock at some point(s) between the medial edge of the greater sciatic foramen to the greater trochanter *(10)*. A few clinical signs and provocative maneuvers that stretch the piriformis muscle and create additional pressure on the sciatic nerve are useful. Lasegue sign is arguably helpful. More consistent is pain on voluntary flexion, adduction, and internal rotation of the hip *(19)*; Freiberg sign is pain on passive internal rotation of the extended thigh *(20)*; Solheim modified this, looking for buttock pain on passive adduction and internal rotation of the flexed thigh, a reliable sign *(2)*. Pace sign, which is also reliable, describes weakness on resisted abduction of the flexed hip with the patient in contralateral decubitus (*see* Fig. 1; ref. 1).

Previously, the diagnosis of PS was thought to be exclusively clinical (1–3, 8, 16, 21). Modern methods of diagnosis began with the work of Fishman and Zybert (11–14) using the H-reflex and EMG in 1987. The H-reflex is essentially an electronic version of the reflex arc responsible for the Achilles tendon reflex, measuring it in millionths of volts and hundred-thousandths of a second. The H-reflex in the unstretched anatomical position is compared with the H-reflex in the flexion adduction and internal rotation (FAIR) test position. In a positive result, the piriformis muscle tightly compresses the sciatic nerve against the underlying structures, causing a statistically significant delay in the H-reflex (*see* Fig. 2).

Since the 1987 study, patients were judged to have PS if they had FAIR test values that were prolonged more than three standard deviations beyond the mean seen in normal controls or in contralateral lower extremities. More than 80% of patients so diagnosed improved 50% or more with conservative therapy aimed at loosening the piriformis muscle in the buttock. The number of people with PS and the recovery rate of patients identified by the FAIR test were greater than what had been seen in patients selected by any other known means *(14)*.

Because of the nature of the syndrome, the test for PS is functional in nature, comparing conduction speed when the sciatic nerve is compressed with values seen in a resting position.

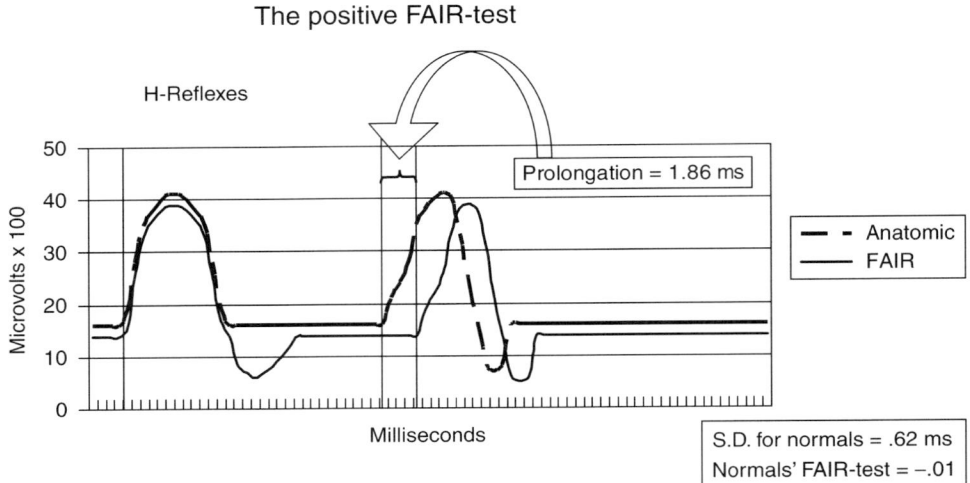

**Fig. 2.** We consider piriformis syndrome confirmed if flexion adduction and internal rotation (the FAIR-test) brings more than three standard deviation delay of the H-reflex (1.86 ms).

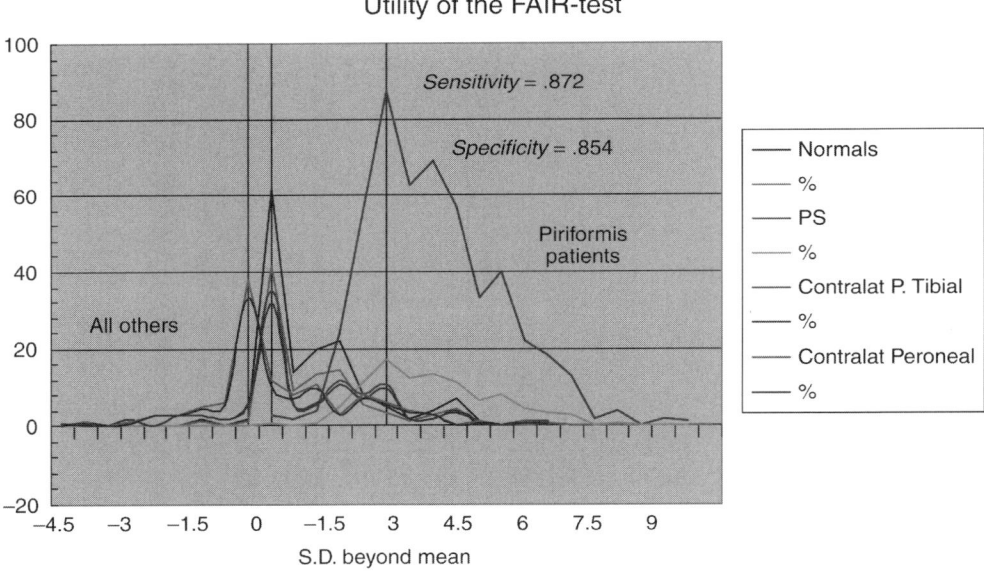

**Fig. 3.** The mean delay of H-reflexes in flexion adduction and internal rotation for patients with clinical signs of piriformis syndrome is nearly five standard deviations beyond what is seen in patients with herinated discs, normal volunteers, and contralateral extremities of patients with piriformis syndrome.

The delay seen in PS is not subtle, because compression in the buttock region affects both the afferent and the efferent limbs of the H-reflex (10–14). The H-reflex delay in PS is reasonably easy to identify (*see* Fig. 3).

Because severe compression or damage may obliterate a reflex, both posterior tibial and peroneal H-reflexes are studied in the anatomical position and the FAIR test position. Therefore, the H-reflex is actually performed four times with each limb that is studied *(11)*.

**Table 1**
**Validity of Pirformis Tests**

| Piriformis syndrome | Specificity | Sensitivity |
|---|---|---|
| Filler et al. | 0.93 | 0.64 |
| Fishman et al. | 0.83 | 0.88 |
| Used together | Higher | Higher |

EMG testing can differentiate PS from other causes of low back pain, including radiculopathy and spinal stenosis. In these cases, the H-reflex without the FAIR test is performed on the unaffected limb for comparison to rule in or out radiculopathy and spinal stenosis, while it is performed with the FAIR test on the affected limb.

Dr. Aaron Filler's group at the University of California, Los Angeles has validated the neural scan method by successfully injecting the piriformis muscle with marcaine and celestone in 136 of 162 PS patients the neural scans identified, using titanium needles and MRI guidance *(15)*. They used 15 to 25 MRI images per patient to ensure proper localization of the muscle for injection. The 62 patients that failed to retain their improvement, or refused injection, went on to surgery. On 26-month follow-up, 76% had good or excellent results *(15)*.

## DOES PS EXIST?

How does one justify introduction of a clinical entity? Give a consistent presentation of signs and symptoms, confirm a pathogenetic mechanism that explains their co-presence and verify that a treatment based on this mechanism helps the people with that constellation of complaints.

In 2003, John Stewart of McGill University set out five criteria for confirming a case of PS *(21)*. The patient must have sciatica, with EMG evidence of neurological injury along the course of the sciatic nerve, normal EMG evaluation of the paraspinal muscles, a normal lumbosacral MRI, and compression confirmed at surgery. Dr. Stewart exaggerates his final criteria by asserting that the patient also must improve with surgical decompression. However, with that line of reasoning, if a patient did not improve after cancer surgery we could conclude that he or she did not have cancer. Even so, between Filler and Fishman, these criteria are well-satisfied:

1. Sciatica. Confirmed in Filler's and Fishman's studies.
2. EMG: Demonstrating involvement of the sciatic nerve, but not the paraspinal muscles. Confirmed in 320 patients in Fishman's study, 239 in Filler's study.
3. Normal lumbosacral MRI.
4. Surgically confirmed compression. Confirmed in 47 of 62 patients in Filler's study and 60 of 85 patients in Fishman's study.
5. Improvement with decompression. Confirmed in 47 of 62 patients in Filler's study and 60 of 85 patients in Fishman's study.

These two types of tests for PS have acceptably high sensitivity and selectivity. Both are significantly higher when the tests are used together (Table 1).

At this writing, both EMG and neural scan have been completed on 19 problematic cases of PS that failed conservative management. Seventeen have been found positive under both sets of criteria.

## PATHOGENETIC MECHANISM

There are essentially three mechanisms by which the piriformis muscle interferes with conduction along the motor and sensory fibers of the sciatic nerve:

1. Overuse leads to spasm. In the case of spasm, there is direct compression of the nerve bundles, through pressure by the muscle on one side and, on the other, by the sharp tendinous edge of the gemellus superior, ischiofemoral ligament, or indirect pressure from the innominate bone.
2. Trauma brings scar formation within 3 to 6 months. Cicatrix, especially on the ventral surface of the piriformis muscle, can place a hardened and irregular object directly in the path of the sciatic nerve, exerting direct mechanical pressure on the nerve, or altering its course, producing high tension within its fibers and/or compressing the vaso nervorum.
3. A number of anatomical and genetic variations are correlated with changes in the physiological and chemical properties of myelin. Leg length discrepancy asymmetrically exercises the piriformis muscles; in high-performance athletes, there is MRI evidence of sciatic nerve thinning and reduced fat-padding at the sciatic foramen. In hereditary neuropathic pressure palsy and Charcot-Marie Tooth, for example, the myelin elements of nerves are particularly vulnerable to the types of forces exerted in numbers 1 and 2 *(22)*.

In the first two cases, PS is associated with denudation of the vaso nervorum, thinning, and/or traumatic alteration of the epineureum. Myelin coverings of individual nerve sheaths are affected in the third.

Several anatomical studies have been taken to precipitate PS with the anomalous anatomical condition in which one or both divisions of the sciatic nerve pass through or even over the piriformis muscle. However, this common anatomical variant does not seem to cause or correlate with PS. These anomalies are almost invariably bilateral, whereas PS is unilateral in 95% of cases. Further, in 72 surgical cases reviewed, only 15% reveal these anatomical variations, the same percentage as is seen in the general population. However, these are rare anatomical causes of PS. We have seen three symptomatic patients with entrapment of the superior gluteal artery, and two in whom some fibers of the piriformis muscle penetrate fascicles of the sciatic nerve.

We believe that the pathogenesis of PS is mechanical pressure of the piriformis muscle against the fibers of the sciatic nerve. The H-reflexes show delay and neural scans reveal dilatation, flattening and inflammation, with signs of compression of the sciatic nerve in patients with PS. If mechanical compression is the true cause, then the amount of delay seen in the FAIR test should reflect the patient's symptoms, and both the delay and the patient's symptoms should decrease proportionately with effective treatment *(see* Fig. 4; ref. *23)*.

## NONOPERATIVE MANAGEMENT

Physical therapy that consists of stretching of the piriformis muscle, using a combination of manual maneuvers and ultrasound treatments, has been a mainstay of the conservative therapeutic approach *(10–14,24,25)*. Five percent of the time, leg-length discrepancies appear, which are treated with in-shoe lifts and pelvic work. In our clinic, we have developed a treatment protocol that is correlated with 60 to 90% improvement, depending on the injection technique that accompanies it *(see* Table 2).

Injections into the minimally land-marked buttock area are generally guided. Several injection methods have been described. The CT-guided approach may be accurate *(26)*. Locating the piriformis muscle by its proximity to the sciatic nerve using a nerve stimulator has also been used *(27,28)*. However, the nerve is adjacent to the gemellus superior, the obturator internis, the

**Table 2**
**Physical Therapy Protocol for Patients Diagnosed With PS[a]**

Place patient in contralateral decubitus and flexion adduction and internal rotation (FAIR) position.[b]

1. Ultrasound 2.0–2.5 watts/cm², applied in broad strokes longitudinally along the piriformis muscle, from the conjoint tendon to the lateral edge of the greater sciatic foramen for 10–14 minutes.[b]
2. Wipe off ultrasound gel.[c]
3. Hot packs or cold spray at the same location for 10 minutes.
4. Stretch the piriformis muscle for 10–14 minutes by applying manual pressure to the muscle's inferior border, being careful not to press downward, rather directing pressure tangentially, toward the ipsilateral shoulder.[d]
5. Myofascial release at lumbosacral paraspinal muscles.
6. McKenzie exercises.
7. Use lumbosacral corset when treating post-surgical patients in the FAIR position.[e]

Duration: two to three times weekly for 1 to 3 months.

[a]Patients usually require 2 to 3 months of biweekly therapy for 60 to 70% improvement.
[b]Because it is painful, patients often subtly shift to prone. This must be avoided because it works to place the affected leg in abduction, not adduction, greatly reducing the stretch placed on the piriformis muscle.
[c]Cavitation is unreported in more than 20,000 treatments.
[d]Unless explicitly stated, therapists may tend to knead or massage the muscle, which is useless or worse. The muscle must be stretched perpendicular to its fibers, in a plane parallel to one that is tangent to the buttock at the point of intersection of the piriformis muscle and the sciatic nerve, but approximately 1 to 1.5 in. deep to the buttock, (i.e., just below the gluteus maximus).
[e]This is particularly important to avoid inducing lumbar hypermobility in patients with histories of laminectomy, fusion, or spondylolisthesis.

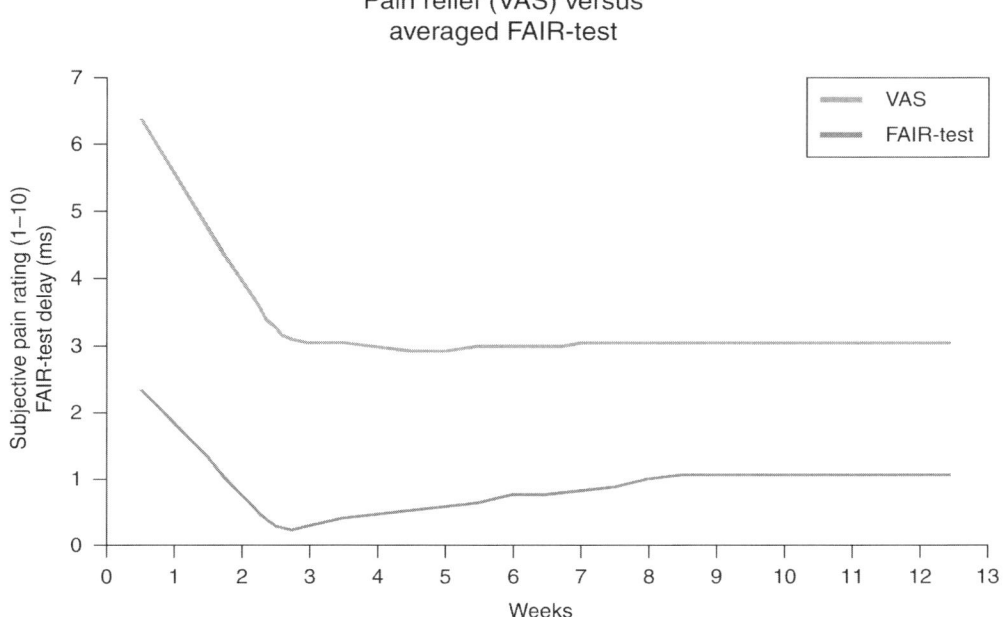

**Fig. 4.** The parallel curves representing patient symptoms and flexion adduction and internal rotation (FAIR) test results suggest that the FAIR test mirrors the pathogenetic mechanism of sciatica in these cases.

gemellus inferior, and very close to the gluteus maximus and quadriceps femoris. A combination of fluoroscopic guidance and needle EMG has been described in which the patient is placed prone and the piriformis muscle is identified by using the greater trochanter of femur and the lateral border of sacrum and the sacroiliac joint as orienting points *(29)*.

Needle EMG and contrast injection have been used together to confirm needle position in the piriformis muscle *(30)*. A similar study using fluoroscopy and nerve stimulator was done by Benzon et al. with good clinical outcome *(31)*. In this method, one first locates the sciatic nerve by inserting the needle at 2 cm lateral and 1 cm caudal to the lower border of sacroiliac joint to a depth of $9.2 \pm 1.5$ cm, then inducing a foot movement response by stimulating the nerve at $0.4 \pm 0.1$ mA, and subsequently extricating the needle 5 cm to avoid direct sciatic nerve injection. Injectable steroid (40 mg triamcinolone acetonide or the equivalent) mixed with normal saline (5–6 cc) is then introduced. Afterwards, the needle is pulled back another 3 to 8 mm to locate it in the belly of the piriformis muscle, where another equal dose of steroid and 7 to 10 cc of 1% lidocaine is instilled *(25)*.

These methods appear to work well. However, the piriformis muscle is at its deepest point medially, and it might be less painful and more accurate to inject further laterally, where the muscle is appreciably closer to the surface. Further, botulinum toxin (BTX) requires multiple injections to medicate as many myoneural junctions as possible. The authors use an EMG-guided approach described in the next section.

The most common substances used for piriformis injections are local anesthetics, injectable steroids and BTX. Several studies using BTX injections in the treatment of piriformis have yielded results that are superior in efficacy and longevity to other injectates. Childers et al. performed a double-blind placebo-controlled crossover study comparing injection of 100 U of BTX type A (BTX-A; Botox®) with saline using a fluoroscopic/EMG-controlled unilateral injection method. This study showed significant benefit of Botox over saline using Visual Analog Scale scores *(30)*.

In another single-center, randomized trial comparing the effects of Botox with steroid methylprednisolone, each administered intramuscularly with 0.5% bupivacaine followed by a course of physical therapy in patients suffering from chronic myofascial pain in the piriformis, iliopsoas, or scalenus anterior muscles, pain severity had decreased significantly from baseline in both treatment groups at 30 days follow-up. However, at 60 days post-injection, the pain severity score for the BTX-treated patients was significantly lower than the pain score for the steroid-treated population *(26)*. A noncontrolled study of BTX-B (Myobloc®) in treatment of PS showed significant symptomatic improvement in patients injected with 5000 U *(32)*. Studies performed by one of the authors demonstrate similar results and are reported in the following paragraphs *(33)*.

## OUR METHOD OF INJECTION

We inject Botox or Myobloc under EMG guidance, selecting four points in the muscle that should reach different myoneural junctions *(see* Fig. 5). Each site receives either 75 U of Botox or 3125 U of Myobloc, adding up to 300 U of Botox or 12,500 of Myobloc. We use a 75- or 80-mm monopolar Teflon-coated 23 gauge injectible monopolar needle (e.g., of the type made by Chalgren Enterprises; *see* Figs. 5 and 6).

We palpate the buttock for the most tender spot, then judge by the greater trochanter and the sciatic foramen where the piriformis muscle's outlines are located. After one has a little experience, the rostral and caudal edges of the muscle are usually identifiable,

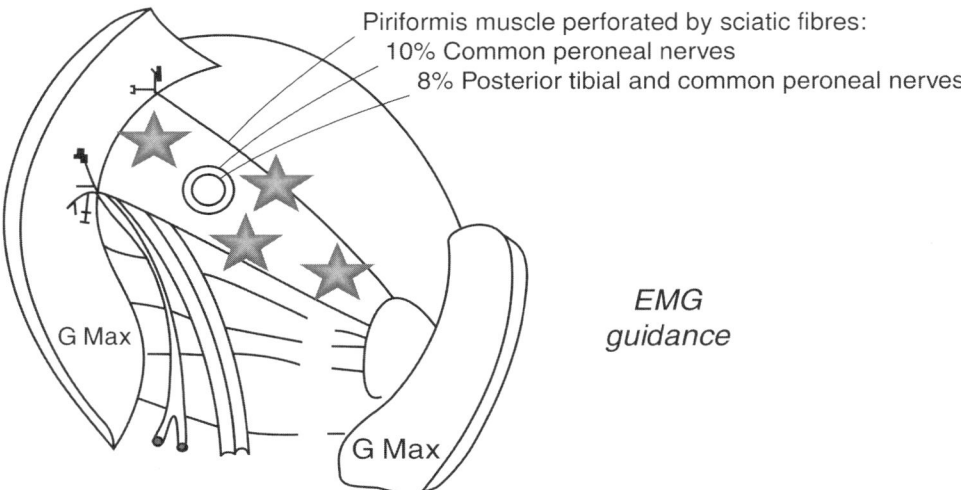

Four doses of 1,250–3,125 U

• Abduction: Piriformis + gluteus maximus respond
• Extension: Only gluteus maximus responds

Piriformis muscle perforated by sciatic fibres:
10% Common peroneal nerves
8% Posterior tibial and common peroneal nerves

G Max

G Max

*EMG guidance*

**Fig. 5.** The piriformis muscle is deeper in more medial sites, but is almost always within reach of a 3.5-in. teflonized EMG-injectible needle.

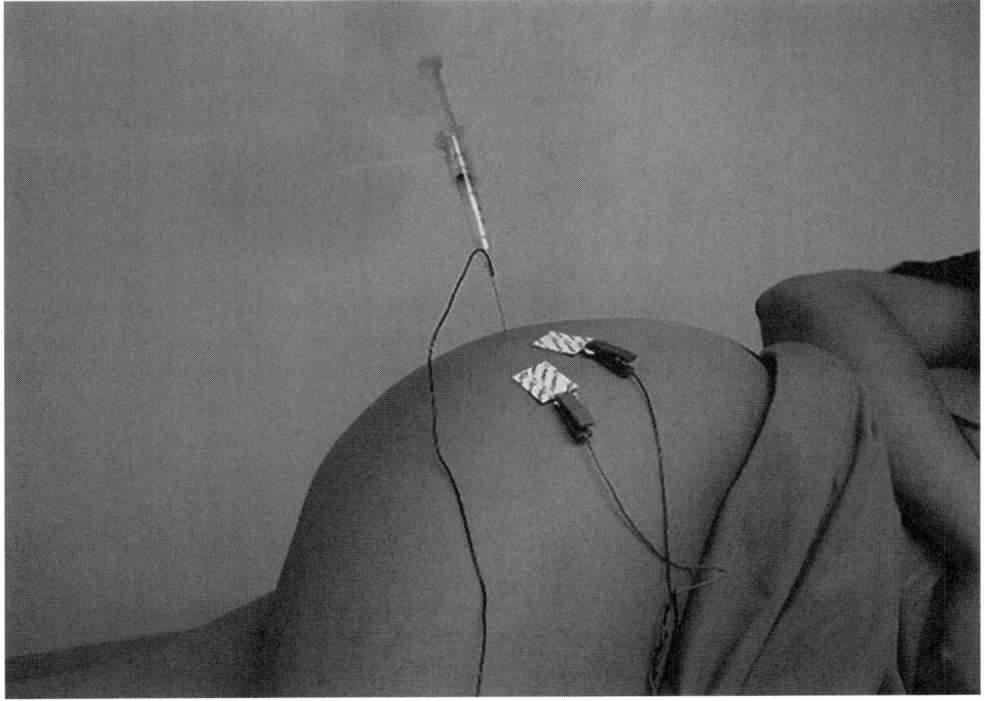

**Fig. 6.** The flexion adduction and internal rotation test position facilitates the injections, and patients have no trouble abducting and extending the leg from it.

because it lies just beneath the gluteus maximus, and often close to 1 in. below the skin at its lateral extreme *(23)*.

We start the series of four injections by positioning the patient in lateral decubitus position with the hips and knees flexed 90°. The first needle is inserted just medial to the musculotendinous junction, inserting the needle approximately 1 in.

Then we go through two maneuvers to be sure the EMG-guided needle is located in the piriformis muscle. First, the patient is asked to abduct the thigh. If we see no interference pattern, then we insert the needle 0.25 in. further and repeat the process until we see a reasonable interference pattern. The interference pattern assures us that we are either in the gluteus maximus or the piriformis muscle.

Second, we ask the patient to extend the leg. If we are in the piriformis muscle, there will be electrical silence, and we can proceed with injecting the BTX. If there is an interference pattern, then the needle tip is in the gluteos maximus; we continue to advance the needle another 1/4 inch and repeat the entire process, beginning with abduction, until we see an interference pattern with abduction, but not with extension.

There are a couple of fine points. In the first maneuver, if the first injection point is particularly lateral, then it is possible that the needle will encounter the gluteus medius or minimus. In that case, one must use external rotation to distinguish these muscles from the piriformis. We ask the patient to keep his or her feet together and raise just the knee in that case, externally rotating instead of abducting the entire leg.

In the second maneuver, when a patient is asked to extend the leg, he or she will almost invariably lift it. This will engage the piriformis muscle as well as any of the glutei. So we place one hand between their knees, and encourage them to squeeze their knees together while extending the hip. We often hold the sole of the affected leg's foot and ask the patient to push that hand away while squeezing our other hand between the knees. This is easy for them to do. Once in a while the patient will try to lift just the ankle, which also has an obscuring effect on the test. We therefore also ask these patients to squeeze their ankles together while extending the upper leg.

After completing both maneuvers and the injection in all four locations, we stress to the patients that it will take anywhere from 5 days to 2 weeks to actually feel the benefits of the injection, and that physical therapy is absolutely necessary if the relief is going to last. We encourage them to learn a short series of yoga poses as well (*see* www.sciatica.org).

A few patients may experience reduced or no responsiveness to BTX following repeated injections. Factors including severity, improper muscle selection, dosing, and genetic characteristics can contribute to ineffectiveness or increased resistance. Although not commonly done in our practice, numerous tests are available to detect antibodies against BTX if resistance is suspected. The simplest and most cost-effective tests are the frontalis antibody test and the unilateral brow injection test. Other tests include mouse protein assay, Western blotting, and enzyme-linked immunosorbent assay. Antibody formation can be limited by using the lowest possible dose in concordance with the longest possible hiatus between injections.

Botox and Myobloc are immunologically distinct. Therefore, if the patient has had Botox, then he or she is still very unlikely to have a reaction to Myobloc unless there is a history of botulism earlier in life. Alternating Botox and Myobloc over time is a wise course if multiple injections are necessary.

However, most patients with PS do not need repeat injections. It is clear from many laboratory tests that the actual neurotoxins inhibit evagination of the acetylcholine vacuoles from the neuron at the myoneural junction for only 2 to 3 months. Nevertheless, these injections frequently result in permanent or at least significantly greater periods of relief. How does this happen? We believe that once the muscle has been lengthened, at least two different mechanisms come into play.

The first mechanism involves the continued denervation of a subset of those muscle fibers initially affected by the injection. We have seen EMG evidence of denervation many months and even years after a single BTX injection. Second, after patients have improved, they incorporate greater movements into their daily lives. It is similar to a frozen shoulder where one works and works until a good range is obtained, but then, upon cessation of therapy, the patient rarely redevelops a frozen shoulder. This commonly happens because the patients' newly acquired extra range is used reaching something on a high shelf, passing the sugar, or playing handball. The same occurs with PS: after stretching the muscle, the patient will elongate that muscle more naturally in getting up from sitting, walking up a flight of stairs, and in other activities.

The injection of Botox for PS is high-dose relative to many of its other uses. Nevertheless, it has resulted in no side effects to date, in more than 500 different instances of these multiple injection patterns.

Myobloc is safe, but we have seen a few side effects with it including dry mouth, rare blurry vision that may last a week or two (2 cases out of 100) and constipation in three cases.

One unexpected beneficial side effect from Myobloc was seen in a patient with severe asthma that frequented emergency rooms four times per year with exacerbations. She surprisingly reported that she had suffered no asthma attacks for nearly 1 year following a Myobloc injection. This may be a parasympathetic effect in that respect similar to the constipation and the dry mouth that are more commonly seen with Myobloc.

Putting no monetary value on patient suffering, loss of work days, and ability to fill societal roles such as parent or spouse, the cost of underdiagnosed and virtually untreated PS, including 1.5 unnecessary MRIs, 0.4 unnecessary surgeries, and visits to 6.5 clinicians per patient is well above $8000 per patient and rising daily *(14)*.

The average cost of proper diagnosis and BTX injection is less than $3000 per patient, but is also susceptible to increases.

## CLINICAL EXPERIENCE

We first used the electrodiagnostic techniques outlined here when standard diagnostic means turned up nothing in patients with severe sciatica. In 1992, after accumulating 34 patients, and following their generally successful surgical course, we published a small article in the *Archives of Physical Medicine and Rehabilitation*.

Possibly because of the preponderant emphasis on intramedullary causes of sciatica, the study was heralded in the New York Times, and expounded in the lay press fairly widely. There were two effects: first, many clinicians in the United States and Europe volunteered their experience in treating the syndrome conservatively. Second, we were deluged with patients.

In the past 14 years more than 9000 patients have presented themselves for diagnosis and treatment of PS. Slightly more than 50% of them have had sufficient clinical and electrophysiological findings to confirm the diagnosis.

Treatment at first was simply physical therapy, informed and enriched by generous and knowledgeable suggestions from the international medical community. In essence, the therapy lengthened the piriformis muscle, reducing spasm and pressure on the descending sciatic nerve, and giving the nerve enough slack to remove itself from harm's way (*see* Table 2 for the specific program). The therapy was helpful, but progress was slow. On the suggestion of Dr. Janet Travell, we began injecting triamcinolone acetonide 20 mg with 1.5 cc of 2% lidocaine into the motor point of the piriformis muscle, just medial to its musculotendinous junction in the lateral buttock.

This had only rare minor and transient side effects on nondiabetics, and shortened the recovery time considerably.

On average 10.2 months follow-up time of 1014 cases of PS, more than 80% of the patients had improved 50% or more within 3 months *(15)*. These patients had suffered from PS for an average of 6.2 years, and had seen an average of 6.5 clinicians before coming to us.

Probably because PS was considered a diagnosis of exclusion, other less important diagnostic entities had received undue attention in these patients. Among these 1014 cases there had been more than 350 spinal, trochanteric and gynecological surgeries, none of which were definitive, more than 1500 imaging studies, of which less than 1 of 5 were relevant, and more than 10,000 appointments with clinicians for diagnostics, epidurals, physical therapy, and alternative methods of pain relief *(14,23,33)*.

More recently, we have conducted several institutional review board-approved studies of specific nerve blocks, using neurotoxins of the botulinum bacterium. In the latest and most successful of these, we have used 300 U Botox or 12,500 U Myobloc. In our latest study with Myobloc, 89% of the patients were at least 50% improved on a visual analog scale of pain within 2 to 3 weeks *(23,33)*.

The use of BTXs has fewer side effects than triamcinolone and lidocaine, being safe for diabetics, anticoagulated patients, and patients with immune deficiencies. BTXs give more relief faster, and appear in our follow-up studies to last longer, with fewer relapses *(33)*. Showing a much more rapid decline in pain levels and normalization of the FAIR test, it obviates physical therapy sessions that surpass the injections in cost.

There are three reasons that 300 U Botox or 12,500 U Myobloc should be considered in the treatment of PS:

1. In clinical experience, the injection of 300 U Botox or 12,500 U of Myobloc are, at this writing, the most effective treatment for PS.
2. More than 5 million currently undiagnosed patients will continue to suffer and consume health care resources in vain unless and until adequate treatment is afforded them.
3. Cost–benefit analysis of current data supports injection of 300 U Botox or 12,500 U Myobloc in the treatment of PS.

Nevertheless, the importance of physical therapy in obtaining lasting relief from PS cannot be overemphasized. Although some otherwise excellent injection studies report only 37% lasting relief *(15)*, we have consistently found at least 79% of the patients to recover after injection and physical therapy. In the long term, we have effectively used a set of yoga exercises that are available in book form *(34)*.

In summary, PS is a commonly underdiagnosed condition that can significantly limit function and the quality of one's life. Patients often seek multiple medical opinions and undergo numerous unnecessary and costly interventions. With proper diagnosis, injection, and physical therapy, PS resolves in a large majority of cases.

## REFERENCES

1. Pace JB, Nagle D. Piriform syndrome. West J Med 1976;124;435–439.
2. Solheim LF, Siewers P, Paus B. The piriformis muscle syndrome. J Orthop Scand 1981; 52:73–75.
3. Syneki VM. The PS; review and case presentation. Clin Exp Neurol 1987;23:31–37.
4. Onions CT, Friedrichsen GWS, Burchfield RW. The Oxford Dictionary of English Etymology. Oxford: Publisher; 1994, p. 797.
5. Mixter WJ, Barr JS. Ruptures of the intervertebral disc with involvement of the spinal canal. N Engl J Med 1934;211:210–211.
6. Patrick DL, Deyo RA, Atlas SJ, Singer DE, Chapin A, Keller RB. Assessing health-related quality of life in patients with sciatica. Spine 1995;20:1899–1909.
7. Agency for Health Care Policy and Research. Acute Low Back Problems in Adults. Clinical Practice Guidelines. Rockville, MD; 1994, p. 14. Publication 95–0642.
8. Sridhara CR, Izzo KL. Peroneal nerve entrapment syndrome. Arch Phys Med Rehabil 1985;66:789–791.
9. Jensen MC, Brant-Zawadzki MN, Obuchowski N, Modic MT, Malkasian D, Ross JS. Magnetic resonance imaging of the lumbar spine in people without back pain. N Engl J Med 1994; 331:69–73.
10. Parziale JR, Hudgins TH, Fishman LM. The PS—a review paper. Am J Orthop 1996;25:819–823.
11. Fishman LM. Electrophysiological evidence of PS. Arch Phys Ed Rehabil 1987;68:670 (abstract).
12. Fishman LM. Electrophysiological evidence of PS II. Arch Phys Med Rehabil 1988;69:300 (abstract).
13. Fishman LM, Zybert PA. Electrophysiological evidence of PS. Arch Phys Med Rehabil 1992;73:359–364.
14. Fishman LM, Dombi GW, Ringel SR, Rosner BH, Rozbruch J, Weber C. PS: diagnosis, treatment and outcome—a ten year study. Arch Phys Med Rehabil. Accepted April, 2001.
15. Filler AG, Haynes J, Jordan SE, et al. Sciatica of nondisc origin and PS: diagnosis by magnetic resonance neurography and interventional magnetic resonance imaging with outcome study of resulting treatment. J Neurosurg Spine 2005;2:99–115.
16. Hallin RP. Sciatic pain and the piriformis muscle. Postgraduate Medicine. 1983;74:69–72.
17. Fishman LM, Schaefer MP. The PS is underdiagnosed. Muscle Nerve 2003;28:626–629.
18. Benzon HT, Katz JA, Benzon HA, Iqbal MS. PS anatomic considerations, a new injection technique, and a review of the literature. Anaesthesiology 2003;98:1442–1448.
19. Robinson D. PS in relation to sciatic pain. Am J Surg 1947;73:355–358.
20. Freiberg AH. Sciatic pain and its relief by operations on muscle and fascia. Arch Surg 1937;34:337–350.
21. Stewart JD. The PS is overdiagnosed. Muscle Nerve 2003;28:644–666.
22. Kemholz J, Awatramani R, Menichella D, Jiang D, Xu W, Shy M. Regulation of myelin-specific gene expression. Charcot Marie-Tooth disorder. In: Shy M, Kamholz J and Lovelace RE (eds.) Annals of the New York Academy of Science. Vol. 883. New York: New York Academy of sciences. 1999, pp. 94–104.
23. Fishman LM, Konnoth C, Rozner B. Botulinum neurotoxin type B and physical therapy in the treatment of PS: a dose-finding study. Am J Phys Med Rehabil 2004;83:42–50.
24. Cameron HU, Noftal F. The PS (editorial). Can J Surg 1998;31:210.
25. Barton PM. PS: A rational approach to management. Pain 1991;47:345–352.
26. Porta M. A comparative trial of botulinum toxin type A and methylprednisolone for the treatment of myofascial pain syndrome and pain from chronic muscle spasm. Pain 2000;85:101–105.
27. Hanania M. New technique for piriformis muscle injection using a nerve stimulator (letter). Reg Anesth Pain Med 1997;22;200–202.
28. Hanania M, Kitain E. Perisciatic injection of steroid for the treatment of sciatica due to PS. Reg Anesth Pain Med 1998;23:223–228.

29. Fishman SM, Caneris OA, Bandman TB, Audette JF, Borsook D. Injection of the piriformis muscle by fluoroscopic and electromyographic guidance. Reg Anesth Pain Med 1998;23:554–559.
30. Childers MK, Wilson DJ, Gnatz SM, Conway RR, Sherman AK. Botulinum toxin type A use in piriformis muscle syndrome: a pilot study. Am J Phys Med Rehab 2002;81:751–759.
31. Benzon HT, Katz JA, Hubert A, Benzon BA, Muhhamad S, Iqbal MD. PS: anatomic considerations, a new injection technique, and a review of the literature. Anesthesiology 2003;98:1442–1448.
32. Lang AM. Botulinum toxin type B in PS. Am J Phys Med Rehab 2004;83:198–202.
33. Fishman LM, Anderson C, Rosner B. Botulinum toxin type A and physical therapy in the treatment of piriformis syndrome. Am J Phys Med Rehabil 2002;81:936–942.
34. Fishman LM, Ardman C. Relief is in the Stretch: Yoga Cures Back Pain. New York: W.W. Norton, 2005.

Mary S. Babcock

## DEFINITION AND ANATOMY

The plantar fascia runs from the medial tubercle of the calcaneus to the transverse ligaments of the metatarsal heads of the foot. The fascia has medial, central, and lateral parts, underneath which lie the abductor hallucis, flexor digitorum brevis, and flexor digiti minimi muscles, respectively. It holds down muscles and tendons in the concave surface of the sole and digits, facilitates excursion of the tendons, prevents excessive compression of digital vessels and nerves, and possibly aids in venous return (1). The origin of this fibrous aponeurosis is rich in sensory innervation and has fibrocartilage with longitudinal collagen fibers that resist tension. This fibrocartilage is also metabolically active in forming cartilage. Overuse of this structure can lead to a condition known as plantar fasciitis. Because fascia has little elastic properties, repetitive stretching can cause microtears at its origin.

Although originally perceived to be an inflammatory condition, histological findings are consistent with a degenerative process. Tissue analysis reveals a thickened fascia (up to 15 mm) as well as fibrocyte necrosis, microtears, chondroid metaplasia, angiofibroblastic proliferation and type I collagen fibers. This myxoid degeneration, which occurs in chronic conditions, replaces the normal cellular matrix and is mechanically inefficient. During the night, as the foot rests in the equinus position, the plantar fascia contracts. Thus, the first step out of bed in the morning abruptly stretches the fascia and causes irritation and pain.

## BIOMECHANICAL FACTORS AND PATHOPHYSIOLOGY

The plantar fascia connects the hind foot to the fore foot, providing stabilization important for stance and gait. When tension increases during the heel-off phase, the plantar fascia stores potential energy and converts that stored tension into kinetic energy as it passively contracts during toe-off, imparting foot acceleration. Because of this windlass effect, the plantar fascia contributes more to the mechanical support of the arch than the spring ligament in gait. Cadaver studies reveal that dissecting the plantar fascia weakens the medial longitudinal support of the arch and increases the tensile forces in other ligaments and the posterior tibial tendon. The pain in refractory plantar fasciitis may be to the result of one or more of the following mechanisms:

1. Irritation of pain fibers by repeated trauma and/or chronic pressure from a thickened plantar fascia (2).
2. Ischemic pain from chronic pressure of thickened fascia against digital vessels.

From: *Therapeutic Uses of Botulinum Toxin*
Edited by: G. Cooper © Humana Press Inc., Totowa, NJ

3. Enhanced effect of local pain neurotransmitters/chemicals such as substance P or glutamate *(3)*, which are shown to accumulate at the site of local trauma.
4. Increased nociceptor sensitivity secondary to inflammation.

Furthermore, in any chronic painful condition, a cascade of events typically occurs, leading to a vicious cycle of pain maintenance *(4)*. These may include central sensitization after peripheral injury in which non-nociceptive spinal cord neurons perceive non-nociceptive peripheral stimuli as painful and sympathetically maintained pain in which an overgrowth of sympathetic nerve fibers occurs into the dorsal root ganglia resulting in persistent pain transmission *(5)*.

## EPIDEMIOLOGY AND RISK FACTORS

Plantar fasciitis is the most common cause of chronic heel pain observed in up to 10% of the general population. A survey among professional team physicians and trainers in 1995 found plantar fasciitis to be among the top five causes of foot and ankle injuries in professional athletes *(6)*. Another study estimated that about one million patient visits per year are for plantar fasciitis *(7)*. It mainly occurs in middle-aged females and male runners younger than 20 years old, although all ages can be affected. The male to female ratio is 1:2 with obesity concomitantly present in 40% of affected males and 90% of affected females. Mortality is low and is associated with fibrosarcoma of the plantar fascia. This rare tumor has an incidence of 30 per year in the United States. Delayed diagnosis leads to a 5-year survival rate of less than 10%.

Proven risk factors include obesity, sedentary lifestyle, repetitive loading, and a mean age of 40 to 50 years old. Decreased healing response, along with decreased tissue elasticity and repetitive tearing have been implicated in the middle-aged population and may be contributing factors. Other factors implicated in this condition include:

1. Pes cavus with a rigid high medial arch.
2. Shoes with stiff soles or poor arch support.
3. Tight calf muscles.
4. Forefoot pronation.
5. Leg length discrepancy.
6. Excessive tibial torsion.
7. Excessive femoral anteversion.

Prichasuk described the mean calcaneal pitch to be significantly lower in symptomatic patients (16 versus 20.5°) than in asymptomatic patients *(7)*. On lateral foot radiographs, the calcaneal pitch (also known as the calcaneal inclination angle) is the angle formed by intersecting a line drawn from the plantar most surface of the calcaneus to the inferior border of the distal articular surface and the transverse plane. Other conditions associated with increased risk for plantar fasciitis include pregnancy, hypothyroidism, and certain arthropathies.

Training errors are also a common cause of plantar fasciitis. Patients often report a recent increase in intensity, duration, or distance during exercise activities. Plyometrics, graded hill workouts, speed workouts, or running on poorly padded surfaces are also high-risk behaviors. Improper shoes also play a role; lightweight shoes with minimal cushion do not adequately decrease the forces impacting the heel during activity. Because shoes rapidly lose their cushioning properties, frequent shoe replacement appropriate to a patient's activity is advocated *(8)*.

## DIFFERENTIAL DIAGNOSIS

Other possible etiologies for pain about the heel include:

1. Tarsal tunnel syndrome.
2. Entrapment of the medial calcaneal branch of the posterior tibial nerve.
3. Irritation of the nerve to the abductor digiti quinti.
4. Stress fracture.
5. Fat pad necrosis.
6. Seronegative arthropathies, such as psoriatic arthritis or ankylosing spondylitis.
7. Sacral radiculopathy.
8. Calcaneal apophysitis in adolescents (Sever's disease).
9. Plantar fascia rupture.
10. Retrocalcaneal bursitis.
11. Tumor.
12. Infection.
13. Foreign body.

## HISTORY AND PHYSICAL EXAMINATION

Pathognomonic for this condition is heel pain that is worst with the first step out of bed in the morning. In severe cases, the pain is sharp and can radiate proximally with an electric-like sensation. During the course of the day, the pain typically decreases with activity only to be re-aggravated after prolonged sitting, standing, or walking long distances. Any sudden changes in weight, exercise, running terrain, or mileage should also be noted. On physical examination, some swelling about the heel in the absence of erythema or warmth may be noted. Other findings may include the following:

1. Palpated taut and tender muscle structures about the arch may also be palpated.
2. Decreased active ankle dorsiflexion of less than 20° may indicate a tight gastroc–soleus complex.
3. Decreased hallux dorsiflexion.
4. Palpable granuloma along the medial fascial origin.
5. A positive windlass test, heel pain reproduced with passive dorsiflexion of the toes, can be elicited. According to De Gareau, performing this test while the patient is weight bearing increases its sensitivity from 13.5 to 31.8%.
6. Heel raises or toe-walking may also reproduce pain.

Shoe wear and gait patterns also supplement the overall biomechanical assessment. Much information can be gained from observing the patient's gait with and without shoes. In-toe walking with or without "kissing patellae" may indicate internal tibial torsion or excessive femoral anteversion. Studying the wear pattern on the soles of their shoes and knowing the terrain they frequent may reveal subtleties that further direct physical exam. For example, a treadmill runner whose shoes are more worn in the anteromedial aspect of the sole may have forefoot pronation. On the other hand, a lateral sole wear pattern may be caused by a rigid pes cavus. A proper shoe evaluation should examine cushioning properties of the shoe, wear pattern, manufacturing quality, and hind-foot stability.

## DIAGNOSIS

Although edema about the plantar fascia insertion may be seen on magnetic resonance imaging and ultrasound, plantar fasciitis is diagnosed clinically. About 70% of patients with this condition also have radiographic evidence for heel spurs *(9)*. However, heel spurs can also be found in asymptomatic patients and recent studies suggest that the bone spurs are more often associated with the flexor digitorum brevis than the plantar fascia. Bone scans are helpful in identifying stress reactions or fractures. Laboratory studies may be useful in elucidating rheumatologic causes of heel pain. However, HLA-B27 has only 65% sensitivity for ankylosing spondylitis and rheumatoid factor has only 50% specificity.

## TREATMENT

Conservative treatment involves a combination of stretching and strengthening exercises. Stretching of the calf and foot intrinsic muscles is a key part of treatment (Figs. 1–8). Each stretch should be held for 15 to 30 seconds per repetition. Wall stretches are done by having the patient lean against a wall while pushing hips into the wall (Figs. 4 and 5). Intrinsic muscle stretching is performed with the patient sitting down and passively stretching their toes into extension (Fig. 2). To strengthen the foot intrinsic muscles, towel curls, marble pickups, and toe tapping can be performed (Figs. 7 and 8).

Modalites found helpful for pain relief in plantar fasciitis include cold therapy in the form of ice massage or ice bath. Ice massage can be conducted using water frozen in a Styrofoam cup. Part of the cup is peeled off and then applied to the heel of the foot in circular motion for 5 to 10 minutes. Iontophoresis, a modality that drives medicine or other charged molecules through the skin using electrical charge, can decrease symptom recovery time *(10)*. Iontophoresis can be done with 0.4% dexamethasone six times over 2 weeks to facilitate symptom relief. However, no long-term improvements were found at 6 weeks *(11)*.

Nonsteroidal anti-inflammatory drugs can decrease pain during therapy, but may not assist with the physiological healing process. Options for nonsteroidal anti-inflammatory drugs to use include:

1. 800 mg Motrin® by mouth three times a day.
2. 500 mg Naprosyn® by mouth twice a day.
3. 200 mg Celebrex® by mouth daily.
4. 15 mg Mobic® by mouth daily.

In cases in which some local neuritis may be present because of fat pad atrophy, tricyclic medications or neuroleptic medications, such as gabapentin or pregabalin, may be helpful.

Orthotics as adjunctive therapy decrease local direct trauma with ambulation, provide some increased stability in stance and gait, and can provide some passive stretch. Heel cups are often prescribed and provide cushioning. Night splints, which keep the foot in slight 5° dorsiflexion, have shown to be helpful. However, patients often complain of difficulty sleeping with splint use, which affects compliance.

Steroid injection is widely used as the first-line invasive treatment. Ten milligrams triamcinolone or 2.5 mg dexamethasone diluted in 1 cc 1% lidocaine plain is injected with a 25-gage needle using the medial approach to avoid the fat pad. Adverse complications can include fat pad atrophy, infection, or plantar fascial rupture from repeated steroid use.

Surgery involves release of the medial plantar fascia with decompression of the abductor digiti quinti with or without heel spur excision. In a retrospective review of 870 patients with plantar fasciitis only 3% required surgery *(12)*. Successful outcomes range from 50 to 90%. However, postoperative rehabilitation is prolonged and involves casting immobilization and crutch use for 3 to 4 weeks followed by about 4 weeks of physical therapy. Potential complications include infection, plantar hypesthesia, plantar fibrosis, and rupture.

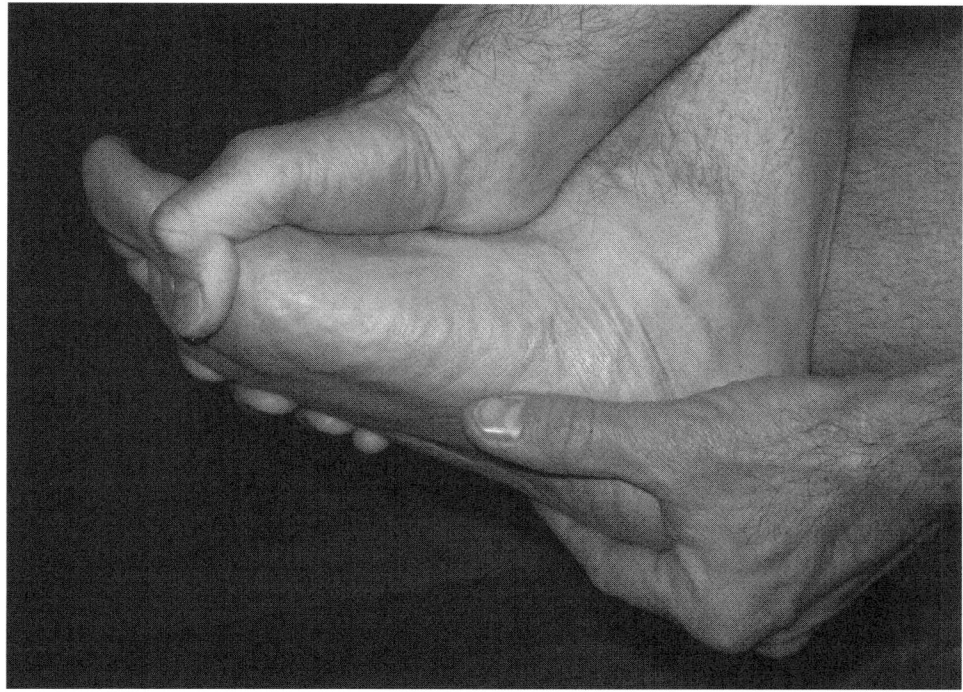

**Fig. 1.** Ankle dorsiflexion stretch.

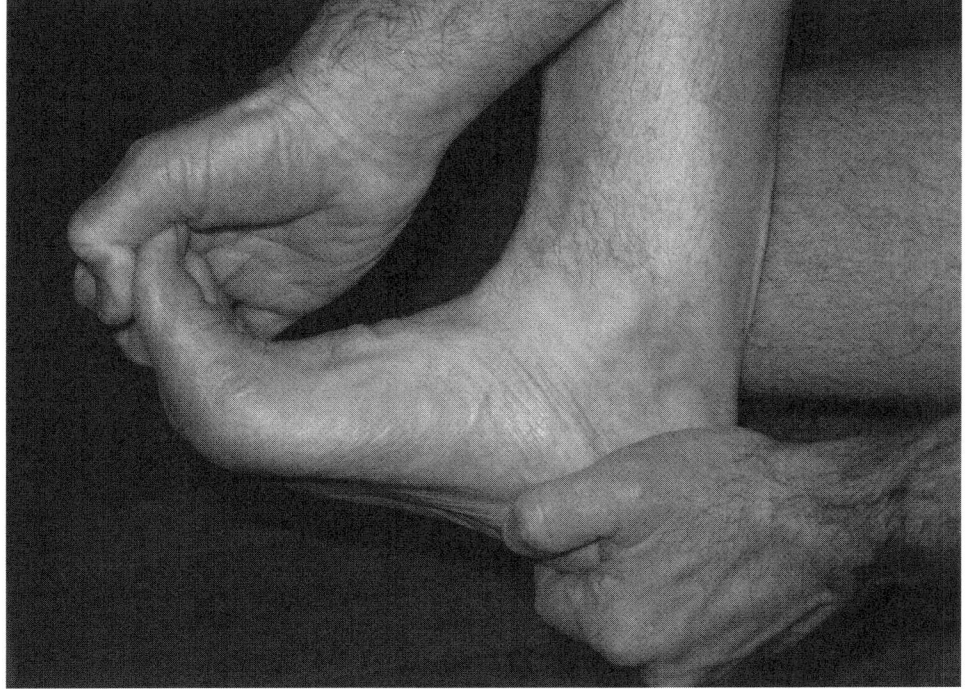

**Fig. 2.** Great toe stretch.

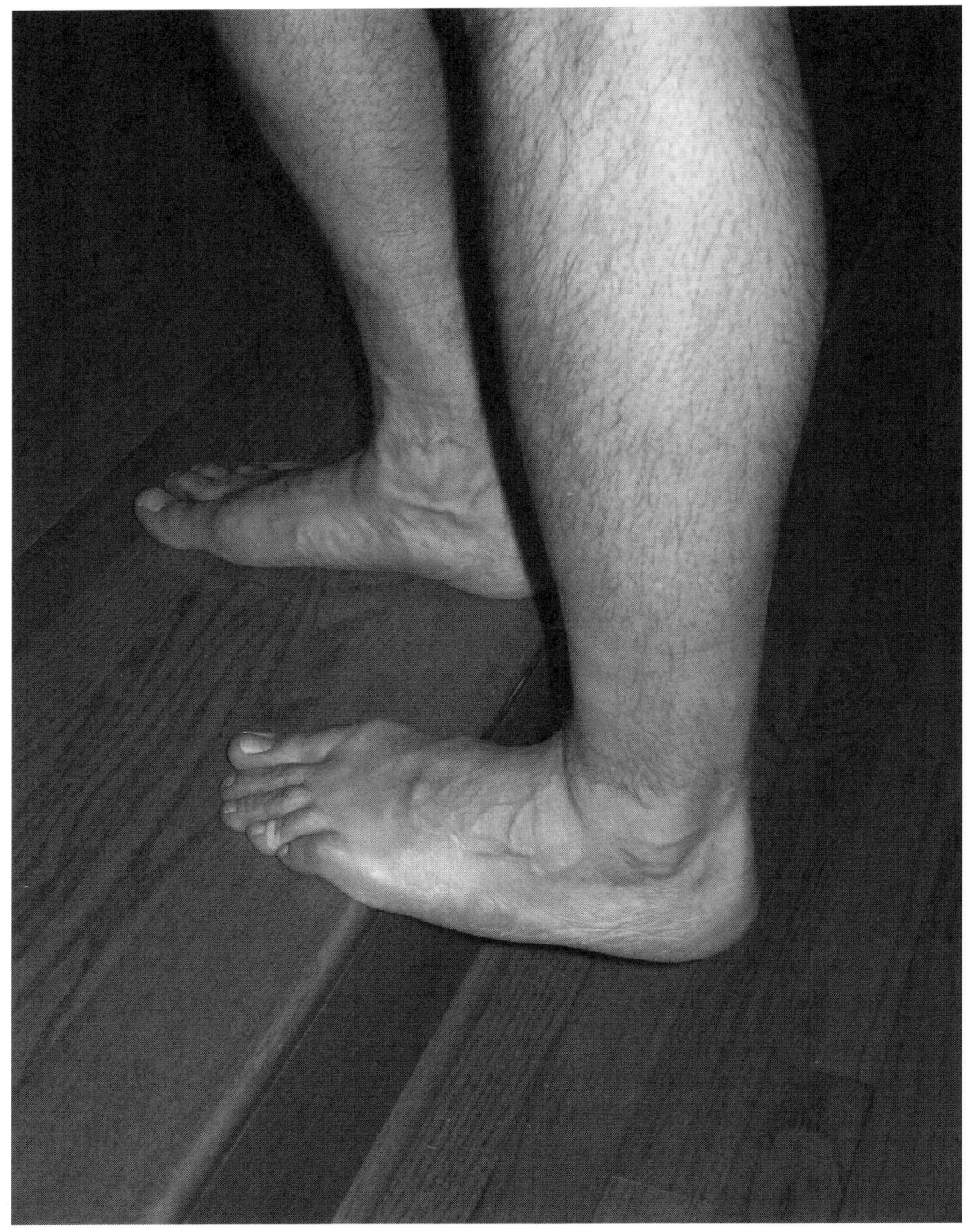

**Fig. 3.** Plantar fascia stretch.

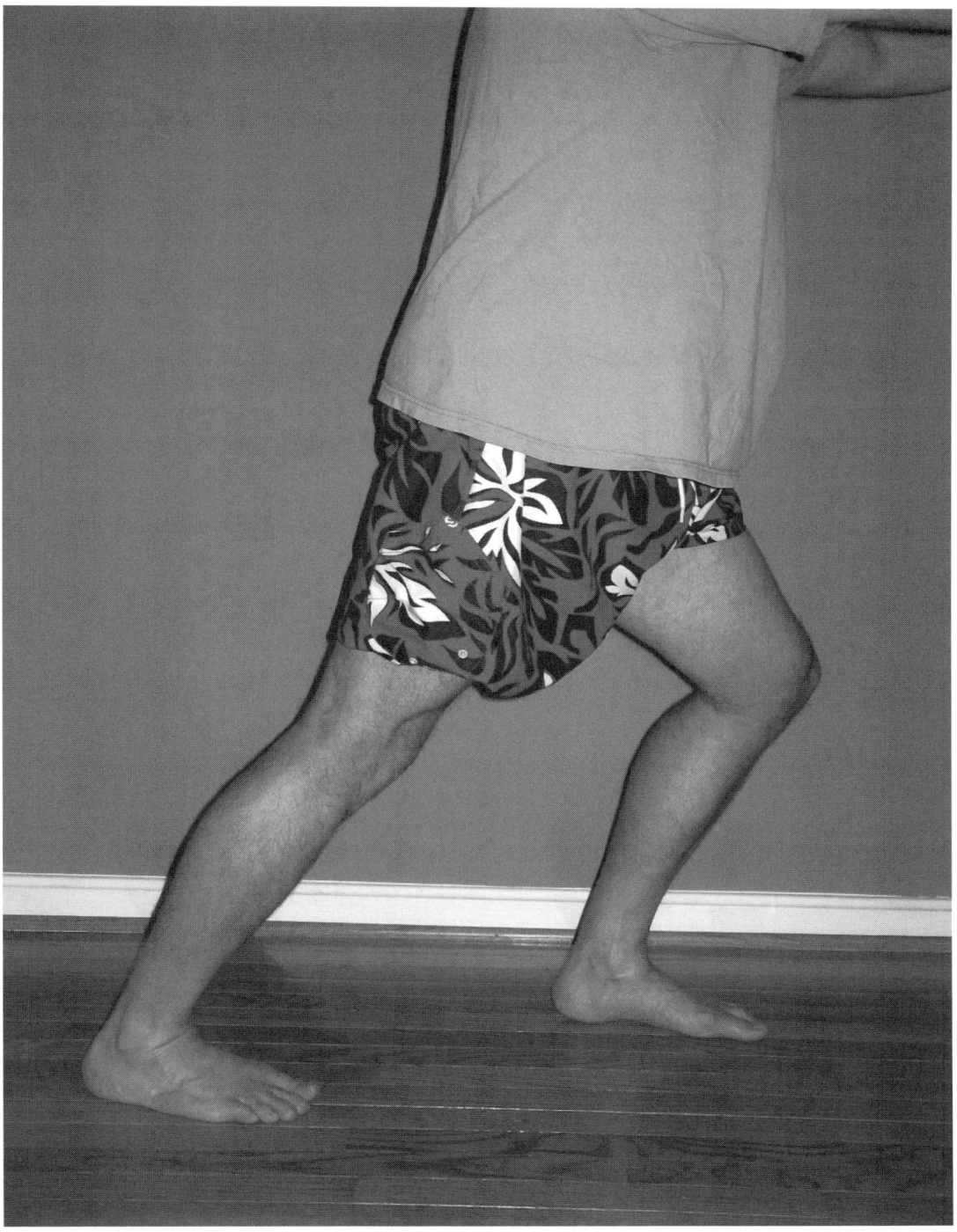

**Fig. 4.** Gastrocnemius stretch.

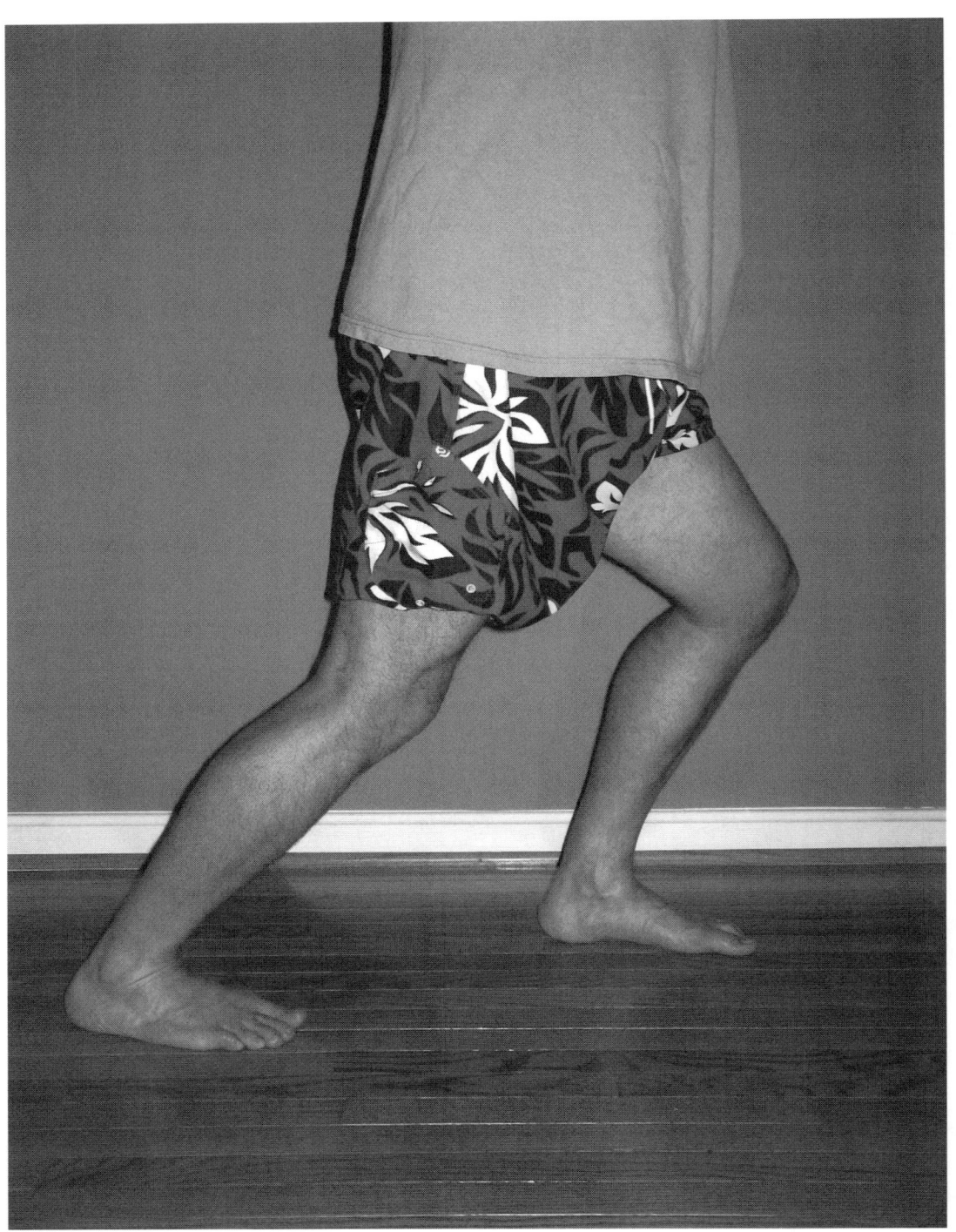

**Fig. 5.** Soleus stretch.

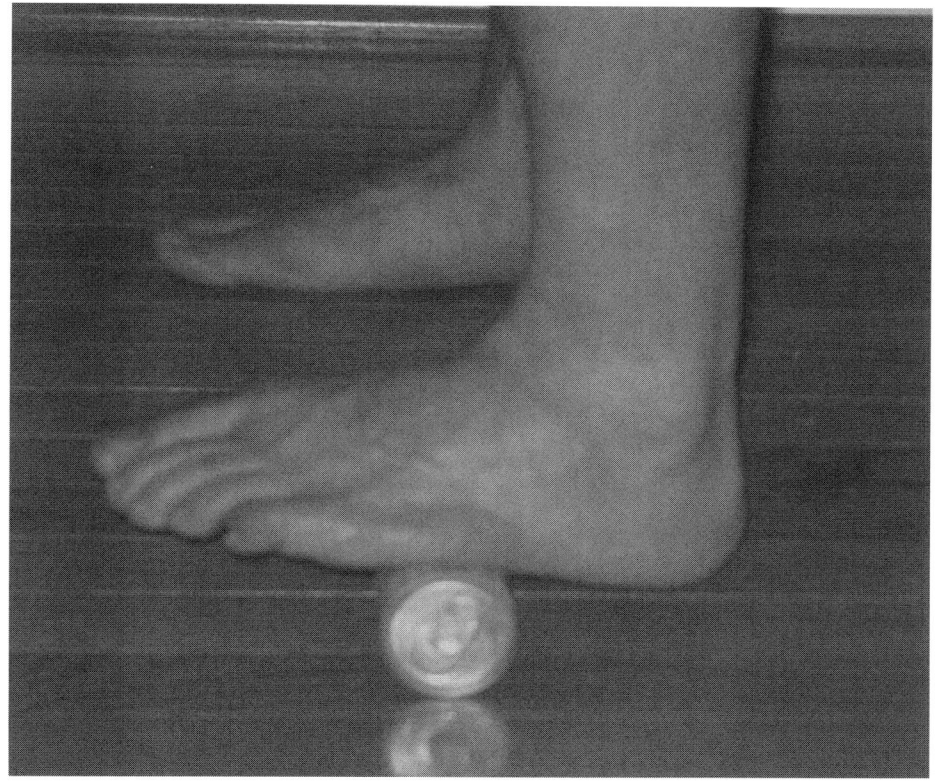

**Fig. 6.** Can roll.

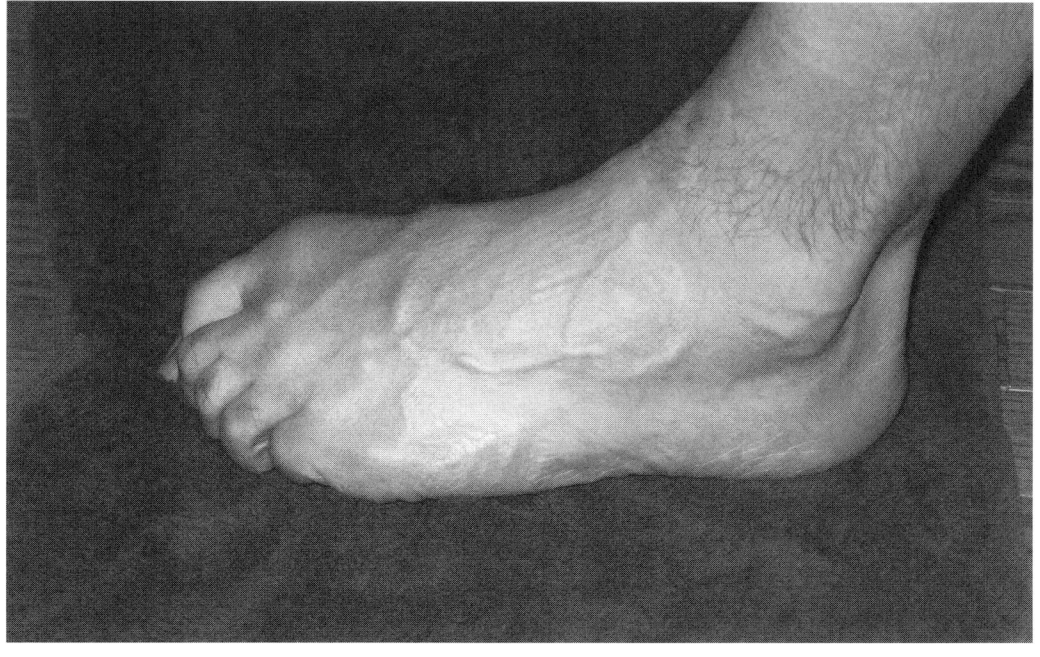

**Fig. 7.** Towel curl, lateral view.

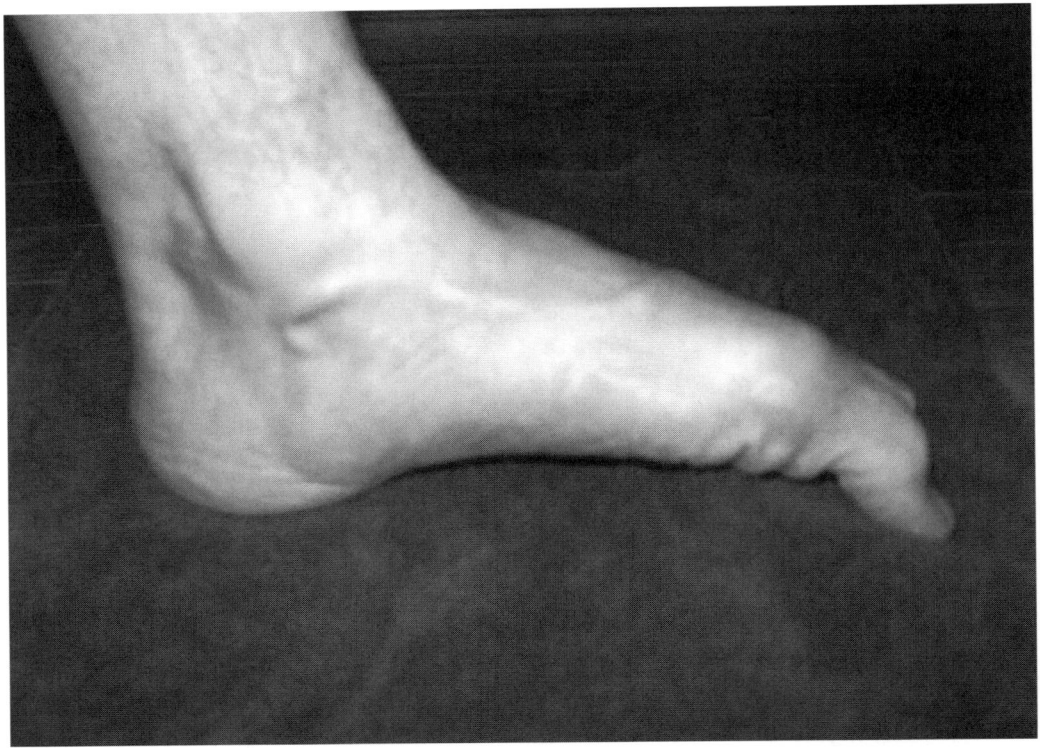

**Fig. 8.** Towel curl, medial view.

Extracorporeal shock wave therapy (ECSWT) has been shown to provide relief in patients showing more than 4 mm fascial thickening by ultrasound. Results seem controversial and are affected by the concomitant use of local anesthetic during this procedure. The application apparatus is expensive and treatment cost ranges from $800 to $3000 depending on the number of treatments. Proper technical application is clouded by the lack of universal consensus of terms such as "high," "medium," or "low" energy. Low-energy ECSWT has been advocated and two classifications have been proposed by Mainz (low = 0.08–0.27 mJ/mm$^2$) and Kassel (low = <0.12 mJ/mm$^2$). However, upon reviewing several randomized, placebo-controlled clinic trials using ECSWT for plantar fasciitis, results were variable for significant difference between treated and placebo groups. These results may be explained by the technical variability regarding machine design, shock-wave intensity, focal energy, geometry of the shock-wave focus, frequency of treatment, and the use of different forms of placebo therapy *(13)*. The accuracy of treatment localization is also variable. High cost and staff expertise prevents routine application of this method.

## BOTULINUM TOXIN TYPE A INJECTION PROCEDURE (FIGS. 9–11)

Over the last several years, botulinum toxin type A (BTX-A) has been increasingly used in the treatment of various medical conditions. Increasing literature supports the role of BTX-A in the treatment of chronic pain syndromes. Blockade of acetylcholine release from the presynaptic membrane plays an important role in relief of muscles spasms and myofascial pain syndromes. However, some animal models suggest alternative mechanisms for the analgesic

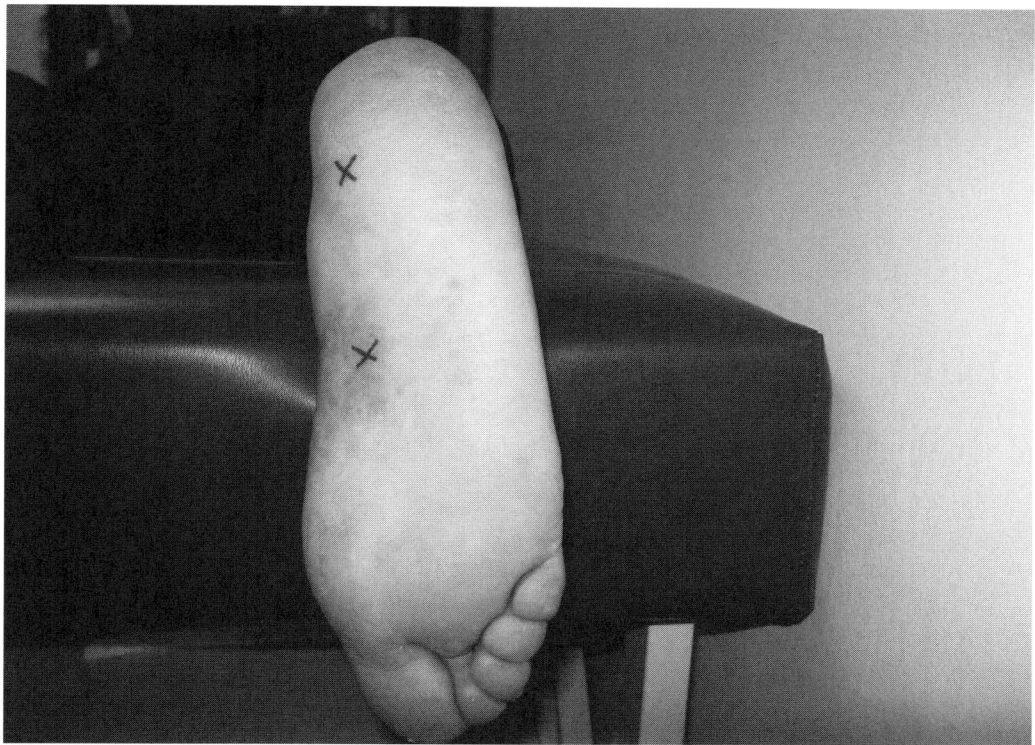

**Fig. 9.** Identify tender lesions on the sole of the foot.

effects of this agent. Some of these mechanisms include action against locally accumulated stimulant neurotransmitters (glutamate, substance P) also pertain to the pathophysiology of plantar fasciitis. This author and colleagues recently published a randomized, placebo-controlled, prospective, short-term clinical trial that studied the effect of BTX-A injection for refractory plantar fasciitis.

The patients with plantar fasciitis had almost all of the aforementioned therapeutic measures with the exception of extracorporeal shock or surgery. The solution of BTX-A (Botox®, Allergan, Inc.) was prepared by mixing 100 U with 1 cc bacteriostatic normal saline. We injected the patients of group A with 70 U BTX-A (0.7 cc) in two divided doses: 40 U (0.4 cc) in the tender region of the heel medial to the base of the plantar fascia insertion and 30 U (0.3 cc) in the most tender point of the arch of the foot (between an inch anterior to the heel to middle of the foot; *see* Fig. 1). A 27-gage, 0.75-inch needle was used for injections. Group B received normal saline at the same locations and with similar volume. In patients with bilateral plantar fasciitis of comparable severity, BTX-A was injected in one foot and saline in the other foot. All patients were also given a handout reviewing a home stretching program targeting the plantar fascia and gastroc/soleus muscle complex. No medication changes were recommended; however, patients were informed that receiving another injection or surgery on their foot would terminate their participation in the study.

Main outcome measures included pain visual analog scale, Maryland foot score, pain relief visual analog scale, and pressure algometry response. Patients were assessed prior to injection, at 3 weeks and at 8 weeks. The study revealed statistically significant changes in the

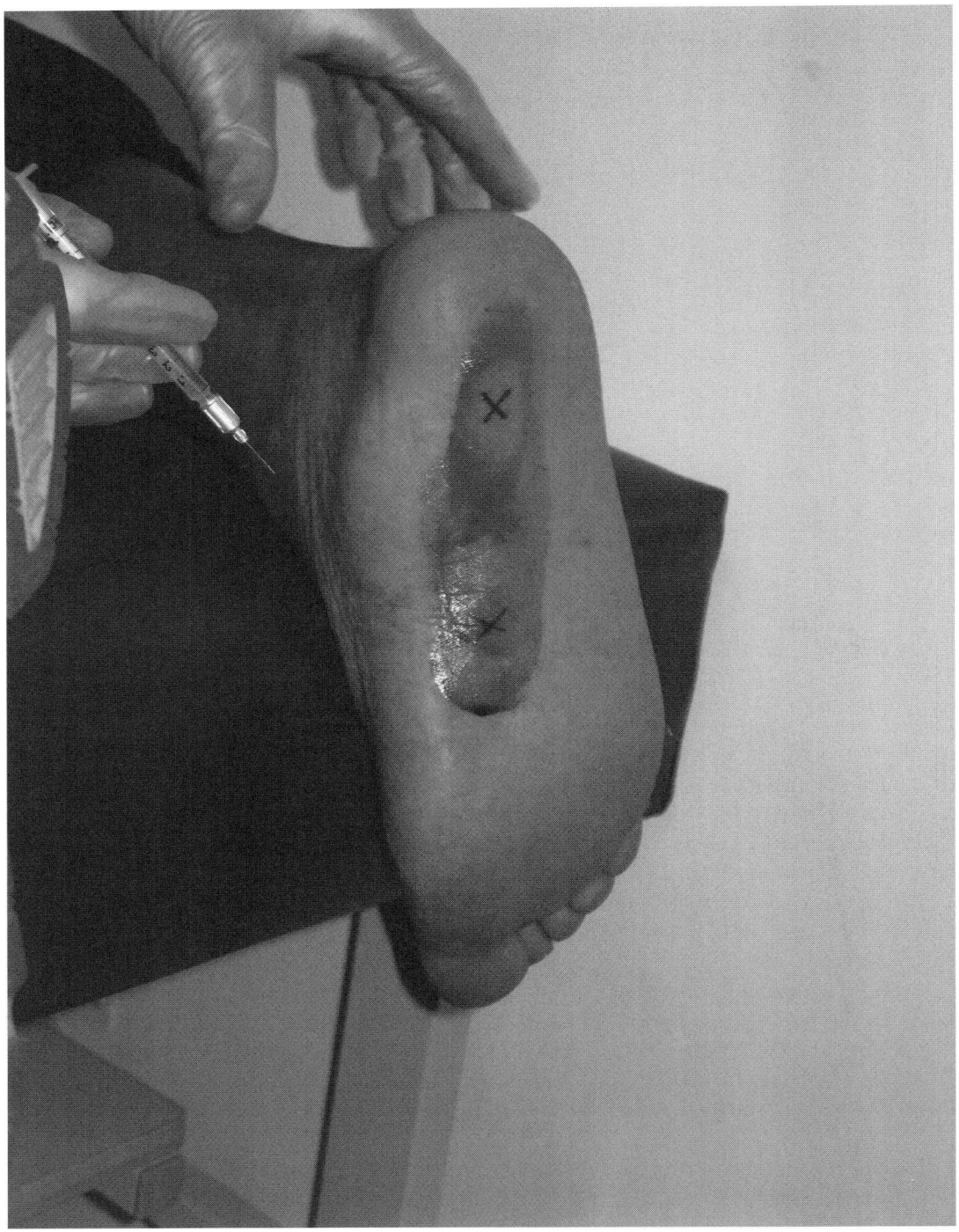

**Fig. 10.** After iodine skin preparation, apply cold mist spray to help numb the foot.

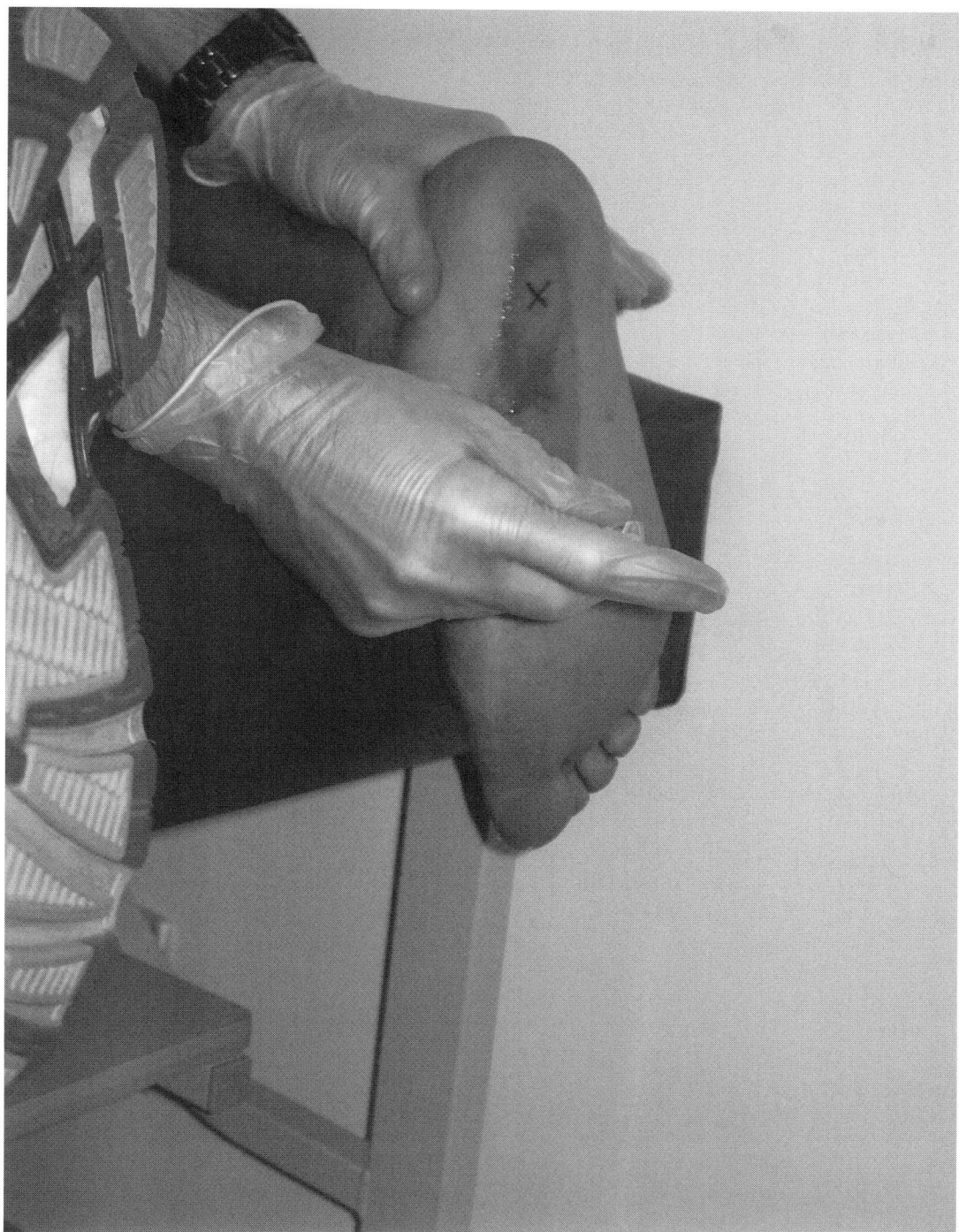

**Fig. 11.** Botulinum toxin type A injected directly into the points with the needle perpendicular to the skin surface.

treatment group. Compared with placebo injections, the BTX-A group improved in all measures: pain visual analog scale ($p < 0.005$), Maryland foot score ($p = 0.001$), pain relief visual analog scale ($p < 0.0005$), and pressure algometry response ($p = 0.003$). No side effects were noted.

The work from animal and human data demonstrates that BTX-A can affect each of the aforementioned mechanisms:

1. Both clinical and experimental data have shown that the introduction of BTX-A into a muscle results in transient loss of muscle volume via induction of muscle atrophy. Considering our injection methodology, it is possible that the subsequent reduction of the size of the intrinsic foot muscles resulted in the relief of pressure on the neurovascular structures trapped under a tight and enlarged plantar fascia.
2. BTX-A has been shown to inhibit the release of substance P from dorsal root ganglia as well as block the release of glutamate from synaptosomes *(14,15)*.
3. Pretreatment with BTX-A in rats results in a decreased local inflammatory response after the administration of formalin *(16)*.
4. Intramuscular injection of BTX-A reduces the discharge of intrafusal muscle fibers, which normally convey large non-nociceptive input (reporting muscle length) to the spinal cord *(5)*. In chronic pain conditions (which may be the case in our subjects who all complained of symptoms for >6 months), reduction of this input theoretically can reduce the level of central sensitization. In animals, administration of BTX-A reduces the discharge of sympathetic neurons *(17)* and thus can reduce the role of the sympathetic system in pain maintenance.

Our injection technique aimed to treat both the plantar fascia and the underlying muscles in case that both fascia and muscle contributed to the patients' pain. In the fascia, we hoped BTX-A to reduce inflammation and in the underlining muscles we hoped to see a positive effect on heel pain via muscle relaxation and loss of muscle volume. Yet other suggested BTX-A actions (decreased central sensitization, decreased sympathetic activity, and reduced accumulation of substance P and glutamate) could have worked at the level of both structures. In our clinical practice, BTX-A injection into the arch of the foot with a 27-gage, 0.75-in. needle often relieves painful flexor toe spasms in patients with stroke, head injury, cerebral palsy and multiple sclerosis. We chose to treat preferentially the tender points in our patients because previous reports in myofascial pain syndromes have linked success in pain relief to this approach *(18,19)*.

Although most of our responders revisited us at 6 months, only a few could be followed for 12 months because of the moving nature of our studied population (mostly young military soldiers) and the fact that the study was conducted at the time of a major military mobilization (2002–2004). Those who visited at 6 months and a few who were seen at 12 months had no recurrence of symptoms. Several subjects were able to return to full duty as military police, or return to activities such as bowling, tennis, and running. One patient was able to mow the lawn after an inability to perform this chore for 10 years. A few subjects with bilateral plantar fasciitis requested that their placebo foot be injected with BTX-A. They also had similar results. These limited long-term results are encouraging but need to be reproduced in a prospective study of a larger number of patients.

The results of our study demonstrate that the injection of BTX-A into the plantar region significantly improves the pain of recalcitrant plantar fasciitis at both 3 and 8 weeks after treatment. Although the exact mechanism of action has yet to be elucidated, several theories presented may explain the positive effect. Furthermore, blinded studies are necessary to confirm these results, which bear significant implications in caring for patients suffering from this disorder. Long-term prospective studies are also necessary to show if these positive effects can be sustained with repeated treatments. According to the American Society for

Aesthetic Plastic Surgery, the average cost of BTX-A injection ranges from $300 to $500. Compared with ECSWT, which may require multiple sessions, BTX-A injection for plantar fasciitis is, for the most part, a one-time procedure. Treatment of plantar faciitis with BTX-A should be considered for those patients who have failed standard modes of treatment.

## ACKNOWLEDGMENTS

Special thanks to my husband, Richard Babcock, and William Deas for their cooperation and collaboration. A note of thanks to Leslie Foster, DO and Bahman Jabbari, MD for their mentorship.

## REFERENCES

1. De Maio M, Paine R, Maaangine RF, et al. Plantar fasciitis. Orthopedics 1993;16:1153–1163.
2. Akfirat M, Sen C, Gunes T. Ultrasonographic appearance of the plantar fasciitis. Clin Imaging 2003;27:353–357.
3. Alfredson H, Lorentzon R. Chronic tendon pain: no sign of inflammation but high concentration of glutamate. Implications for treatment? Curr Drug Targets 2002;3:43–54.
4. Rand MJ, Whaler RC. Impairment of sympathetic transmission by botulinum toxin. Nature 1965; 206:588–591.
5. Sanchez-Prieto J, Sihra TS, Evans D, Ashton A, Dolly JO, Nicholls DG. Botulinum toxin A blocks glutamate exocytosis from guinea-pig cerebral cortical synaptosomes. Eur J Biochem 1987;165:675–681.
6. Moseley JB Jr, Chimenti BT. Foot and ankle injuries in the professional athlete. In: Baxter DE, ed. The Foot and Ankle in Sports. St. Louis, MO: Mosby; 1995, pp. 321–328.
7. Prichasuk S, Subhadrabandhu T. The relationship of pes planus and calcaneal spur to plantar heel pain. CORR 1991;266:185–196.
8. Reid DC. Running: injury patterns and prevention. In: Sports Injury Assessment and Rehabilitation. New York, NY: Churchill Livingstone; 1992, p. 1158.
9. Young C, Rutherford D, Niedfeldt M. Treatment of plantar fasciitis. Am Fam Physician 2001; 63:467–474, 477–478.
10. Gibbon WW, Long G. Ultrasound of the plantar aponeurosis. Skel Raiol 1999;28:21–26.
11. Gudeman SD, Eisele SA, Heidt RS Jr, et al. Treatment of plantar fasciitis by iontophoresis of 0.4% dexamethasone. A randomized, double-blinded, placebo-controlled study. Am J Sports Med 1997;25:312–316.
12. Sammarco GJ, Helfrey RB. Surgical treatment of recalcitrant plantar fasciitis. Foot Ankle Int 1996;17:520–526.
13. Speed CA. Extracorporeal shock-wave therapy in the management of chronic soft-tissue conditions. JBJS(Br) 2004;86:165–171.
14. Ondo W, Vuoung K, Derman H. Botulinum toxin A for chronic daily technique: a randomized, placebo-controlled parallel design study. Cephalgia 2004;24:60–65.
15. Cheshire WP, Abashian SW, Mann JD. Botulinum toxin in the treatment of myofascial pain syndrome. Pain 1994;59:65–69.
16. Welch MJ, Purkiss JR, Foster KA. Sensitivity of embryonic rat dorsal root ganglia neurons to Clostridium botulinum neurotoxins. Toxicon 2000;38:245–258.
17. Cui ML, Khanijou S, Rubino J et al. Botulinum A toxin effects on rat jaw muscle spindles. Acta Otolaryngol 1993;113:400–404.
18. Lang AM. A pilot study of botulinum toxin type A (Botox), administered using a novel injection technique, for the treatment of myofascial pain. Am J of Pain Mgmt 2000;10:105–109.
19. Wheeler AH, Goolkasian P, Gretz SS. A randomized, double blind, prospective pilot study of botulinum toxin injection for refractory, unilateral, cervicothoracic, paraspinal, myofascial pain syndrome. Spine 1998;23:1662–1666.

# 7
# Headache

## Jerome S. Schwartz, Phillip Song, and Andrew Blitzer

### INTRODUCTION

Headaches are one of the most common patient complaints to primary care physicians in the United States. The debilitating nature of many headache disorders often results in significant loss of productivity, social engagement, and quality of life. Although the overwhelming majority of headache disorders are benign in nature, patients often fear the worst case scenario, such as an aneurysm or brain tumor. To compound the situation, physicians, particularly those who are unfamiliar with headache management, often needlessly resort to extensive diagnostic examinations in search of organic pathology, thereby creating additional anxiety and financial burden.

This chapter describes the most common headache disorders with particular attention to migraine and tension-type headaches (TTHs). Because many of the routinely prescribed medications have inadequate efficacy and significant adverse effects, alternative treatment regimens are under investigation. Botulinum neurotoxin (BoNT) injection is becoming an accepted adjunct to the medication algorithm with which to treat these disorders. The proposed mechanism of action, pharmacokinetics, dosing, and safety profiles as well as injection techniques to treat common headache disorders are to be discussed in detail.

### BACKGROUND

Headaches have plagued humans since the beginning of time. The earliest reference to a migraine-like headache was found among the Sumerian poems, dated to around 3000 BCE, which described an individual as being "sick-headed" (1). Hippocrates first described the phenomenon of a visual aura, and later, during the second century CE, Aretaeus of Cappadocia reported the symptom structure of what we now refer to as migraine with aura (2). In more modern times, various theories to explain the pathophysiology of migraine headaches have emerged. Liveing is credited with the origination of the neural theory, purporting that certain "disturbances" within the autonomic nervous system may play a role in migraine (1). Dey subsequently described the phenomenon of cyclical pituitary growth with intermittent compression of the trigeminal nerve as a plausible cause for pain production (1). During the last century, Harold Wolff, through experimental evidence, illustrated a cycle of extracranial vascular dilatation and constriction, which formed the basis for the vasogenic theory of migraine (2).

From: *Therapeutic Uses of Botulinum Toxin*
Edited by: G. Cooper © Humana Press Inc., Totowa, NJ

**Table 1**
**First Level of the International Classification of Headache Disorders, Second Edition**

Part one: the primary headaches

 1. Migraine.
 2. Tension-type headache.
 3. Cluster headache and other trigeminal autonomic cephalalgias.
 4. Other primary headaches.

Part two: the secondary headaches

 5. Headache attributed to head and/or neck trauma.
 6. Headache attributed to cranial or cervical vascular disorder.
 7. Headache attributed to non-vascular intracranial disorder.
 8. Headache attributed to a substance or its withdrawal.
 9. Headache attributed to infection.
10. Headache attributed to disorder of homoeostasis.
11. Headache or facial pain attributed to disorder of cranium, neck, eyes, ears, nose, sinuses, teeth, mouth, or other facial or cranial structures.
12. Headache attributed to psychiatric disorder.

Part three: cranial neuralgias, central and primary facial pain, and other headaches

13. Cranial neuralgias and central causes of facial pain.
14. Other headache, cranial neuralgia, central or primary facial pain.

The term *headache* is often used as a descriptive term, a symptom, and a disorder. Certain headaches can be attributed to known inciting factors; however, many headaches are of unclear etiology. The need for a formal headache classification schema arose to facilitate the diagnostic evaluation, communication, and effective therapeutic modalities. In 1988, the International Headache Society published a classification system, the International Classification for Headache Disorders (ICHD)-1, which lists the major headache groups, and distinguishes primary from secondary headache disorders *(3)*. Revised in 2003, the ICHD-2 (*see* Table 1) defines primary headache disorders as those for which no identifiable structural or organic cause is known (e.g., migraines and TTHs). In a secondary headache disorder, the headache arises as a symptom, secondary to a known structural or systemic etiology *(4)*. Although the ICHD classification system has undergone much scrutiny and re-evaluation, it nevertheless provides a basic structure to initiate a rational approach to headache management. Table 2 lists diagnostic criteria for migraines and TTHs by the International Headache Society.

## EPIDEMIOLOGY/SYMPTOMATOLOGY

### Migraine Headache

Nearly 27.9 million, or 10 to 15% of Americans suffer from moderate to severe migraine headaches, accounting for nearly 10 million physician visits yearly *(5,6)*. Headaches account for nearly 1 to 2% of all emergency room visits, with migraines making up nearly 40% of headache-related visits *(7)*. Migraines affect nearly 18% of women and 6% of men; however, these estimates may underreport the true incidence of the disease, because many patients go undiagnosed. The disorder most commonly affects individuals between the ages of 25 and 55 *(8)*.

**Table 2**
**Diagnostic Criteria for Migraine and Tension-Type Headache**

1. Migrain (code 1.1)
    a. At least five attacks fulfilling items b through d.
    b. Attacks last from 4 to 72 hours.
    c. Headache has at least two of the following characteristics:
        i.   Unilateral location.
        ii.  Palsating quality.
        iii. Moderate or severe intensity.
        iv.  Aggravation by routine physical activity.
    d. During headache, at least one of the following:
        i.  Nausea and/or vomiting.
        ii. Phtophobia *and* phonophobia.
2. Tension-type headache (code 2.1)
    a. At least 10 episodes fulfilling items b through d.
    b. Episodes that last from 30 minutes to 7 days.
    c. Headache has at least two of the following characteristics:
        i.   Pressing or tightening quality.
        ii.  Mild or moderate intensity.
        iii. Bilateral location.
        iv.  No aggravation by routine physical activity.
    d. During headache, both of the following:
        i.  No nausea or vomiting.
        ii. Photophobia *or* phonophobia.

Adapted from ref. *3*.

Migraine is considered a leading cause for missed days at work in the United States. Lost productivity at work or school, impaired quality of life, and disruptions in family and social life increase the risk of affective disorders among these patients *(9,10)*.

Migraine presents as a paroxysmal headache disorder, with periods of relative quiescence between episodes. Headaches typically manifest as a unilateral, throbbing head pain lasting hours to days. Associated symptoms may include anorexia, nausea, vomiting, malaise, photophobia, phonophobia, or blurred vision. Migraine with aura presents with peculiar, transient neurosensory perceptions before or concomitant with the pain phase. Headaches may be precipitated by food intake (meats and cheeses with high nitrites, nuts, chocolate, alcohol ingestion), caffeine withdrawal, menstruation, bright lights, and exercise. Patients will often seek a dark, quiet room to help relieve the symptoms.

## Tension-Type Headache

TTH is the most common type of primary headache disorder with an estimated prevalence of between 31 and 74% of people in the United States *(11)*. The disorder presents more frequently in women, tense and anxious individuals, and in those whose work or posture requires sustained contraction of posterior cervical, frontal, or temporal muscles. TTHs are most prevalent among the 30- to 39-year-old age group. There is a positive correlation between TTH prevalence and level of education, with up to 45% of post-graduate school individuals affected *(11)*.

TTHs may be difficult to distinguish from migraine headache on initial presentation. They have been recently subcategorized according to the frequency of episodes as infrequent episodic TTH (ETTH), frequent episodic headache, and chronic TTH *(12)*. Infrequent ETTH is the most prevalent subtype, presenting as a constant, pressing, mild to moderate, bilateral headache lasting between 30 minutes and several days for less than 1 day per month (<12 days per year). Frequent ETTH is defined as headaches occurring more frequently than 1 day but less than 15 days per month, whereas chronic TTH is reserved for headaches more frequent than 15 days per month. The pain is often described as a bilateral "hatband" extending from the forehead across the sides of the head to the back of the neck *(13)*. There is an absence of nausea or vomiting, and photophobia is rare. The symptoms may be precipitated by fatigue and anxiety.

## PATHOPHYSIOLOGY

### Migraine Headache

The pathophysiology of migraine headache is not completely understood. Clinical experimental evidence suggests that at least three mechanisms are involved in the pathogenesis of the migraine headache: extracranial arterial vasodilation, extracranial neurogenic inflammation, and decreased inhibition of central pain transmission. Research advances using transcranial stimulation and biochemical analysis have provided convincing evidence that no theory alone can yet explain the onset, maintenance, and resolution of migraine headaches.

The classic vasospasm–vasodilatation theory suggests that changes in both intra- and extracranial arterial diameter mediate the symptoms of migraine. Oligemia to extracranial blood vessels (i.e., the frontal branch of superficial temporal artery) occurs during the headache prodrome and persists into the headache phase. Blood vessel diameter and cerebral blood flow are markedly diminished during the aura phase of migraine. As the pain phase begins, a reversal occurs, whereby vessel diameters and cerebral blood flow increase. The resulting hyperemia persists throughout the duration of the pain phase. Manual compression of the superficial temporal or carotid arteries during an acute episode results in mild relief of headache symptoms. This headache model warranted the use of vasoconstricting agents as a pharmacological means to control migraine-induced pain. Vasoconstrictors such as caffeine, serotonergic 5-HT1B/1D receptor agonists (triptans), and the nonselective serotonergic agonists (ergot alkaloids) have all been used with variable success in treating migraines.

A second theory suggests that dysfunction of the trigeminoneurovascular system mediates migraine pain. The trigeminoneurovascular system describes a neuronal reflex arc originating at the trigeminal nerve afferents. The trigeminal nerve transmits abnormal pain signals from the extracranial soft tissues to the central nervous system (CNS). The signal then follows the autonomic pathways via the facial nerve efferents. Parasympathetic fibers from the facial nerve, mediated through the pterygopalatine and otic ganglia, alter the extracranial vascular tone resulting in vasodilation.

Numerous neuropeptides released from parasympathetic nerve terminals are believed to affect vascular smooth muscle contraction. Of these, vasoactive intestinal polypeptide (VIP) has been histologically demonstrated within the terminal nerve endings associated with extracranial vessels supplying the tongue, salivary gland, and nose *(14,15)*. Antibodies directed against VIP appear to block the neurogenic vasodilatory response following electrical stimulation of the locus ceruleus or pterygopalatine ganglion. In addition, VIP release into the extracranial circulation has been observed following trigeminoneurovascular stimulation *(16)*.

Neuromodulators have also been found in the cell bodies of trigeminal nerve afferents, particularly near the trigeminal ganglion. Substance P and calcitonin gene-related peptide (CGRP) are among those that have been studied extensively *(17)*. Serum levels of CGRP taken from the external jugular vein during the headache phase of migraine are elevated *(18)*. Similarly, stimulation of the trigeminal ganglion as well as the superior sagital sinus (both of which induce headache when stimulated) releases CGRP into plasma *(19)*.

Central pain modulators in the CNS also appear to be involved. The exact mechanism is unclear; however, it appears that neurotransmitter release may lower the pain threshold by increasing the response to afferent sensory signals. There are also reports of relative serotonergic hyperactivity in the CNS, possibly modulating pain processing in the brainstem *(20)*. It is likely that a combination of events are involved, ultimately resulting in neurovascular irritation and CNS signal modification.

### Tension Headache

Like migraine, the pathophysiology of tension headache is unclear. The belief for many years that TTH was simply a disorder of increased muscle tension appears to be only partly true. Studies examining the myogenic potentials of the frontalis muscle using electromyography have demonstrated no differences in myogenic activity among TTH sufferers compared with controls *(21)*. However, recent studies have suggested an increase in muscle "hardness" and tenderness in both the frontalis and trapezius muscles among patients with headaches compared to patients without headaches *(22)*.

Even less is known about the biochemical mediation of TTH. Nitric oxide, an endogenous vasodilator, appears to influence certain aspects of headache. Infusion of nitric oxide has been shown to reproduce headache in patients diagnosed with TTH, whereas the blockade of nitric oxide production relieves muscle "hardness" and tenderness in those patients *(23,24)*. Neurotransmitter function in the CNS, particularly that of norepinephrine, epinephrine, and serotonin, may be altered. In one study, serum levels of catecholamines were significantly lower, and serotonergic levels higher in patients with TTH compared with controls *(25)*.

## CLINICAL DIAGNOSIS

### History

Reaching a correct diagnosis for patients presenting with chronic head and facial pain can be difficult. Global anxiety, feelings of helplessness, and other mood disorders often co-exist among patients and obscure the physician's ability to acquire the necessary information to form a rational differential diagnosis. A careful interview and documentation of the complete headache history can help establish the correct diagnosis.

The interview should begin with the history of present illness. The anatomic location of headache onset, region of distribution, and temporal or spatial progression of the pain are important descriptors for mapping. The patient should be able to recall the approximate age of symptom onset, and describe the course of progression through the present time. A detailed account of the frequency and timing of attacks, with reference to any known inciting factors should be elicited. The patient should be asked to recall whether the onset of headache is correlated to head or neck position, chewing, stress, consumption of certain foods (e.g., chocolate, nuts, meats or cheeses, alcohol, or caffeine), menstruation, weather changes, or sleep disturbances. A detailed medication history including any newly prescribed medications, changes in drug dosing, or other noted adverse drug effects should be recorded. The duration of each attack as well as quality of the pain (e.g., dull, sharp, throbbing, aching, electrical, pressure sensation) provide important clues to differentiate between myogenic and neuropathic pain. Finally, the patient should be asked about mitigating or alleviating measures, including medications, stress relief, sleep, or preference for a dark, quiet location.

The physician must be aware that headaches may impact other bodily systems other than the head and neck. Rarely is head or facial pain the sole manifestation of the disorder, and associated signs and symptoms should be thoroughly investigated. The patient should be questioned about symptoms, including nausea, fever, visual changes or diplopia, syncope, lacrimation, nasal congestion, photophobia, or phonophobia, either before or during an episode. Migraine headaches may be preceded or accompanied by a reversible aura, consisting of visual, sensory, motor, or brainstem disturbances, such as bizarre scotomata, numbness or tingling of the fingers, feet or lips, and weakness or nausea. In addition, certain headache disorders are heralded by "warning" phenomena or premonitory symptoms, characterized by vague complaints such as hyper- or hypoactivity that may occur hours to days before the onset of pain *(3)*.

Clinical information from the past medical history supplies additional indicators to narrow the diagnostic investigation. A history of trauma, intracranial disease (e.g., meningitis or subarachnoid hemorrhage), or craniofacial surgery may imply a secondary headache disorder. Systemic illness attributable to hypertension, diabetes, venereal disease, or psychiatric illness may warrant additional clinical testing and medical optimization to avoid incorrect treatment of the headache. A comprehensive analysis of all prescription and nonprescription medications taken, with concern for potential adverse effects, is essential. Vasodilators and vasoconstrictors may alter cerebral or extracranial blood flow contributing to headache pathogenesis. Any allergic reactions to medications, foods, or other environmental agents should be clearly documented.

Certain headache disorders appear to relate to the "nature versus nurture" hypothesis with evidence to support both heritable and acquired etiologies. The family history should include both: headache and systemic medical disorders through second-degree relatives. Assessment of familial migraine, TTH, temporomandibular joint disease, intracerebral neoplasia, psychiatric illness, and substance abuse may suggest a congenital headache disorder. Alternatively, the patient's social history may unearth a pattern of maladaptive behaviors that may influence the headache symptomatology. A discussion of smoking, alcohol, and drug use is recommended, in addition to day-to-day stressors such as occupation, finances, marriage, and family.

*Physical Examination*

The physical examination for headache evaluation is guided by the history and pain description; however, a complete physical examination is warranted on the initial visit. Cardiovascular, neuromuscular, and ophthalmological examinations may reveal abnormal findings often missed when examining only the areas of perceived pain. The ears, nose, throat, scalp, and neck should be thoroughly examined as well.

Specific aspects of the physical examination that may reveal subtle findings to help narrow the differential diagnosis include *(26)*:

1. Vital signs.
2. Heart and lung evaluation.
3. Auscultation of the carotid and vertebral arteries, cranium, and orbits for bruits.
4. Range of neck motion for evidence of meningeal irritation.
5. Palpation of the head, neck, and back for trigger points, masses, bruises, or thickened or tender blood vessels.

6. Assessment of the temporomandibular region for tenderness, decreased mobility, asymmetry, clicking, or adjacent muscle hypertrophy.
7. Examination for evidence of papilledema and focal neurological signs indicating possible secondary cause (could include visual field deficits, pupillary asymmetry, sensory deficits of the face, trunk or extremities, asymmetric gait, or motor weakness).

## Diagnostic Evaluation

The correct diagnosis of headache is fundamental to implementing an effective treatment regimen and avoiding persistent patient disability. Often the diagnosis will be clear following a thorough patient history, although occasionally additional testing is required. This is especially true when focal neurological signs are found, and a secondary headache disorder is suspected. On occasion, testing is warranted for patients who are disabled by their fear of serious pathology, or when the physician has concerns despite the lack of organic pathology indicators. Nevertheless, various guidelines have been put forth to assist the physician in deciding whether additional diagnostic testing is indicated.

Neuroimaging in the form of computed tomography (CT) or magnetic resonance imaging (MRI) may be useful in the evaluation of headache to assess for structural pathology. Certain headache indicators have been shown to increase the likelihood of an abnormal finding on cranial imaging, including rapidly increasing headache frequency, history of coordination difficulty, focal neurological signs or symptoms, and headache awakening one from sleep *(27)*. According to the American Academy of Neurology, for those patients with a chronic headache disorder, "with no recent change in pattern, no history of seizures, and no other focal neurological signs or symptoms, the routine use of neuroimaging is not warranted" *(28)*. When the headache presentation is atypical or accompanied by seizure, CT or MRI may be indicated.

The electroencephalogram (EEG) has been used historically as an adjunct to neuroimaging in the diagnostic evaluation of headache. It was suggested that EEG may identify structural abnormalities in the brain among certain individuals with headache, warranting further diagnostic evaluation. An evidence-based review of the literature by the American Academy of Neurology failed to find sufficient evidence supporting its utility in the routine evaluation of headache *(29)*. If the purpose of the EEG is to exclude an underlying structural lesion, such as a neoplasm, CT or MRI is far superior.

Lumbar puncture is indicated in headache evaluation under certain conditions, such as a first or worst migraine or a crash migraine to exclude subarachnoid hemorrhage or meningitis. Lumbar puncture can also be diagnostic of meningeal carcinomatosis or lymphomatosis, and high or low cerebrospinal fluid pressure *(30)*. The cerebrospinal fluid is usually normal in patients with migraine, although in rare cases, the protein concentration may be increased because of an altered blood–brain barrier when the migraine is frequent and severe or associated with cerebral infarction *(31)*. Radiographic imaging to rule out any cause for asymmetric cerebral pressures should precede lumbar puncture.

## TREATMENT APPROACH

### Migraine

The effective treatment of migraine headache involves implementing an abortive therapy for the acute attack (acute therapy), as well as developing a rational strategy to prevent or minimize future migraine episodes (preventative therapy; ref. *32*). Acute therapy aims to rapidly and effectively lessen the severity of the acute migraine and restore patient comfort and function. The goals of preventative therapy are to reduce the severity, frequency, and duration of future episodes. In addition, preventative therapy should help increase responsiveness to acute medications, improve patient function, and reduce disability from disease *(32)*. Preventative therapy should be implemented if any of the following conditions are met: poor response to acute therapy alone, adverse reaction or contraindication to acute therapy, exhaustion of acute therapy modalities, severe functional disability from recurrent episodes, high frequency of recurrent episodes, or the presence of a comorbid condition requiring long term migraine control. A comprehensive approach generally includes both pharmacological and non-pharmacological therapy, such as avoidance and biofeedback.

*Abortive Therapy*

Abortive therapy aims to provide full relief of symptoms within a few hours of initiation of treatment. The acute treatment serves both a humanistic and a medical role. From a humanistic perspective, abortive therapy eases patient suffering and reduces the strain on interpersonal relationships and professional productivity. From a medical perspective, it appears to interrupt the progression from the acute migraine headache to a chronic debilitating disorder *(33)*.

One commonly used pharmaceutical regimen involves a stepwise trial of medications, beginning with the lower potency formulations. Should the patient's symptoms require additional therapy, a more potent therapeutic agent is prescribed until maximal benefit is achieved or serious adverse effects arise. Commonly used abortive medications include the following:

1. Nonsteroidal anti-inflammatory drugs (NSAIDs):
   a. Ibuprofen.
   b. Aspirin.
   c. Sodium naproxen.
2. Analgesics:
   a. Opiates/barbiturates.
   b. Acetaminophen.
3. Vasoconstrictors:
   a. Caffeine.
   b. Sympathomimetics:
      i. Isometheptine
   c. Serotonergics:
      i. 5HT1B/1D selective (triptans).
      ii. Nonselective (ergots alkaloids).

The following sequence outlines a typical stepwise treatment protocol for migraine *(33)*:

1. A nonsteroidal anti-inflammatory analgesic.
2. Step 1 plus a mild vasoconstrictor.
3. Steps 1 and 2 plus codeine or a barbiturate or a change of analgesic.
4. Oral triptan.
5. Intranasal or subcutaneous triptan.
6. Alternatively, use an intranasal, rectal, or subcutaneous ergot.

*Preventative Therapy*

The goal of headache prevention therapy is to limit the severity, duration, and frequency of episodes, which ultimately should improve quality of life. Both pharmacological and non-pharmacological interventions play a role. The choice of which agent or combination of agents to use depends on the patient's comorbid medical conditions, adverse effect profile, physician preference, and cost.

1. Group 1:
   a. Divalproex sodium (anticonvulsant).
   b. Propranolol, timolol (β-blocking agents).
   c. Amitriptyline (tricyclic antidepressant).
2. Group 2:
   a. Atenolol, metoprolol, nadolol (β-blocking agents).
   b. Nimodipine, verapamil (calcium channel blockers).
   c. Aspirin, naproxen, naproxen sodium, mefenamic acid (NSAIDs).
   d. Gabapentin (GABA receptor blocker), guanfacine (α2-receptor agonist).
   e. Feverfew, magnesium, and vitamin B2.
3. Group 3:
   a. Nortriptyline, protriptyline, doxepin, and imipramine (tricyclic antidepressants).
   b. Fluvoxamine, paroxetine, and sertraline (selective serotonin reuptake inhibitors).
   c. Bupropion, mirtazepine, trazodone, and venlafaxine (miscellaneous antidepressants).
4. Group 4:
   a. Methysergide, dihydroergotamine (serotonin antagonists).

Nonpharmacological approaches, including exercise, dietary adjustment, and biofeedback therapy, continue to play an important role in migraine management. They are not only effective for headache prevention, but may also reduce the impact of comorbid psychological disturbances.

### Tension-Type Headaches

Treatment for TTHs follows the same principles as for migraine headache. Acute episodes are treated rapidly to restore patient function and comfort. Medications shown to be effective include analgesics and opiates. TTHs are commonly associated with affective, anxiety, and sleep disorders. Medications demonstrating efficacy for these disorders appear to be effective in the management of TTH. Prophylactic therapeutics commonly prescribed for TTH include: tizanidine (α-2 adrenergic agonist), tricyclic antidepressants, selective serotonin reuptake inhibitors, neuronal stabilizing agents, buspirone, and venlafaxine *(13)*.

Psychological and biofeedback therapy are useful treatment adjuncts, stressing the importance of treating the range of comorbid psychological disorders simultaneously.

### How BoNT Fits In

#### Rationale for Usage

The current pharmaceutical agents available to treat migraine are unsatisfactory because of limited efficacy, severe adverse effects, and drug interactions. BoNT-A is a paralytic neurotoxin that inhibits acetylcholine release at the neuromuscular junction. Although it has been approved for treating blepharospasm, strabismus, cervical dystonia, hyperfunctional glabellar lines, and hyperhidrosis, it has been safely used for various dystonias, spasticity, and tremor of the head and neck. The indication that BoNT-A may be effective for treating headache disorders was derived from anecdotal reports among patients being treating for hyperfunctional facial lines. Incidentally, these patients reported marked reductions in the frequency and severity of headache episodes and facial tension *(34)*. These findings have been reproduced in several clinical studies for migraine headache *(35–37)*.

BoNT-A has also been shown to block acetylcholine release at parasympathetic nerve terminals, and is currently also being used to treat sialorrhea and hyperhydrosis, as well as various other conditions. The mechanism by which BoNT-A relieves headache is unclear; however, various suggestions have been put forth. These suggestions include direct effects at the neuromuscular junction and direct antiproprioceptive effects on nerves of the head and neck. Recent evidence suggests that BoNT-A may also inhibit the release of various neuropeptides and neuromodulators and block the transmission of afferent neuronal signals *(38)*.

*Technical Aspects*

DOSAGE AND DILUTION

There are currently four formulations of BoNT-A (Botox®, Dysport®, Linurase™, Xeomin™, and Chinese toxin) and one type B complex (Myobloc®) approved for clinical use. Only Botox and Myobloc are currently available in the United States for injection. The three products have different dosing, safety, and efficacy characteristics and familiarity with each complex is essential before administration. There are no well established methodologies to calculate equivalent doses *(39)*.

Lyophilized BoNT-A (Botox, Allergan, Inc., Irvine, CA) is the only type A toxin currently available in the United States. Each vial contains 100 U of BoNT-A and requires dilution with 0.9% non-preserved saline. The authors typically dilute each vial with either 2 or 4 mL saline to prepare a 5.0 or 2.5 U per 0.1 mL stock, respectively. BoNT-B (Myobloc, Solstice Neurosciences, Inc., South San Francisco, CA) is available in 2500 and 5000 U/mL vials prediluted with 0.05% human serum albumin.

Although there is no consensus regarding dilution of BoNT for headache disorders, our experiences have indicated a greater overall response using lower concentrations at multiple sites with larger injection volumes (e.g., 2.5 U/0.1 mL) as opposed to higher concentrations at fewer sites with smaller injection volumes *(40)*. Affected areas may remain untreated if an inadequate number of injection sites are infiltrated, resulting in an incomplete response. Total dose administration is often individualized, taking into consideration the severity of symptoms, body habitus. and headache type.

INJECTION TECHNIQUE

BoNT injection for headache is administered using either a fixed-position or follow-the-pain technique depending on the headache type and physician's examination. Migraine headaches typically respond well to the fixed-position technique, whereas TTHs, because of the variability in presentation, are often treated with the follow-the-pain approach *(35)*. Patients exhibiting mixed features of migraine and TTH often required a combination of both techniques.

Following appropriate dilution, the toxin is drawn from the stock vial into a 1-mL syringe and a 30-gage needle is attached. Sterile technique is used both during toxin preparation and administration. The patient is placed in either a sitting or supine position and the skin cleansed with alcohol to remove debris and contaminants. Injections should be placed intramuscularly. By limiting injections to the subcutis or muscle belly, injection-related pain and risk of bruising is lessened, and effect is maintained. Injecting into the periosteum on the forehead or glabella often causes unnecessary pain *(41)*.

The target muscles for the fixed-site approach include those of the glabellar region, forehead, temporal area, and occipital region (if occipital pain is present). Specifically, the procerus, corrugator, frontalis, and temporalis muscles are isolated. Our protocol for BoNT-A

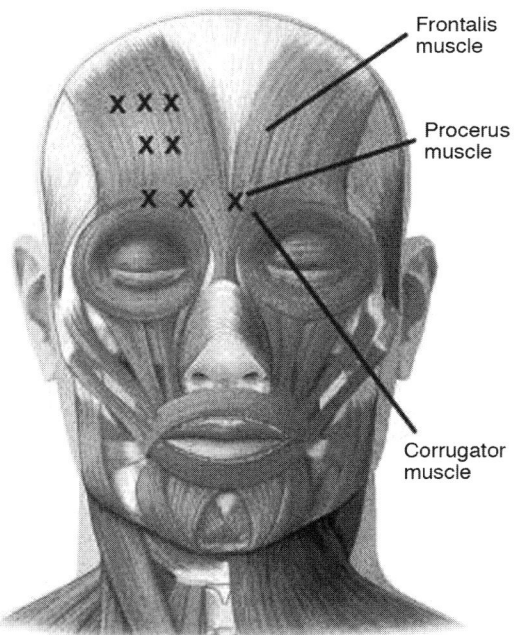

**Fig. 1.** Injection sites: glabellar and frontal regions. Reprinted from ref. *48*, © 2004, with permission from Elsevier.

injection includes the procerus muscle (5 U, one site), corrugator muscle (2.5 U each site, two sites [medial and lateral] on each side), frontalis (2.5 U each site, five sites on each side) and temporalis muscle (2.5 U each site, four sites on each side; *see* Figs. 1 and 2; ref. *36*). When using the follow-the-pain approach, we typically inject the frontalis, temporalis (doses as above), and, depending on pain localization, the trapezius (7–15 U on each side), splenius capitis/semispinalis capitis (5–15 U per side, one to two sites on each side), and occipitalis (2.5–5 U per side) muscles (*see* Fig. 3; refs. *35* and *42*). In addition, patients with temporomandibular disorder or anterocollis may benefit from BoNT-A injection to the masseter or sternocleidomastoid muscles, respectively.

Injections of the forehead and glabellar region should be performed symmetrically, using smaller injection volumes, to avoid facial asymmetry or diffusion to unintended sites. Intramuscular injections of the temporalis, occipitalis, masseter, sternocleidomastoid, and paraspinal muscles are often larger injection volumes, need not be symmetric, and are typically guided by patient symptomatology.

ANATOMICAL CONSIDERATIONS

*Procerus Muscle.* This small inverted-triangular muscle is continuous with the inferior extension of the frontalis muscle in the midline. It passes from the lower forehead over the bridge of the nose, where it attaches to the skin over the glabella. It is responsible for medial eyebrow depression, producing a typical horizontal frown line over the nasal bridge. Injections are directed in the midline toward the muscular base.

*Corrugator Supercilii Muscle.* This muscle lies over the supra-orbital rim in an oblique direction toward the nasal dorsum. It serves to depress the medial brow and is responsible for

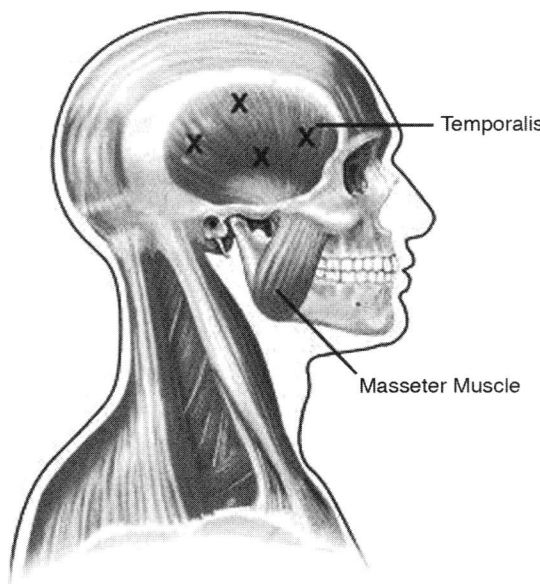

**Fig. 2.** Injection site: temporalis and masseter muscles. Reprinted from ref. *48*, © 2004, with permission from Elsevier.

creating vertical frown lines over the glabellar region. Deep to the lateral aspect of the muscle, the supra-orbital neurovascular bundle exits the skull, while the supratrochlear nerve and vessels exit medially. By having the patient frown, the muscle can be identified, and the physician's thumb and finger can then grasp the muscle belly to facilitate a precise injection. Poor technique can result in extravasation of toxin toward the eyelid, causing lid ptosis.

*Frontalis Muscle.* This large broad muscle extends over the cranium from the supra-orbital rim to the parietal region. Hyperfunctional frontalis muscles create horizontal forehead lines, most notable during eyebrow elevation. Proper injection technique involves broad application to the superior and middle aspects of the muscle. Injections directed toward the lower lateral portion of the frontalis may result in brow ptosis. Should injection into this region be required, the patient should be informed about mild brow ptosis. Additional injections to the lateral infrabrow portion of the orbicularis oculi muscle may reduce the degree of ptosis.

*Temporalis Muscle.* This large fan-shaped muscle covers the lateral aspect of the cranium, originating from the temporal line and inserting to the coronoid process of the mandible. While palpating the temporal area, having the patients clench their teeth enables localization for injection. Injections are usually administered as 5 U in 0.2-mL aliquots at four distinct sites. Because of the large size of the muscle, a larger volume may be administered without affecting adjacent structures *(42)*.

*Other Muscles.* Muscles of the posterior scalp, cervical region, and back are addressed based on patient report and the finding of tenderness on palpation. Pain may be present at the occipital region (lateral to the protuberance), yet more often is located in the paraspinal area adjacent to the nuchal line. Within this region, the trapezius muscle, splenius capitis, and semispinalis muscles converge. Precision is not crucial within this region, and injections should be correlated with areas of maximal tenderness. Larger doses (5–15 U per area) and larger injection volumes are acceptable, because extravasation will enhance the toxin's regional penetrance.

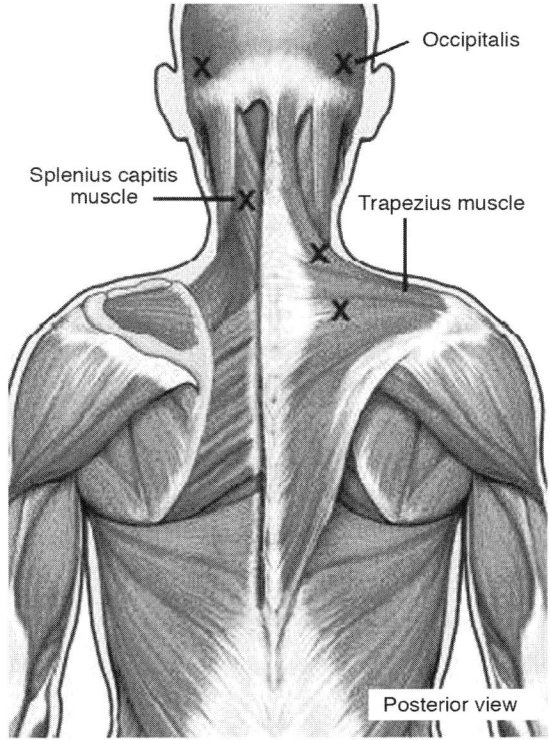

**Fig. 3.** Injection site: occipital, suboccipital, and trapezius muscles. Reprinted from ref. *48*, © 2004, with permission from Elsevier.

## RISKS AND HAZARDS

Adverse effects are often mild or transient, and can usually be minimized through proper injection technique. The most significant adverse effects involve sequelae of weakening or paralyzing muscles at or near the injection site. Most local complications are cosmetic in nature; however, inactivation of periorbital muscles when treating the glabella and forehead may result in visual disturbances. Very few of the complications reported during cosmetic BoNT-A administration have been noted when treating headache disorders. Adverse effects reported during the treatment of headache disorders include blepharoptosis, brow ptosis, diplopia, and muscle weakness at the site of injection *(43)*. Various minor sequelae associated with needle injections are also discussed.

### Eyelid Ptosis (Blepharoptosis)

Although relatively few occurrences of eyelid ptosis have been reported during BoNT-A treatment for migraine headaches, the physician should be aware of this potential complication when injecting the corrugator muscles. Eyelid ptosis occurs when toxin extravasates through the superior aspect of the orbital septum, causing paralysis of the levator palpebrae superioris muscle. The risk of eyelid ptosis increases if injections are placed at or under the middle of the eyebrows in the vicinity of the mid-pupillary line *(44)*. Caution is advised in elderly patients with areas of reduced orbital septum. The onset of ptosis may occur between 2 and 10 days following injection and persist for 2 to 4 weeks. Proper injection technique, including using small injection volumes, maintaining digital pressure at the superior orbital rim during injection, and placing injections at least 1 cm above the supraorbital rim at the mid-pupillary line, significantly reduces the risk of ptosis *(41)*. Treatment involves the use of mydriatic eye drops (e.g., 2.5% phenylephrine hydrochloride) three times daily until symptoms resolve *(45)*.

## Brow Ptosis

Transient brow ptosis has been infrequently reported following treatment of migraine headache with BoNT-A. This complication arises secondary to inferolateral frontalis muscle weakness (lateral brow ptosis) or supraorbital frontalis weakness (middle brow ptosis). The frontalis muscle is the major muscle involved in brow elevation, hence, weakening of this muscle can result in brow droop. Proper injection technique is essential to avoiding brow ptosis. In general, BoNT-A injections should be performed at least 2 cm above the supraorbital rim, and up to 4 cm in patients with low set brows *(41)*. Not rendering the frontalis muscle completely immobile but weakened can achieve a comparable goal while maintaining some forehead movement. Correction involves BoNT-A injection to either the ipsilateral superolateral orbicularis oculi muscle (lateral depressor) or corrugator and superomedial orbicularis oculi muscles (medial depressors) depending on the presentation.

## Diplopia

Diplopia is a disabling but fortunately rare complication that can be avoided through cautious BONT-A infiltration. Double vision may occur from inadvertent extravasation of toxin beyond the orbital septum to the lateral rectus muscle within the orbit. Most cases have occurred during treatment of the orbicularis oculi muscle with BoNT-A. The orbicularis oculi muscle surrounds the palpebral fissure circumferentially, and extends beyond the orbital rim just deep to the subcutaneous tissue. Diplopia may be prevented by injecting just below the epidermis, 1 cm outside the orbital rim or 1.5 cm lateral to the lateral canthus *(41)*. The needle should be directed away from the orbit to prevent extravasation of the toxin toward the globe. Should diplopia arise, immediate referral to an ophthalmologist is recommended.

## Minor Sequelae

Minor sequelae that can occur secondary to BONT-A injection at any site include pain, edema, erythema, ecchymosis, and short-term hypoesthesia. Ice applied immediately after injection reduces pain, edema, and erythema associated with an intramuscular injection. Ecchymosis can be minimized by having the patient avoid aspirin, NSAIDs *(41)*, and vitamin E for 7 days before injection. Careful attention to small subcutaneous vessels or palpation of larger vessels can help avoid ecchymosis and intravascular injection. Pain associated with injections can be minimized by infusing slowly with a 30- or 32-gage needle directly into the muscle belly avoiding the periosteum.

## POST-INJECTION MANAGEMENT

The headache relief from BoNT-A may take several weeks to reach maximal effect. Patients should maintain an accurate headache diary during the course of botulinum injections, documenting the time, severity, duration, location, and frequency of all headache events *(42)*. Any medications taken to relieve acute breakthrough headaches should be noted. The patient should return for reevaluation at 4 to 6 weeks following the previous injection to document any adverse effects or suboptimal responses. Additional BoNT-A may be administered at that time as dictated by the clinical examination.

## FREQUENCY OF INJECTIONS

Repeated injections are necessary as the botulinum effect subsides. There is tremendous variation among patients with respect to optimal dosing frequency. Some patients experience relief well beyond the predicted pharmacokinetic duration of the drug. This suggests a possible neuromodulating effect of the toxin at the CNS level. In addition, the response to toxin injection may change over time, with some patients reporting greater therapeutic effect with repeat injections *(46)*. Although the majority of patients require repeat injections at 3- to 4-month intervals, the headache diaries serve as a useful guide for the physician to direct future treatment.

## SUCCESS WITH BoNT

Clinical evidence overwhelmingly supports the use of BoNT injections for headache disorders, especially migraine. In one open-label study, 51% of migraine sufferers treated with prophylactic therapy reported complete responses, and an additional 38% reported partial responses. Complete responders reported a mean benefit of 4.1 months, while partial responders benefited for 2.7 months. Furthermore, 70% of patients treated acutely for migraine pain reported complete response *(37)*. In another study, patients were categorized according to headache type, including migraine, ETTH, mixed headache and chronic daily headache. Patients were treated with prophylactic BoNT injections in the manner previously described. Overall, the number of headache days per month was reduced 56%, the headache intensity score dropped 25%, and 86% of patients reported improvement in headache intensity and frequency *(35)*.

Prophylactic treatment of headache disorders may have a significant impact on medication costs and requirements. Blumenfeld performed a cost analysis comparing the annualized cost of treatment before and following the initiation of BoNT injection therapy *(47)*. Annualized medication costs (excluding BoNT-A) were reduced between $670 and $3524 during BoNT-A therapy. Taking into consideration the annual costs of BTX-A treatment ($666–$1480 per year), the overall annualized medication cost was decreased in three out of five patients. Patients, therefore, are likely to require less medication and, in certain cases, to avoid the need for additional medication while undergoing prophylactic BoNT therapy.

## CONCLUSIONS

Headache is a leading cause of disability among patients in the United States. Chronic pain and associated symptoms significantly interfere with interpersonal relations, professional duties, and overall quality of life. Patients suffering from chronic headaches have an increased risk of developing psychiatric disorders, particularly affective disorders such as depression. The treating physician has the unique opportunity to diagnose and treat headache disorders, and ease patient suffering. A detailed examination with appropriate diagnostic testing often allows the physician to classify the specific disorder and initiate an effective therapeutic plan.

The medications currently available to treat headache disorders have variable efficacy and an often unacceptable adverse effect profile. BoNT, through poorly understood pathways, provides significant relief from headache pain and reduces intensity, frequency, and duration of recurrent episodes when properly administered. Injection protocols, including fixed-site and follow-the-pain techniques, have provided lasting relief up to 4 months in patients with migraines, ETTHs, and chronic daily headaches. The adverse effects from BoNT are often mild, transient, and limited to adjacent muscle weakness, which can often be avoided through the use of proper injection technique. Although not yet approved by the Food and Drug Administration for this indication, BoNT therapy provides a safe and effective means by which to treat certain headache disorders.

## REFERENCES

1. Silberstein SD, Silberstein MM. Clinical symptomatology and differential diagnosis of migraine. In: Tollison CD, Kunkel RS, eds. Headache: Diagnosis and Treatment. Baltimore: Urban and Schwarzenberg; 1993, pp. 59–75.
2. Critchley M. Migraine: from cappadocia to queen square. In: Smith R, ed. Background to Migraine, vol 1. London: Heinemann, 1967.
3. International Headache Society. Classification and diagnostic criteria for headache disorders, cranial neuralgias, and facial pain. Cephalalgia 1988;8:1–96.
4. Silberstein SD, Young WB. Headache and facial pain. In: Goetz CG, ed. Textbook of Clinical Neurology, 2nd ed. Philadelphia: Saunders; 2003, p. 1187.
5. Goldstein M, Chen TC. The epidemiology of disabling headache. Adv Neurol 1982;33:377–390.
6. Lipton RB, Stewart WF, Diamond S, Diamond ML, Reed M. Prevalence and burden of migraine in the United States: data from the American Migraine Study II. Headache 2001;41:646–657.
7. Leicht MJ. Non-traumatic headache in the emergency department. Ann Emerg Med 1980;9: 404–409.
8. Stewart WF, Lipton RB, Celentano DD, Reed ML. Prevalence of migraine in the United States. JAMA 1992;267:64–69.
9. Solomon GD. Treatment considerations in headache and associated medical disorders. J Pain Symptom Manage 1993;8:73–80.
10. Lipton RB, Silberstein SD. The role of headache related disability in migraine management: implications for headache treatment guidelines. Neurology 2001;56:S35–S42.
11. Schwartz BS, Stewart WF, Simon D, Lipton RB. Epidemiology of tension-type headache. JAMA 1998;279:381–383.
12. Headache Classification Committee of the International Headache Society. The international classification of headache disorders. Cephalalgia 2004;24:1–160.
13. Krusz JC. Tension-type headaches: what they are and how to treat them. Prim Care 2004;31:293–311.
14. Jia X. Immunohistochemical study on the distribution and coexistence of SP, VIP and NPY in the rat submandibular gland. Zhongguo Yi Xue Ke Xue Yuan Xue Bao 1997;19:107–109.
15. Yoshida K. Colocalization of acetylcholinesterase and vasoactive intestinal peptide (VIP) in nicotinamide adenine dinucleotide phosphate diaphorase (NADPH-d) positive neurons in the intralingual ganglia and perivascular nerve fibers around lingual arteries in the porcine, monkey and canine tongue. Neurosci Lett 1997;222:147–150.
16. Goadsby PS, Macdonald GJ. Extracranial vasodilation mediated by vasoactive intestinal polypeptide. Brain Research 1985;329:285–288.
17. May A, Goadsby PJ. The trigeminovascular system in humans: pathophysiologic implications for primary headache syndromes of the neural influences on the cerebral circulation. J Cereb Blood Flow Metab 1999;19:115–127.
18. Goadsby PJ, Edvinsson L, Ekman R. Vasoactive peptide release in the extracerebral circulation of humans during migraine headache. Ann Neurol 1990;28:183–187.
19. Goadsby PJ, Edvinsson L, Ekman R. Release of vasoactive peptides in the extracerebral circulation of humans and the cat during activation of the trigeminovascular system. Ann Neurol 1988;23: 193–196.

20. Raskin NH. Headache, 2nd ed. New York: Churchill Livingston; 1988.
21. Sutton EP, Belar CD. Tension headache patients versus controls: a study of EMG parameters. Headache 1982;22:133–136.
22. Ashina M, Bendtsen L, Jensen R, et al. Muscle hardness in patients with chronic tension-type headache: relation to actual headache state. Pain 1999;79:201–205.
23. Ashina M, Bendtsen L, Jensen R, Olesen J. Nitric oxide-induced headache in patients with chronic tension-type headache. Brain 2000;123:1830–1837.
24. Ashina M, Lassen LH, Bendtsen L, Jensen R, Olesen J. Effect of inhibition of nitric oxide synthase on chronic tension-type headache: a randomised crossover trial. Lancet 1999;353:287–289.
25. Castillo J, Martinez F, Leira R, Lema M, Noya M. Plasma monoamines in tension-type headache. Headache 1994;34:531–535.
26. Taylor, FR. Diagnosis and classification of headache. Prim Care 2004;31:243–259.
27. Silberstein SD. Practice parameter: evidence-based guidelines for migraine headache (an evidence-based review): report of the Quality Standards Subcommittee of the American Academy of Neurology. Neurology 2000;55:754–762.
28. American Academy of Neurology. Practice parameter: the utility of neuroimaging in the evaluation of headache in patients with normal neurologic examinations (summary statement). Report of the Quality Standards Subcommittee of the American Academy of Neurology. Neurology 1994;44: 1353–1354.
29. American Academy of Neurology. Practice parameter: the electroencephalogram in the evaluation of headache (summary statement). Report of the Quality Standards Subcommittee of the American Academy of Neurology. Neurology 1995;45:1411–1413.
30. Evans RW. Diagnostic testing for headache. Med Clin North Am 2001;85:865–885.
31. Welch KMA. Cerebral metabolic and cerebrospinal fluid studies. In: Olesen J, Welch KMA, Tfelt-Hansen P, eds. The Headaches, 2nd ed. Philadelphia: Lippincott Williams & Wilkins; 2000, pp. 293–299.
32. Silberstein SD, Freitag FG. Preventative treatment for migraine. Neurology 2003;60:S38.
33. Spierings EL. Migraine mechanism and management. Otolaryngol Clin North Am 2003;36: 1063–1078.
34. Carruthers A. Improvement of tension-type headache when treating wrinkles with botulinum toxin A injections. Headache 1999;39:662–665.
35. Blumenfeld A. Botulinum toxin type A as and effective prophylactic treatment in primary headache disorders. Headache 2003;43:853–860.
36. Blumenfeld A. Botulinum toxin type A (BOTOX) as en effective prophylactic treatment in headache. Cephalagia 2002;22:20.
37. Binder WJ, Brin MF, Blitzer A, et al. Botulinum toxin type A (BOTOX) for treatment of migraine headaches: an open label study. Otolaryngol Head Neck Surg 2000;123:669–676.
38. Volknandt W. Commentary: the synaptic vesicle and its targets. Neuroscience 1995;64:277–300.
39. Jankovic J, Brin MF. Botulinum toxin: historical perspective and potential new indications. Muscle Nerve Suppl 1997;6:S129–S145.
40. Blumenfeld A, Binder WJ, Blitzer A, et al. The emerging role of botulinum toxin type A in headache prevention. OP Tech Otolaryngol Head Neck Surg 2004;15:90–96.
41. Klein AW. Complications with the use of botulinum toxin. Dermatol Clin 2004;22:197–205.
42. Blumenfeld AM, Binder W, Silberstein SD, et al. Procedures for administering botulinum toxin type A for migraine and tension-type headache. Headache 2003;43:884–891.
43. Silberstein S, Mathew N, Saper J, et al. Botulinum toxin type A as a migraine preventative treatment. For the BOTOX Migraine Clinical Research Group. Headache 2000;40:445–450.
44. Klein A. Cosmetic therapy with botulinum toxin: anecdotal memoirs. Dermatol Surg 1996;22: 757–759.
45. Burns RL. Complications of botulinum exotoxin. Presented at the 25th Annual Clinical and Scientific Meeting of the ASDS. Portland, OR: May 13–17, 1998.

46. Mathew NT, Kaup AO. The use of botulinum toxin type A in headache treatment. Curr Treat Options Neurol 2002;4:365–373.
47. Blumenfeld AM. Impact of Botulinum toxin type A treatment on medication costs and usage in difficult-to-treat chronic headache: case studies. Headache Q 2001;12:241–244.
48. Blumenfeld AM, Dodick DW, Silberstein SD. Botulinum neurotorin for the treatment of migraine and other primary headache disorders. Dermatol Clin 2004;22:167–175.

## SUGGESTED FURTHER READING

1. Blumenfeld A, Binder WJ, Blitzer A, et al. The emerging role of botulinum toxin type A in headache prevention. OP Tech Otolaryngol Head Neck Surg 2004;15:90–96.
2. Dodick DW. Botulinum neurotoxin for the treatment of migraine and other primary headache disorders: from bench to bedside. Headache 2003;43:S25–S33.

# 8

# Spasmodic Dysphonia

## Jerome S. Schwartz, Phillip Song, and Andrew Blitzer

## INTRODUCTION

Spasmodic dysphonia (SD) is a focal laryngeal dystonia characterized by involuntary, action-induced spasms of the muscles controlling vocal fold motion. The laryngeal adductor muscles (lateral cricoarytenoid [LCA], interarytenoid, and possibly the cricothyroid and thyroarytenoid [TA]), abductor muscle (posterior cricoarytenoid [PCA]), or rarely both groups of muscles may be affected. Adductor SD is characterized by a harsh, strangled, or effortful voice (glottal fry) with irregular phonatory breaks secondary to vocal fold hyperadduction or spasm. The supraglottic structures may be hyperfunctional as well. Abductor SD presents as a breathy, effortful, hypophonic voice with irregular breaks following consonant voicing secondary to vocal fold hyperabduction. Although the exact etiology of SD is unclear, SD is now recognized as a neurological disorder of central processing.

Botulinum toxin (BTX) has become one of the most important pharmacological agents to treat the symptoms of laryngeal dystonia. Although not curative, BTX may significantly ameliorate the muscle spasms and restore patient function and quality of life. Although oral pharmacological therapy is often beneficial in reducing the severity of multifocal or generalized symptoms, its effect on focal dystonias is modest at best when used as a single modality. Combination therapy incorporating both oral pharmacological agents and BTX injection may be efficacious in certain cases. BTX injection for the treatment of SD is an off-label indication; however, its excellent efficacy, duration, safety profile, and ease of administration render it a useful therapeutic for the management of SD.

This chapter focuses on the diagnosis and management of SD with particular attention to the use of BTX. The proposed mechanism of action, pharmacokinetics, dosing, and safety profiles as well as injection techniques to treat SD are discussed in detail.

## BACKGROUND

Dystonias are neuromuscular disorders that manifest as involuntary, repetitive muscular contractions producing a twisting or squeezing movement or altered posture. In primary (idiopathic) dystonia, there is no evidence of underlying organic pathology, such as neurological illness or exposure to drugs known to cause acquired dystonia (e.g., phenothiazines). In addition, there must be normal cognitive, pyramidal, and cerebellar examinations in order to classify a dystonia as primary (1,2). Secondary dystonias are associated with a known underlying organic illness. Dystonias may occur at rest, during position changes (postural), or while

From: *Therapeutic Uses of Botulinum Toxin*
Edited by: G. Cooper © Humana Press Inc., Totowa, NJ

performing a specific muscular activity (action-induced or task-specific; refs. *3* and *4*). Dystonias may also be described in relation to the anatomic region affected. Generalized dystonias involve the whole body, multifocal dystonias may affect multiple non-adjacent sites (e.g., larynx and hand), segmental dystonias involve contiguous body parts (e.g., face, neck, and shoulder), and focal dystonias manifest among one anatomic region (e.g., larynx or periocular muscle [blepharospasm]).

Although the clinical presentation of dystonias may appear heterogeneous, there are certain clinical attributes common to most dystonias that may help the examiner establish the correct diagnosis. First, dystonic symptoms tend to start in one site irrespective of the ultimate presentation. Second, the earlier the onset of symptoms (e.g., childhood-onset), the more likely the dystonia is to affect other regions. Similarly, many adult-onset dystonias remain relatively well localized. Third, dystonias tend to exhibit diurnal variation with mild symptoms in the morning after awakening and more severe symptoms toward the evening as the day progresses. Fourth, dystonic symptoms may lessen following the use of various sensory "tricks" or "gestes antagonistique," such as relieving jaw spasms by placing a finger in the corner of the mouth. Finally, many patients exhibit a tremor (dystonic tremor) in the regions affected by dystonia, which is exacerbated as the patient attempts to resist the muscle spasms. Careful attention to these details may help the clinician establish the proper diagnosis *(4)*.

SD ("spastic dysphonia") was historically considered a disorder of unknown etiology. Many considered it to be a disorder of unclear psychogenic origin similar to a hysterical reaction *(5)*. Patients with SD could often sing or shout normally, yet developed symptoms while engaging in normal conversation. In addition, some patients were noted to mitigate their symptoms through the use of various sensory tricks (such as laughing or yawning when beginning to speak). Similarly, stress appeared to exacerbate the patients' symptoms, whereas sedatives (alcohol or tranquilizers) often improved the symptoms. Although current clinical evidence has improved our understanding of this neurolaryngological disorder, the pathophysiology remains poorly understood.

In a treatise detailing the manifestations of laryngeal typhus, Traube described in 1871 what is currently believed to be the first account of SD. His patient was a young girl, believed to have been suffering from hysteria, who presented with a hoarse, nearly aphonic voice. Only with great strain could she produce a high-pitch whistling sound *(6)*. A similar description was presented by Critchley in 1939, who noted a peculiar, forced quality of speech as though his patient were trying to talk while being choked *(7)*.

In the latter half of the 20th century, evidence supporting a neurological basis for SD was emerging. The association of other movement disorders with SD, including tremor and other cranial dystonias, led Aronson (1968) to believe that SD may in fact be of neurogenic origin. Furthermore, SD patients did not differ significantly from non-dysphonic patients on routine psychological testing *(8)*. In 1976, Dedo described a cohort of patients with adductor SD who experienced symptomatic improvement following lidocaine injections to the recurrent laryngeal nerve (RLN). He subsequently introduced the surgical technique of RLN transection to relieve vocal fold spasms *(9)*. Dedo noted a profound improvement in voicing following surgery, further suggesting an organic rather than psychogenic etiology for SD.

## EPIDEMIOLOGY/SYMPTOMATOLOGY

SD is a rare disorder, with an estimated incidence of 1 case per 100,000 *(10)*. The true incidence of the disorder may be greater, because the diagnosis is often missed. Because of its heterogeneous presentation and paucity of expert laryngeal clinicians, epidemiological data, such as age of onset, race and ethnic prevalence, regional variation, and risk factors, have been difficult to assess.

SD is an example of a focal dystonia, a disorder of muscle tone affecting one specific anatomic site. Other focal forms of focal dystonias include blepharospasm, torticollis (cervical dystonia), oromandibular dystonia, and writer's cramp. Focal dystonias have an estimated prevalence of 30 cases per 100,000 population *(11,12)*. Of the focal cranial dystonias, SD is the third most prevalent form; cervical dystonia affects nearly 5.4 per 100,000 and blepharospasm 3.1 per 100,000 *(13)*. The average age of onset ranges from 39 to 45 years, and there is a 63 to 79% female predominance *(14,15)*. Between 0 and 12% of patients report a history of dystonia within first- or second-degree relatives. Many patients report a history of an upper respiratory tract infect (30%) or major stressful event prior to the onset of symptoms *(14–16)*.

Blitzer and Brin *(15,17)* published one of the largest clinical studies of SD with more than 900 patients treated with BTX injections. In their series, 82% of patients had the adductor subtype of SD, 17% had abductor SD, and 1% demonstrated a rare adductor breathing dystonia characterized by involuntary vocal fold spasms and stridor during inspiration. Seventy percent of patients had a focal dystonia only involving the larynx, while 30% demonstrated dystonic involvement of other anatomic areas as well. Of patients presenting initially with symptoms limited to the larynx, 16% eventually manifested signs of dystonia in other areas of the body. Patients with SD should be warned of the possibility of spread and be routinely examined for signs of extralaryngeal involvement *(1,15)*.

## PATHOPHYSIOLOGY

SD, like other focal dystonias, is believed to be a movement disorder caused by dysfunction of the central nervous system (CNS). As a task-specific dystonia, the dysfunction in SD may involve the volitional centers (cerebral cortex) or more likely the modulating centers (basal ganglia, midbrain, and reticular formation) of the CNS. An understanding of the anatomic pathways and neuromodulators that influence the transmission of neural signals to the vocal folds may provide some insight into the pathophysiology of the disorder.

The production of speech involves a complex, highly coordinated sequence of events, ultimately resulting in the expulsion of subglottic air through adducted vocal folds. Rudimentary vocal function has been studied in cats following transection of the cortex, cerebellum, and subcortical forebrain. These animals maintained the ability to produce vocalizations. Based on these studies, it is believed that innate vocal patterns are mediated through the motor neurons in the brainstem (e.g., nucleus ambiguus); the reticular formation of the brainstem, which coordinates the motor neuron with respiration; the solitary tract nucleus, which receives sensory input from the larynx; and the periaqueductal grey matter of the midbrain, which triggers and modulates vocalizations *(18)*.

Learned vocalizations require additional signal generation from the cerebral cortex. The primary motor cortex receives input from various cortical sites and then transmits neural signals to the brainstem through the corticobulbar tracts. Cortical structures that influence the primary motor region include the premotor cortex, the supplementary motor area, the primary somatosensory cortex, and the insular gyrus *(19)*. The primary laryngeal motor cortex *(20)* appears to integrate these signals and sends output signals to the reticular formation either via a direct connection through the pyramidal tract or an indirect connection via the putamen and substantia nigra. It is well-known that basal ganglia regions (e.g., putamen and substantia nigra) contain a large number of dopaminergic receptors, which may explain why certain forms of dystonia may respond to the administration of dopamine agonists.

Additional studies suggest that SD may be considered a disorder of sensory gating. The larynx is exquisitely sensitive to a variety of mucosal stimuli. Sensory fibers from the glottis and supraglottis are carried in the internal branch of the superior laryngeal nerve (SLN) and terminate in the brainstem at the solitary tract nucleus *(21)*. Interneurons then appear to relay the sensory signal to the nucleus ambiguus where the motor fibers of the RLN descend to the larynx. Abnormal processing of the sensorimotor signal in the brain stem is believed to mediate disorders such as chronic cough (abnormal laryngeal adductor reflex) and tic doloureux. Similarly, a reduced inhibition of the laryngeal adductor response to SLN stimulation has been reported among both adductor and abductor SD patients *(22,23)*. Further investigations using animal models, functional imaging modalities, and electroencephalography/electromyography (EMG) may help identify specific abnormalities within the central and peripheral nervous systems that contribute to laryngeal dystonias.

## CLINICAL DIAGNOSIS

The diagnosis of SD relies on clinical history, voice analysis, and a thorough physical examination including flexible fiberoptic laryngoscopy. Patients often first notice their symptoms following an illness or during a period of increased stress. The majority of patients complain of symptom exacerbation while speaking on the telephone. Speech fluency is often best early in the morning after awakening, with a progressive decline throughout the course of the day. Although symptoms may wax and wane, there is almost always a constant presence of the disorder. Certain words or phrases will be more difficult to vocalize depending on the type of SD. Individuals often report that shouting, laughing, and singing are unaffected and deny any difficulty with swallowing and coughing.

Patients with adductor SD have a characteristic strained, strangled, and effortful speech pattern with both vocal breaks and frequency shifts. There is often a reduction in loudness. Vocal tasks, which include sentences containing a predominance of voiced consonants and vowels such as "we eat eels every day" or counting from 80 to 90, help to elicit the phonatory breaks. Flexible fiberoptic laryngeal exam should reveal a normal laryngeal anatomy during quiet respiration. Glottic motion during sniffing, coughing, and swallowing are similarly normal. When the patient is asked to perform a specific vocal task, the characteristic findings include intermittent and irregular excessive glottal closure with false vocal fold approximation.

Patients with abductor SD have a breathy, effortful vocal quality with aphonic breaks in connected speech. Breaks are typically noted when the patient attempts to phonate a vowel after a voiceless consonant such as /p/, /f/, /t/, /s/, /d/, /k/, or /h/. Functionally, the vocal folds are unable to transition from an abducted position during the consonant phase to the adducted position during the vowel phase. Phrases such as "the puppy bit the tape" and "Harry's hat" elicit the breathy breaks. Flexible fiberoptic examination of the larynx reveals a delay in vocal fold closure during vocal tasks. The vocal folds and arytenoids appear to "hang" for a brief period prior to appropriate adduction.

Any patient with clinical findings suggestive of SD should be evaluated by a neurologist and an otolaryngologist familiar with movement disorders. It is essential to determine whether there is dystonic involvement of other anatomic regions of the body. A thorough examination should also assess for neurological signs suggestive of a causative disorder, such as Wilson's disease, multiple sclerosis, or glycogen storage disease.

## ANATOMICAL LANDMARKS

The larynx is a specialized upper airway organ designed to permit phonation and respiration as well as protect the lower airways from swallowed food and foreign bodies. It rests atop the upper trachea in the anterior neck, measuring approximately 5 cm in vertical dimension. The laryngeal skeleton consists of nine major cartilages joined by membranes and ligaments. Inferiorly, the cricoid cartilage forms a complete ring, with its posterior lamina being much thicker and taller than the anterior arch. Situated above the cricoid is the shield-shaped thyroid cartilage. The thyroid cartilage articulates posteriorly with the cricoid via the cricothyroid joint. Two quadrilateral laminae, adjoined in the midline, form the anterior and lateral regions, with a characteristic notch located superiorly in the midline. Two projections, the superior and inferior cornua, extend from the posterior edge. The arytenoids are paired pyramidal-shaped cartilages that rest on the superior surface of the posterior cricoid lamina, articulating at the cricoarytenoid joints. These joints allow for both gliding and rotational motion. The epiglottis is a leaf-shaped cartilage originating deep in the thyroid cartilage that extends superior toward the tongue base. It attaches to the inner thyroid lamina through the thyroepiglottic ligament, to the hyoid bone via the hyoepiglottic ligament, to the tongue base via the glossoepiglottic ligament, and to the arytenoid cartilages via the aryepiglottic folds. The epiglottis functions as a valve to close off the laryngeal inlet during swallowing. Two smaller structures, the corniculate and cuneiform cartilages, lie within the aryepigglotic folds and are believed to assist with laryngeal closure during swallowing.

Laryngeal motion is a highly coordinated and complex function involving multiple muscle groups. The extrinsic muscles of the larynx control laryngeal position in the neck and are divided into the suprahyoid (mylohyoid, geniohyoid, digastric, and stylohyoid) and infrahyoid (sternohyoid, sternothyroid, thyrohyoid, and omohyoid) muscles. The intrinsic laryngeal muscles are much smaller and control vocal fold position and/or tension. Anteriorly, the paired cricothyroid muscles originate from the anterior cricoid arch and insert on the thyroid laminae. They lie just superficial to the cricothyroid membrane. By virtue of their action on the thyroid cartilage, they indirectly lengthen and tense the vocal folds, which is important for pitch modulation. They are the only intrinsic laryngeal muscles innervated by the external branch of the SLN. The remainder of the intrinsic muscles are innervated by the RLN. The TA muscles form the bulk of the vocal fold and run in an anterior to posterior direction from the inner thyroid lamina to the vocal process of the arytenoid cartilages. TA contraction results in vocal fold thickening and relaxation. The LCA muscles arise from the lateral aspects of the cricoid cartilage and insert into the muscular processes of the arytenoid cartilages. Their contraction causes the arytenoids to rotate medially resulting in vocal fold adduction. Adduction is also accomplished by the action of the transverse arytenoid or interarytenoid muscle. This muscle extends from the posterior surface of one arytenoid cartilage to the other, and acts to pull the arytenoids together. Finally, the PCA muscles originate from the posterior surface of the posterior cricoid lamina and insert upon the muscular processes of the arytenoid cartilages. PCA contraction results in lateral rotation of the arytenoids resulting in vocal fold abduction.

The soft tissue spaces of the interior larynx are divided into three regions from superior to inferior. The vestibule of the larynx extends from the false vocal folds (vestibular folds) upward. The lateral aspects of the vestibule are bounded by the mucosal-lined quadrangular membranes. Inferior to each vestibular fold is a lateral recess known as the laryngeal ventricle. It forms a sinus from which the saccule of the larynx passes between the vestibular fold and the thyroid cartilage. The infraglottic cavity extends from the true vocal folds inferiorly to the cricoid cartilage, and is bounded laterally by the conus elasticus.

## TREATMENT APPROACH

### BTX: Rationale for Use

The pharmaceutical agents currently available to treat dystonias are limited by partial efficacy, unwanted adverse effects, and drug interactions. Although commonly employed either alone, or in combination with BTX administration to treat segmental, multifocal, or generalized dystonias, pharmacological agents such as anticholinergics, benzodiazepines, and baclofen have demonstrated only partial benefit when used to treat focal dystonias alone. These medications, however, may be useful as an adjunct to BTX injection in SD to prolong the duration of improvement.

Voice therapy is generally unsuccessful as a single modality therapy for SD. Nevertheless, voice therapy plays an important role in the diagnosis of SD as well as in the prevention of adverse vocal behaviors. Because many patients with SD attempt to overcome their dysphonia by means of behavioral alterations, they may develop poor compensatory laryngeal behaviors. In training patients on proper vocal technique, voice therapy can minimize the compensatory responses and improve the overall benefit of BTX therapy.

Surgical therapies to treat SD include RLN section, anterior commissure retrodisplacement, nerve reinnervation or stimulation, and LCA myectomy. Although the technical aspects of these procedures are beyond the scope of this book, surgical treatments to improve the symptoms of SD have either failed to demonstrate prolonged vocal benefit or are still under investigation *(24)*.

BTX type A (BTX-A) is a paralytic neurotoxin that inhibits acetylcholine release at the neuromuscular junction. Specifically, BTX-A is a zinc-dependent metalloprotease that cleaves the synaptosome-associated protein-25 docking protein, causing an inhibition of acetylcholine exocytosis at the terminal nerve ending, preventing synaptic transmission *(25)*. BTX injection results in a dose-related muscle weakness that can be used to manage hyperfunctional disorders of the head and neck. Although it has been approved for treating blepharospasm, strabismus, cervical dystonia, hyperfunctional glabellar lines, and hyper-hidrosis, BTX has been safely used to treat various other dystonias of the head and neck and is the treatment of choice for SD.

In the early 1980s, Alan Scott *(26)* developed the toxin as a therapeutic modality for the treatment of strabismus, and later for blepharospasm. In 1984, the senior author [AB] *(1)* first treated a patient who had SD and blepharospasm with laryngeal intramuscular injections of BTX. Doses administered to the vocal folds were increased until vocal fluency was achieved. Other authors initially reported similar results using BTX injections for SD *(27,28)*. Since that time, our group has treated more than 1100 patients with good results and few adverse effects.

### Technical Aspects

#### Dosage and Dilution

There are currently five formulations of BTX-A (Botox®, Dysport®, Linurase™, Xeomin® and Neuronox®) and one type B complex (Myobloc®) approved for clinical use. Only Botox and Myobloc are currently available in the United States for injection. The three products have different dosing, safety, and efficacy characteristics and familiarity with each complex is essential prior to administration. There are no well-established methodologies to calculate equivalent doses *(29)*.

Lyophilized BoNT-A (Botox, Allergan, Inc., Irvine, CA) is the only type A toxin currently available in the United States. Each vial contains 100 U of BTX-A, and requires dilution with 0.9% non-preserved saline. The authors typically dilute each vial with either 2 or 4 mL saline to prepare a 5.0 or 2.5 Botox U per 0.1 mL stock, respectively. Further dilutions are performed by adding additional saline, keeping a uniform volume of 0.1 mL. BTX-B (Myobloc, Solstice Neurosciences, Inc., South San Francisco, CA) is available in 2500 and 5000 U/mL vials prediluted with 0.05% human serum albumin.

Dosage determination is complicated by the variability in both physiological BTX response and patient preference. Individual doses of BTX-A for adductor SD may range from 0.005 to 30 U Botox per TA muscle, and the authors generally begin treatment at 1 U Botox per vocal fold. Subsequent doses are determined from the prior response, including maximal effect (using a Likert scale from 0 to 100%), duration, and side effect profile. The majority of patients will remain well controlled for 3 months or more with injections of 0.625 to 2.5 U Botox per side. Additional smaller doses a few weeks after the initial one may be added if the voice does not become fluent. Most patients benefit from bilateral TA injections, however, some patients may not tolerate the initial degree of breathiness often resulting from this technique. As such, some patients require staggered doses, others have unilateral smaller doses, and still others benefit from mini-doses bilaterally that are administered more frequently. For abductor SD, injections are routinely administered to one PCA muscle per session, either the right or left, to prevent a life-threatening airway obstruction from over-medialization of both vocal folds. The authors' average starting dose for abductor SD is 3.75 U Botox to the PCA muscle. Subsequent injections are determined by the functional status of the vocal folds as documented on flexible fiberoptic laryngoscopy. Occasionally, patients will fail to respond to even high doses of BTX-A, possibly secondary to antibody-mediated resistance, and require BTX-B administration. In a study comparing the effects of BTX-B injections with BTX-A injections for patients with adductor SD, Blitzer *(30)* reported a conversion ratio of 52:1 U of BTX-B:BTX-A. This dose adjustment has been used for both laryngeal and other dystonias of the head and neck with good overall results.

*Injection Technique*

BTX injection into the laryngeal muscles requires more precision than injections into the larger, palpable muscles of the face and neck. Similarly, unlike the static position of most muscles of the head and neck, the laryngeal muscles are constantly in motion, both during respiration and phonation, therefore the timing of laryngeal BTX injection becomes important. EMG guidance assists the physician in identifying the location of the deep, small muscles of the larynx that are impossible to palpate. While targeting the electrically active muscle belly, the physician avoids accidental injection of toxin into the laryngeal lumen or adjacent soft tissue structures. EMG can help maximize the therapeutic benefit by directing the injection toward the motor endplates, allowing for a smaller dose and less volume to be administered *(31)*. A 27-gage Teflon-coated hollow-bore needle with an EMG interface is attached to a 1-mL syringe for injection. The needle functions as a monopolar electrode and is used for both adductor and abductor types of SD. Two skin electrodes, a reference and a ground, are placed

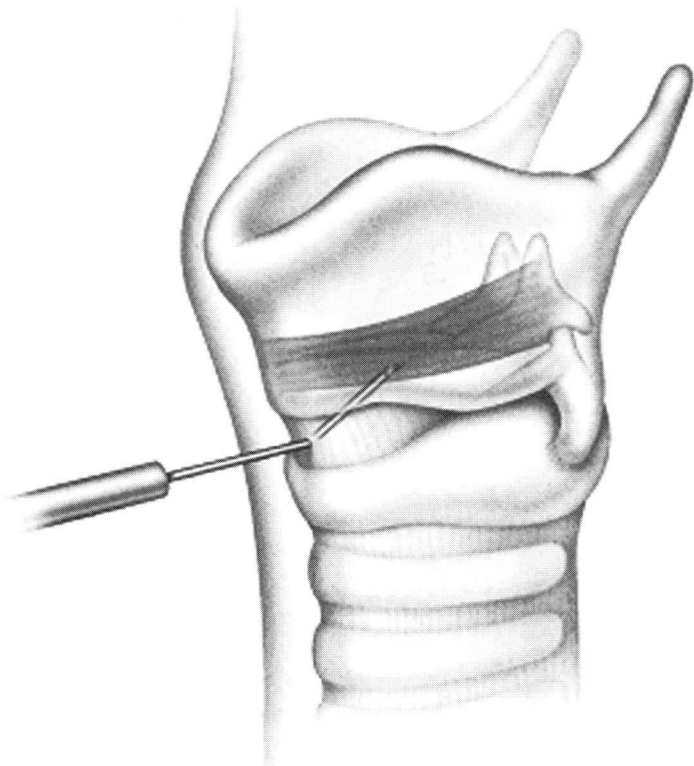

**Fig. 1.** Botulinum toxin injection to the thyroarytenoid muscle through a trans-cricothyroid puncture for adductor spasmodic dysphonia. Reprinted from ref. *31*, © 2004, with permission from Elsevier.

on the neck or jaw away from the injection site. A computer utilizing EMG-specific software displays the electrical myogenic potentials, while a sound speaker allows for auditory perception of the needle's location.

A transcricothyroid approach is used when treating patients with adductor SD. The patient is placed supine with a small shoulder roll to assist with neck extension. The skin is cleansed with alcohol to remove debris and contaminants. Local or intratracheal anesthesia is often unnecessary, and may interfere with EMG signal transmission *(32)*. If needed, 0.3 mL 2% lidocaine may be injected through the cricothyroid membrane into the subglottic airway. This usually stimulates the cough reflex, which sprays the anesthesia to the vocal fold mucosa. Palpation of the space between the anterior cricoid lamina (below) and inferior thyroid lamina (above) denotes the location of the cricothyroid membrane. The needle is curved slightly to allow a more anterior placement, and is inserted percutaneously through the cricothyroid membrane toward the TA muscle *(see* Fig. 1).

Often, as the needle is advanced superiorly and laterally, a characteristic "buzz" from the EMG speaker indicates that the needle is within the intraluminal airway medial to the vocal fold. Entering the tracheal or laryngeal lumen may be irritating to the patient, causing a coughing spasm or swallow. By guiding the needle slowly, in a superolateral direction along the inner thyroid lamina, the injector can usually avoid the airway and minimize

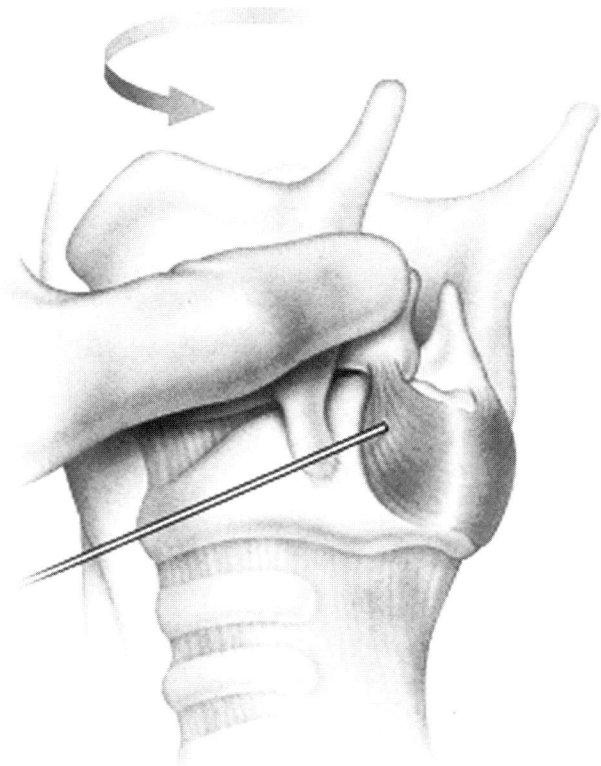

**Fig. 2.** Laryngeal rotation technique for botulinum toxin injection to the posterior cricoarytenoid muscle for abductor spasmodic dysphonia. Reprinted from ref. *31*, © 2004, with permission from Elsevier.

patient discomfort. The needle is advanced until either a "crackling" sound or motor unit potential waveform appears on the monitor, confirming proper muscle belly penetration. The patient is asked to phonate and an EMG interference pattern should result, signifying TA motor unit recruitment during contraction. The toxin may then be safely delivered to the vocal fold. If bilateral vocal fold injections are required, the needle may be removed, allowing the patient to cough or swallow, before the second injection is administered.

Abductor SD is characterized by breathy phonatory breaks resulting from hyperfunction of the PCA muscles, the sole abductor muscle group of the larynx. The PCA muscle may be approached in two ways. Most commonly, the injector places his or her thumb at the posterior border of the thyroid cartilage lamina using counterpressure with the fingers against the opposite thyroid lamina. The larynx is then rotated away from the injection site to maximize exposure to the posterior aspect (*see* Fig. 2). The needle is then inserted per-cutaneously along the lower edge of the cartilage and advanced until the cricoid cartilage is encountered. The needle is then pulled back slightly, and the patient is asked to sniff. A characteristic interference pattern will be elicited on the EMG, confirming PCA motor end-plate activation. The toxin may then be safely administered. Alternatively, the needle may be inserted through the cricothyroid membrane (as previously described), and advanced

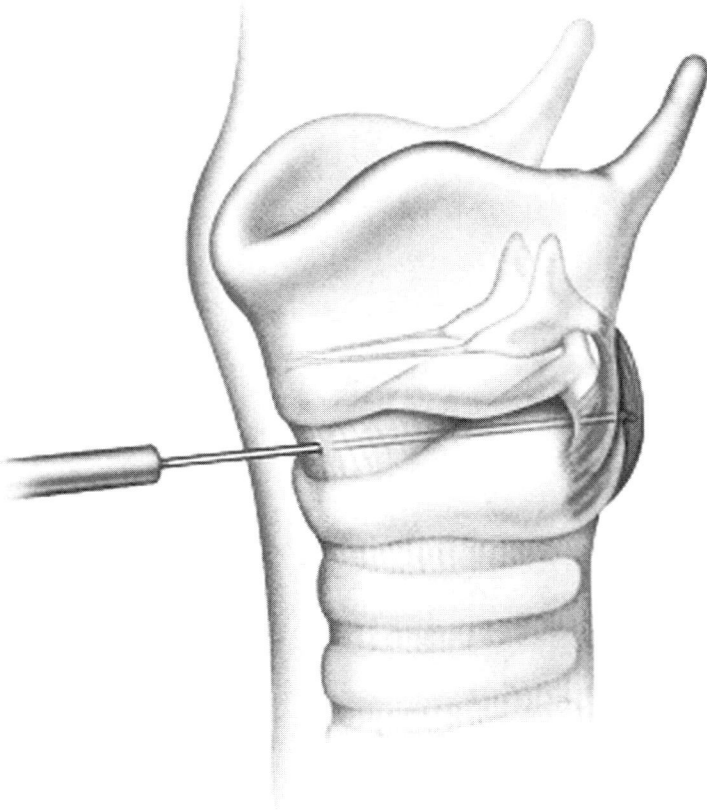

**Fig. 3.** An alternate approach to the posterior cricothyroid muscle through the posterior cricoid lamina. Reprinted from ref. *31*, © 2004, with permission from Elsevier.

through the subglottic air column until the posterior cricoid lamina is reached. With additional pressure, the needle may be advanced through the cricoid cartilage toward the PCA muscle (*see* Fig. 3). Once through the cartilage, the first electrical signal encountered represents the PCA muscle. The patient should be asked to sniff, and the appropriate interference pattern will allow for BTX injection. In our experience, this approach is most useful in younger patients in whom the cricoid cartilage has not yet undergone significant calcification.

Alternatives to EMG-guided injection include a variety of visually guided approaches. BTX may be injected percutaneously, as previously described, using flexible fiberoptic laryngoscopy guidance (*33*). BTX may also be delivered transorally with a curved injector under endoscopic or mirror observation (*34*) or through the instrument channel of a flexible fiberoptic laryngoscope (*35*). Any method that enables the clinician to achieve reliable chemodenervation with minimal patient discomfort can be used to deliver BTX.

### Risks and Hazards

BTX treatment of the larynx often results in an initial period of significant vocal muscle weakness lasting several days, followed by a period of moderate motor weakness, which constitutes the principal therapeutic effect. As a result, the majority of patients who complain of an adverse effect from the toxin usually demonstrate symptoms that tend to resolve within 1 to 2 weeks following injection. In his series, Blitzer *(17)* reported mild breathiness in 35%, mild choking on liquids in 15%, and local pain or sore throat in less than 1% of his patients treated for adductor SD. Breathiness arises from the early effects of chemodenervation manifesting as mild glottal insufficiency. Some patients tolerate this transient phase of dysphonia without requiring dose modification. When intolerable, breathiness can be limited by lowering the dose of toxin administered, which in effect may reduce the overall efficacy and duration of benefit for treating SD. Alternatively, the treatment protocol may be changed to an alternating-side injection strategy, which leaves one vocal fold less denervated than the other. Many patients have been managed successfully with such a strategy.

Dysphagia is also a transient effect, and many patients will make changes to the consistency of their food intake to compensate until swallowing function returns to normal. When treating abductor SD, it is believed that some of the toxin may diffuse to adjacent pharyngeal constrictor muscles, causing this phenomenon. With routine use of the EMG and small injection volumes, the clinician can target the region of muscle with greatest activity and reduce the frequency of constrictor muscle chemodenervation. The physician must recognize the importance of an individualized plan of care. Each individual may have different vocal demands, adverse effect thresholds, and requirements for drug effect, which affect the physician's decision regarding an optimal therapeutic approach.

### Frequency of Administration

The response to BTX injection of the laryngeal muscles varies and the physician must be prepared to treat each patient individually. The average onset of action following vocal fold injection for adductor SD is 2 to 3 days, with a peak effect at 9 to 10 days. Most patients enjoy symptomatic benefit for approximately 3 to 4 months before effortful phonation resumes. The pharmacokinetic profile and duration of action for abductor SD injections are similar; however, the decision to re-inject is influenced by the functional status of the vocal fold as seen during flexible laryngoscopy. Airway obstruction can be precipitated if both abductor muscles (PCAs) are weakened simultaneously. We generally alternate PCA injections between the right and left on subsequent visits, and may withhold an alternate injection if there is a significant residual weakness from the prior intervention.

The treating physician must be aware of the variability in his or her patients' vocal demands and personal preferences. Some patients cannot tolerate the return of mild symptoms and require more frequent dosing, whereas others may allow symptoms to become severe prior to requiring re-injection. Certain patients cannot tolerate the breathiness associated with bilateral injections and require alternate injections to the left and right vocal folds. In order to provide a smooth, constant effect, the physician may need to provide more frequent therapy.

### Success With BTX

Since the first laryngeal injection of BTX in 1984, patients have continued to report significant improvements in disease-specific quality of life. Neither oral pharmacological agents, voice therapy, nor surgery has been shown to affect vocal quality or quality of life to the same degree. In the largest SD series to date, Blitzer *(17)* reported an average improvement in function of 37.3% following BTX injection. He also noted that there was a learning curve in obtaining good responses, as demonstrated by a downward trend in dosing and side effects during the 12-year study. Damrose *(36)* assessed vocal quality in 102 subjects with SD who were treated with serial BTX injections for up to 2 years. Patients demonstrated a significant improvement over baseline at all time points. Until a CNS-specific therapy is found, local injections of BTX provide a safe and effective means of controlling patient symptoms.

## CONCLUSIONS

SD is a task-specific, focal laryngeal dystonia believed to originate from altered signal processing in the brainstem. The adductor type presents as an effortful, strangled vocal quality resulting from intermittent hyperadduction of the vocal folds and supraglottic structures resulting in phonatory breaks. The abductor type presents as an effortful, breathy vocal quality because of hyperabduction of the vocal folds also resulting in phonatory breaks. BTX, by virtue of a chemical denervation, can be injected into specific hyperfunctional laryngeal muscles (PCA or TA) and weaken them. When SD accompanies other forms of dystonia, additional oral pharmacological agents may be useful. BTX injections to the larynx are currently the accepted standard of care for laryngeal dystonias. Delivery of the toxin is facilitated with EMG guidance, which may improve both the safety and effect of therapy.

## REFERENCES

1. Blitzer A, Brin MF. Laryngeal dystonia: a series with botulinum toxin therapy. Ann Otol Rhinol Laryngol 1991;100:85–89.
2. Marsden CD, Sheehy MP. Spastic dysphonia, Meige disease and torsion dystonia. Neurology 1982;32:1202–1203.
3. Stacy M, Jankovic J. Differential diagnosis and treatment of childhood dystonia. Pediatr Ann 1993;22:353–358.
4. Jankovic J. Movement disorders. In: Goetz CG, ed. Textbook of Clinical Neurology, 2nd ed. Philadelphia: Saunders; 2003, pp. 725–727.
5. Heaver L. Spastic dysphonia: a psychosomatic voice disorder. In: Barbara DA, ed. Psychological and Psychiatric Aspects of Speech and Hearing. Springfield, IL: Charles C. Thomas; 1960, pp. 250–253.
6. Traube L. Zur Lehre von den larynxaffectionen beim ileotyphus. Verlag Van August Hisschwald: Berlin; 1871, pp. 674–678.
7. Critchley, M. Spastic dysphonia "inspiratory speech." Brain 1939;62:96–103.
8. Aronson AE, Brown JR, Litin EM, Pearson JS. Spastic dysphonia. I. Voice, neurologic and psychiatric aspects. J Speech Hear Disord 1968;33:203–218.
9. Dedo HH. Recurrent laryngeal nerve section for spastic dysphonia. Ann Otol Rhinol Laryngol 1976;85:451–459.
10. Castelon Konkiewitz E, Trender-Gerhard I, Kamm C, et al. Service-based survey of dystonia in Munich. Neuroepidemiology 2002;21:202–206.
11. Nutt JG, Muenter MD, Aronson A, et al. Epidemiology of focal and generalized dystonia in Rochester, Minnesota. Mov Disord 1988;3:188–194.
12. Le KD, Nilsen B, Dietrichs E. Prevalence of primary focal and segmental dystonia in Oslo. Neurology 2003;61:1294–1296.
13. Pekmezovic T, Ivanovic N, Svetel M, et al. Prevalence of primary late-onset focal dystonia in the Belgrade population. Mov Disord 2003;18:1389–1392.
14. Schweinfurth JM, Billante M, Courey MS. Risk factors and demographics in patients with spasmodic dysphonia. Laryngoscope 2002;112:220–223.
15. Brin MF, Fahn S, Blitzer A, et al. Movement disorders of the larynx. In: Blitzer A, Brin MF, Sasaki CT, Fahn S, Harris K, eds. Neurological Disorders of the Larynx. New York: Thieme; 1992, pp. 240–248.

16. Greene P, Kang UJ, Fahn S. Spread of symptoms in idiopathic torsion dystonia. Mov Disord 1995;10:143–152.
17. Blitzer A, Brin MF, Stewart CF. Botulinum toxin management of spasmodic dysphonia (laryngeal dystonia): a 12-year experience in more than 900 patients. Laryngoscope 1998;108:1435–1441.
18. Jurgens U. Neural pathways underlying vocal control. Neuroscience Biobehav Rev 2002;26: 235–258.
19. Simyon K, Jurgens U. Cortico-cortical projections of the motorcortical larynx area in the rhesus monkey. Brain Res 2002;949:23–31.
20. Simonyan K, Jurgens U. Efferent subcortical projections of the laryngeal motorcortex in the rhesus monkey. Brain Res 2003;974:43–59.
21. Sessle BJ. Excitatory and inhibitory inputs to single neurons in the solitary tract nucleus and adjacent reticular formation. Brain Res 1973;53:333–342.
22. Ludlow CL, Schulz GM, Yamashita T, et al. Abnormalities in long latency responses to superior laryngeal nerve stimulation in adductor spasmodic dysphonia. Ann Otol Rhinol Laryngol 1995; 104:928–935.
23. Deleyiannis FW, Gillespie M, Bielamowicz S, et al. Laryngeal long latency response conditioning in abductor spasmodic dysphonia. Ann Otol Rhinol Laryngol 1999;108:612–619.
24. Aronson AE, DeSanto LW. Adductor spastic dysphonia: three years after recurrent laryngeal nerve resection. Laryngoscope 1983;93:1–8.
25. Binz T, Blasi J, Yamasaki S, et al. Proteolysis of SNAP-25 by types E and A botulinal neurotoxins. J Biol Chem 1994;269:1617–1620.
26. Scott AB. Botulinum toxin injection of eye muscles to correct strabismus. Trans Am Opthalmol Soc 1981;79:734–770.
27. Ludlow CL, Naunton RF, Sedory SE, et al. Effects of botulinum toxin injections on speech in adductor spasmodic dysphonia. Neurology 1988;38:1220–1225.
28. Miller RH, Woodson GE, Jankovic J. Botulinum toxin injection of the vocal fold for spasmodic dysphonia: a preliminary report. Arch Otolaryngol Head Neck Surg 1987;113:603–605.
29. Jankovic J, Brin MF. Botulinum toxin: historical perspective and potential new indications. Muscle Nerve Suppl 1997;6:S129–S145.
30. Blitzer A. Botulinum toxin A and B: A comparative dosing study for spasmodic dysphonia. Otolaryngol Head Neck Surg 2005;133:836–838.
31. Sulica L, Blitzer A. Botulinum toxin treatment of spasmodic dysphonia. Op Tech Otolaryngol Head Neck Surg 2004;15:76–80.
32. Chitkara A, Meyer T, Cultrara A, et al. Dose response of topical anesthetic on laryngeal neuromuscular electrical transmission. Ann Otol Rhinol Laryngol 2005;114:819–821.
33. Green DC, Berke GS, Ward PH, et al. Point-touch technique of botulinum toxin injection for the treatment of spasmodic dysphonia. Ann Otol Rhinol Laryngol 1992;101:883–887.
34. Ford CN, Bless DM, Lowery JD. Indirect laryngoscopic approach for injection of botulinum toxin in spasmodic dysphonia. Otolaryngol Head Neck Surg 1990;103:752–758.
35. Rhew K, Fiedler DA, Ludlow CL. Technique for injection of botulinum toxin through the flexible nasolaryngoscope. Otolaryngol Head Neck Surg 1992;111:787–794.
36. Damrose JF, Goldman SN, Groessl EJ, Orloff LA. The impact of long-term botulinum toxin injections on symptom severity in patients with spasmodic dysphonia. J Voice 2004;18:415–422.

# 9

# Sialorrhea and Frey's Syndrome

## Phillip Song, Jerome S. Schwartz, and Andrew Blitzer

## INTRODUCTION

With the widespread use of botulinum toxin (BTX) and greater appreciation of its safety, physicians are increasingly aware of potential applications beyond dystonias, spasticity, and cosmetic denervation. Although most applications for BTX have focused on muscular denervation, autonomic denervation is currently being explored for a variety of clinical problems including excessive drooling, gustatory sweating, and hyperlacrimation. This chapter focuses on the role of BTX for uncontrolled salivation and gustatory sweating.

## SIALORRHEA

BTX can reduce excessive or uncontrolled salivation (sialorrhea) and ptyalism (drooling) via autonomic denervation rather than muscular denervation. By impairing acetylcholine release in the neural junction, parasympathetic activity can be prevented. Localized injection of BTX is specific and regional. This ability to target secretary glands is a significant advantage over oral medications that are used to control salivation, such as glycopyrrolate and scopolamine, which produce systemic anticholinergic side effects.

Acetylcholine is the neurotransmitter that regulates the parasympathetic side of the autonomic nervous system (ANS) and is also present on sweat glands in the skin that are regulated by the sympathetic side of the ANS. BTX inhibits cholinergic transmission by blocking the presynaptic release of acetylcholine. There are seven recognized serotypes of BTX (A, B, C, D, E, F, and G) and four (A, B, E, and F) are poisonous to humans. The toxin binds to the presynaptic nerve terminal and is internalized into the cytoplasm where it binds to SNARE proteins. SNARE proteins form a complex that mediates vesicle release of acetylcholine. BTX protealyses the SNARE proteins and prevents acetylcholine release and subsequent neural transmission (1).

Autonomic denervation by BTX has been used for intractable drooling and control of salivation. Excess drooling can be socially crippling and affects the quality of life of people with orofacial dysmotility and swallowing difficulties. Loss of fluid and electrolytes can result in serious dehydration and metabolic derangements. In addition, problems such as cheilitis, dental caries, poor oral health, halitosis, aspiration, and skin maceration can occur. Drooling occurs when salivary production exceeds the ability to handle secretions. Almost any disorder that disrupts orofacial movement or swallowing function can result in drooling.

From: *Therapeutic Uses of Botulinum Toxin*
Edited by: G. Cooper © Humana Press Inc., Totowa, NJ

In most instances of drooling, the primary problem is not hypersalivation but insufficient elimination of secretions. This can occur because of poor muscular control of the tongue, pharynx, larynx, mouth, and lips or poor sensory feedback in the oral cavity or oropharynx. In addition, impaired swallowing can result in excessive buildup of saliva with spillage. Upper esophageal sphincter dysfunction can impair swallowing, resulting in pooling of saliva in the hypopharynx and aspiration. Inadequate neck muscle coordination, as seen in people with cerebral palsy, can result in head-down position with pooling in the anterior oral cavity, producing inadvertent spillage of saliva. Many dental problems such as dental caries, oral infections, foreign bodies, epulis, and oral ulcers can result in hypersalivation and impaired swallowing. Neurological conditions including Parkinson's disease, stroke, cerebral palsy, mental retardation, facial palsy, and amyotrophic lateral sclerosis are frequently associated with sialorrhea.

Saliva is produced by the paired major salivary glands composed of the parotid, submandibular, and sublingual glands. In addition, there are several hundred minor salivary glands scattered throughout the upper aerodigestive tract. Approximately 1 to 1.5 L saliva is produced daily. Baseline flow rate is typically 0.001 to 0.2 mL/minute. When stimulated, flow can run from 0.18 to 1.7 mL/minute. The average flow rate during the course of the day is approximately 1 mL/minute *(2)*. The minor salivary glands and submandibular gland provide much of the saliva at rest, while the parotid gland is responsible for the majority of salivary production during stimulation. The parotid and submandibular glands produce approximately 87% of total salivary flow. The sublingual gland contributes about 5%. The submandibular glands are responsible for most baseline salivary production (about two-thirds), while the parotid glands are responsible for two-thirds of the stimulated salivary production.

Swallowing is a complex coordinated function that relies on the interaction of multiple muscle groups in a systematic controlled fashion. There are six active valves that control food and saliva movement through the upper esophagus. These valves are the lips, tongue, glossopalatal valve, velopharynx, larynx, and upper esophageal sphincter. Dysfunction at any of these levels can result in accumulation and spillage of saliva and food. Although the tongue and lips are under cortical control, pharyngeal swallow is accomplished by a brainstem-mediated response via the nucleus solitarius and nucleus ambiguus. Anatomic variances such as macroglossia and hypertrophic tonsils can impair swallowing and result in sialorrhea. In addition, head and neck position as well as gravity, can affect bolus transport and salivary loss.

Saliva plays an important role in swallowing, preserving and maintaining healthy tissue in the mouth. Saliva wets and prepares the bolus of food during the oral phase of swallowing. The amylase begins to break down the carbohydrates, softening the bolus. Saliva buffers and protects the oral cavity from drying out. Also, saliva contains important ions for preventing tooth decay such as calcium, fluoride, phosphate, and magnesium as well as anti-microbials and immunoglobulins.

Both sympathetic and parasympathetic nerves supply the major salivary glands. The stimulation of salivary gland secretion is regulated primarily by the parasympathetic system that is carried through the cranial nerves. The parotid gland receives parasympathetic innervation through the glossopharyngeal nerve. Branches off the glossopharyngeal nerve (lesser superficial petrosal nerve) travel to the otic ganglion. From the otic ganglion, nerve fibers join the auriculotemporal nerve to diffuse into the parotid gland. The submandibular and sublingual glands receive parasympathetic innervation from the chorda tympani of the facial nerve. Chorda tympani fibers then join the lingual nerve and the autonomic fibers synapse at the submandibular ganglion.

There are no true synapses between postganglionic nerves and glands. Stimulation of glandular secretion is achieved via passive diffusion. Acetylcholine is released by postganglionic parasympathetic nerve fibers in close proximity to the target gland. Muscarinic receptors in salivary tissue respond to acetylcholine release through passive diffusion rather than synaptic activation.

The parotid gland is the largest major salivary organ and is located anterior to the ear. Superiorly, the parotid gland is bordered by the zygoma. Posterior landmarks include the external auditory canal and mastoid tip. The styloid process, styloid muscles, the internal carotid artery and jugular veins are inferior to the parotid. The masseter muscle forms the deep margin. The facial nerve courses through the body of the gland, dividing it into a deep and superficial lobe. The parotid gland is composed of serous glands that provide the bulk of salivary flow during eating.

The submandibular glands lie in the anterior triangle of the neck. The boundaries of the submandibular triangle are the anterior and posterior bellies of the digastric muscle and the inferior margin of the mandible. The gland forms a "C" shape as it passes the mylohyoid muscle, forming a deep and superficial lobe. Both serous and mucinous glands are present in the submandibular glands.

Sublingual glands and minor salivary glands also contribute to salivary flow. There are approximately 600 to 1000 minor salivary glands that line the oral cavity. The bulk of these glands are concentrated in the mucosa of the cheeks, lips, palate, and tongue. The sublingual glands lie in the floor of mouth just lateral to the tongue midline. The gland is bordered by the mandible laterally and the mylohyoid muscle inferiorly.

## Epidemiology/Symptomatology

Drooling is the spillage of saliva from the mouth. It is a frequent complaint in patients with neurological impairment. Drooling is also commonly seen in children younger than 4 years old. As children develop better orofacial control and socialization skills, sialorrhea generally ceases.

Surveys and cross-sectional analysis of different populations with neurological impairment show that salivary problems are common. Medical problems among the neurologically impaired include aspiration, local skin maceration, fluid loss, poor dental hygiene, and poor feeding. Drooling can adversely affect self-image, socialization, and quality of life. It also necessitates additional nursing and caretaking needs.

The Oxford Feeding Study was a cross-sectional population analysis of children with neurological impairment. The study found that children with cerebral palsy and other neurological disabilities had a high prevalence of feeding difficulties, including swallowing problems, prolonged feeding times, and poor nutrition, that significantly affected quality of life. More than one-fourth (28%) of respondents reported continuous drooling as a serious condition *(3)*. In a different survey, 37.4% of children with cerebral palsy were found to have severe problems with drooling *(4)*.

A survey of cerebral palsy patients demonstrated a 58% prevalence of drooling and excess salivation, with 33% describing their condition as "severe" *(5)*. In patients with Parkinson's disease, 46.5 to 78% complained of drooling and 18.8% felt that drooling was socially disabling *(6,7)*. Even in early Parkinson's disease, 15% of patients suffered from nocturnal drooling *(8)*. Twenty percent of patients afflicted with bulbar amyotrophic lateral sclerosis reported problems with drooling *(9)*.

Primary hypersalivation is an uncommon problem and is often clinically not evident when swallowing function is intact. Some of the common causes for hypersalivation are inflammation secondary to teething, poor oral health, dental caries, oral cavity infection, gastroesophageal reflux, toxin exposure, and rabies. Excess saliva production can also be seen as side effects of certain medications such as tranquilizers and anticonvulsants.

## Clinical Diagnosis

### History

A complete history and physical examination with a focus on the head and neck and assessment of swallowing and orofacial function are important prior to treatment initiation. Important aspects of the history include the frequency of drooling, whether it is intermittent or constant, and exacerbating factors such as meals, dental infections, and daytime variation. Evidence of recent weight loss or dehydration is also important. Impact on the quality of life needs to be assessed, including prolonged feeding times and frequency of changing clothes secondary to salivary soiling.

Soliciting patient history about dry mouth, dysphagia, aspiration, pneumonias, voice, and swallowing difficulties are also important. Past treatments such as radiation, surgery, and medications should be elicited. Other medical conditions, such as cranial neuropathies, stroke, sensory and motor dysfunction, aspiration, cricopharyngeal dysfunction, decreased mental awareness, cervical instability, and psychological conditions such as depression, are relevant aspects to the patient's history. Intake of systemic medications such as tranquilizers and anticonvulsants that may cause hypersalivation should be ascertained. Dental history and health should also be examined.

The care environment is highly pertinent. The level or absence of patient independence and level of care available will be strongly considered in treatment recommendations. The neurological status and awareness ability of the patient to social stigma is essential, and level of socialization and personal interaction play a key role in the patient's decision and motivation to undertake treatment. The role of treatment is predicated on the individual needs of both the patient and caregiver.

Multiple tools have been developed to assess drooling in a quantifiable manner. Subjective reporting scales such as the teacher drooling scale (TDS) have been designed to assess drooling severity and frequency. The TDS assigns a numerical value (between 1 and 5) for the assessment of drooling. A score of 1 is no drooling, 2 is a small amount of infrequent drooling, 3 is intermittent drooling, 4 is frequent drooling, and 5 is constant drooling. Thomas and Greenberg advocate describing severity and frequency separately on a number scale. Severity is measured on a scale of 1 to 5 with 1 being dry and 5 being profuse wetness. Frequency is measured on a scale of 1 to 4 with 1 being never and 4 being constant *(10)*. The drooling quotient is a validated, semi-quantitative, direct observational method *(11)*. Scoring is based on direct observation of saliva on the lip or chin during two periods of 10 minutes each. Fifteen-second intervals within a 10-minute period are observed for the presence of drooling. The calculated quotient is the percentage of observed episodes of drooling divided by the total number of observations.

*Clinical Examination*

A full physical and neurological examination should be performed for evaluation of the drooling patient beginning with a general overall assessment of global function, health status, and care including grooming, appearance, and affect. The head and neck evaluation should include an assessment of the cranial nerves, oral cavity, inspection of the skin around the mouth, lips, chin, and neck for evidence of maceration or inflammation. Candidal infection of the skin is common because of the impaired skin barrier. Macroglossia and hypertrophic tonsils and adenoids can also contribute to swallowing difficulty and salivary spillage.

Dental evaluation should be performed to look for evidence of dental caries and oral infections. Because most therapies for sialorrhea will dry out the mouth and reduce the protective effects of saliva on dentition, dental examinations at regular intervals are important.

*Diagnostic Evaluation*

Although the importance of diagnostic tests in the treatment of sialorrhea is not well studied, various tools are available to assess swallowing function and salivary function.

Salivary flow studies are generally not useful because most patients do not have dysfunctional glands and the production of saliva is highly variable. Various methods for measuring salivary flow exist, such as weighing cotton pledgets, spitting into cups, various dental and oral devices, and salivary duct stents. However, normative values can be highly variable and generally do not correlate with patient complaints.

Functional endoscopic evaluation of swallowing is useful for evaluating swallowing dysfunction, sensory testing, and risk of aspiration. The test allows direct evaluation of the nasopharyx, oropharynx, and hypopharynx during swallowing. Palate function, laryngeal elevation, and base of tongue control are assessed with the fiberoptic endoscope. Using colored foods of varying consistency, the ability of the oropharynx and hypopharynx to clear boluses is assessed. Airway penetration can be directly visualized. Use of sensory testing with calibrated air puffs can measure the degree of sensory dysfunction in the larynx.

Videoflouroscopy and modified barium swallow (capturing real-time movement of oral boluses) can evaluate the different components of swallowing function as well as evaluate for aspiration. Videoflouroscopy involves the visualization of radio-opaque materials mixed with foods swallowed under fluoroscopy. Different consistencies can be tested as well as the effectiveness of various therapeutic maneuvers and head and neck positions on swallowing. This test is useful in localizing areas of the swallowing cascade that are dysfunctional.

### Treatment Approach

Multiple treatments have been explored for ptyalism. Treatment is individually tailored to the patient's needs. These patients frequently have multiple comorbidities and treatment should take into account the needs of caretakers. Specialized multidisciplinary clinics for the treatment of salivary problems are being developed to address the complexity of these problems with general practitioners, neurologists, otolaryngologists, oral surgeons, dentists, and speech and swallowing therapists.

Speech pathologists employ a variety of techniques that can improve swallowing, decrease aspiration and airway penetration, and decrease salivary loss. Speech training and swallow therapy, changes in head position and support, and specialized orofacial and swallowing techniques are effective and noninvasive ways to improve symptoms.

Medications such as atropine, scopolamine, and methscopolamine have been used as antisialagogues. Scopolamine and glycopyrrolate have been shown to be effective at reducing salivary loss with prospective clinical trials *(12,13)*. However, these medications often have significant anticholinergic systemic side effects, including blurred vision, cardiac arrhythmia, and urinary retention. As a result, noncompliance rates among patients range from 20 to 40%. These medications are poorly tolerated in the elderly or debilitated patients. Anticholinergic effects can be compounded by many common medications, such as antihistamines, neuroleptics, and sedatives. These medications can exacerbate certain medical conditions and should not be used in patients with obstructive uropathy, gastrointestinal motility problems, glaucoma, or myasthenia gravis.

Numerous surgical strategies have been developed for reducing salivary flow. Parasympathetic denervation by severing the tympanic nerve contribution from the glossopharyngeal nerve in the temporal bone has been performed with variable results. Generally, short-term results are successful at reducing salivary flow; however, long-term results have been marginal, possibly secondary to redirected innervation pathways through the greater superficial petrosal nerve *(14)*. Side effects include altered or deceased taste sensation.

Various surgical options directed at the submandibular and parotid glands are effective in reducing salivary production *(14a)*. Rerouting and excision of the submandibular glands is effective at reducing salivary flow especially if drooling is constant and not significantly exacerbated with meals *(15)*. If salivation is primarily during meals, the parotid gland should be addressed. Parotid duct rerouting into a position more posterior in the oral cavity has also been explored as a method of redirecting salivary flow without eliminating the multiple benefits of saliva on dentition. Parotid duct ligation can also be performed and is effective for reducing stimulated salivary flow. The most severe cases of drooling can be treated by addressing both sets of glands *(16)*. The potential complications of surgery include nerve damage, sialoceles, ranulas, and the potential for anterior dental caries *(17)*.

Radiation therapy has also been used to reduce salivary function. Radiation is successful at reducing salivary flow and can be dose-adjusted to produce the desired level of clinical effect. However, overtreatment can produce xerostomia, dental caries, skin hyperpigmentary changes and burns, and mucositis. There is a long-term increased risk of developing malignancy that is estimated to take place 10 to 15 years after treatment. Because of these shortcomings, radiation therapy is often restricted to elderly patients with severe drooling who are not candidates for surgery and can not tolerate medications *(18)*.

BTX type A (BTX-A) is a safe, effective, and selective method of reducing salivary flow. BTX injection is less invasive than surgery and lacks the anticholinergic side effects of medications. Injections are usually well tolerated, even among children. The main disadvantage is cost. The effects are not permanent and injections need to be repeated generally every 3 to 4 months. Other disadvantages include the lack of standardized injection techniques and dosages.

Large-scale, randomized clinical trials comparing BTX to other modalities have not yet been performed, however, in a prospective trial comparing scopolamine with injection, BTX was found to be tolerated better and as equally effective as transdermal scopolamine *(19)*.

*Technical Aspects*

There are currently multiple serotypes available for denervation. Each serotype binds to a specific acceptor site on presynaptic nerve terminals. Although these serotypes are similar in their chemodenervation properties, pharmacological properties may vary. Studies comparing

BTX-A and BTX-B suggest that BTX-B may have greater affinity for the ANS. A report comparing the two serotypes for the treatment of cervical dystonias showed that BTX-B had a significantly higher rate of dry mouth as a side effect *(20,21)*. BTX-B cleaves vesicular-associated membrane protein, whereas BTX-A cleaves synaptosome-associated protein-25.

There are many reported techniques for BTX injection into the salivary glands. The parotid and submandibular glands are selected for autonomic denervation as these two glands represent almost 90% of total salivary production. Blind injection using knowledge of anatomy and palpation has been performed; however, increasing numbers of practitioners are using ultrasound to localize the glands. The authors recommend the use of ultrasound for accurate localization and delivery of toxin based on the belief that greater accuracy enables more efficient use of toxin, producing better results and fewer side effects. Because the majority of side effects occur from diffusion of the toxin to surrounding structures, using small amounts of toxin minimizes spread.

## Dosing

The literature reports a range of different dosages used for sialorrhea from 5 to 150 U with Botox® and from 250 to 1000 U of Myobloc®. Given our knowledge of botulinum effects in other body systems, individuals have different responses to toxin dosages. Injection technique also affects the dosages used. In our practice, we generally use a conservative dose of BTX for the initial dose (25 U Botox for the submandibular gland and 50 U for the parotids) with a follow-up dose as needed 2 weeks later. Patients and caretakers are advised to keep records of drooling as well as side effects. Treatment schedules are individualized to the patient needs. Although the biochemical effects of the toxin last 3 months, the range of therapeutic efficacy can vary considerably. Reported durations range from 1 to 7 months *(7)*. In a report on 33 patients treated for salivary flow, Ellies et al. reported that the effects last about 3 months. Ellies used 22.5 U Botox in each parotid gland and 10 U in each submandibular gland delivered without local anesthesia under ultrasound guidance *(22)*.

## Adverse Reactions

Saliva has multiple beneficial properties and control of drooling is balanced with maintaining a healthy, moist oral environment. The most frequently reported side effects of injection into the salivary glands include overly dry mouth, pain, infection, transient dysphagia, and weak jaw opening and closing. For submandibular injection, diffusion into the lingual muscles can weaken tongue movement and cause dysphagia. For parotid injection, diffusion into the surrounding facial muscles can result in facial weakness and asymmetry. The majority of side effects are transient and normal baseline function will return as the SNARE proteins regenerate. Because most salivary problems are not from hypersalivation but poor handling of secretions, any treatment that results in dry mouth must be balanced with preserving oral health.

## Success

BTX for reduction for sialorrhea has reported successful results in two-thirds of patients treated *(22)*. Success can be determined by subjective patient ratings of drooling severity, objective measurements of salivary flow by sialometry or weight of dental rolls. Because the salivary flow rates vary throughout the day and are affected by multiple factors, quantitative measurements of salivation reduction are limited. Turk and Odderson measured reduction of salivation in a single patient who underwent BTX injection in to both parotids and submandibular glands. They demonstrated an 85.8% reduction salivary flow in the submandibular glands and 23.8% reduction in the parotid gland *(23)*.

In a prospective, controlled clinical trial of drooling in 45 children with cerebral palsy, Jongerius et al. reported a significant improvement in drooling quotient and TDS scores after BTX-A injection into the submandibular glands. Clinical efficacy equaled systemic treatment with transdermal scopolamine. The authors noted that 40% of participants reported significant side effects with scopolamine, including xerostomia, restlessness, somnolence, blurred vision, and confusion. Approximately 7% of the study population was unable to tolerate 48 consecutive hours of the patch and subsequently dropped out of the study. Taking into account the communication difficulties of this population, the side effects were likely under-reported. The study noted one episode of local swelling after injection and one episode of transitory difficulty swallowing that lasted 10 days and was attributed to local diffusion into tongue muscles. They reported about 64% of the patients responded to BTX (as defined by a two point reduction in TDS) after 2 weeks. Twenty-four weeks after injection, 48.7% of patients still reported improvement in salivation *(19)*.

Ellies et al. published the results of a retrospective chart review of 33 patients treated with BTX for drooling, salivary fistulas, and sialadenitis. On average, each submandibular gland was treated with 10 U and each parotid was injected with 22.5 U Botox. Seventy-nine percent of treated patients reported subjective improvement. Salivary flow rates, amylase, thiocyanate, protein, kallikrein, and immunoglobulin A outputs were measured and tracked from 0 to 20 weeks in 31 patients. Salivary rates and thiocyanate level declined to about 50% of baseline beginning 2 weeks after injection and then returned to pre-injection levels after approximately 12 weeks. Amylase increased about twofold several weeks after treatment. Other measures remained constant or increased marginally. However, statistical analysis of significance or power was not performed. He concluded that BTX reliably reduces salivary secretions for 3 to 4 months *(22)*.

## Conclusion

Sialorrhea is a common and debilitating problem for children and adults with a wide range of neurological disorders. Almost any disorder that affects orofacial or swallowing function can result in inadvertent saliva loss. Sialorrhea can have painful social consequences as well as medical problems. The role of BTX for sialorrhea has been in use since 2000. Methodology is still being developed and refined, however, treatment with BTX is very effective and can improve a patient's quality of life.

## GUSTATORY SWEATING

The term hyperhidrosis is used to describe excessive sweating beyond that which is needed to thermoregulate the body. Focal hyperhidrosis affects localized areas such as the palms, soles of the feet, axilla, trunk, and face. Gustatory sweating is a type of focal hyperhidrosis that results in facial sweating with meals. This can occur from aberrant regeneration after parotid gland surgery, sympathectomy, facial trauma, or infection. This section focuses on the role of BTX injection for the treatment of gustatory sweating.

Lucja Frey, a Polish neurologist, described this phenomenon in 1923 and the condition now bears her name *(24)*. Frey's syndrome is thought to be secondary to aberrant innervation of the sweat glands by the postganglionic parasympathetic fibers from the auriculotemporal nerve. After parotid surgery, severed cholinergic nerve fibers connect to sympathetic cholinergic receptors in the skin, resulting in piloerection, sweating, and flushing *(25)*.

Gustatory sweating can also occur in polyneuropathies associated with diabetes mellitus. In this condition, parasympathetic stimulation of the sweat glands may be a response to sympathetic denervation secondary to diabetic neuropathy. This may affect the skin in the distribution of the facial nerve and the auriculotemporal nerve resulting in sweating and flushing in the scalp, face, and neck (25). Bilateral involvement of the face and neck is common in gustatory sweating secondary to diabetes. There is often concurrent systemic sensory neuropathy and nephropathy. Another hypothesis is that gustatory sweating is a physiological compensatory response to anhidrosis induced by diabetic autonomic neuropathy.

BTX was first described as a treatment for Frey's syndrome by Drobik et al. in 1995 (26). Using 0.5 U/cm$^2$ intracutaneously, he reported a 12-month period of relief from gustatory sweating. Since this initial report, numerous studies have shown excellent efficacy in the use of BTX for this condition. Botox has been approved for on-label use for focal hyperhidrosis.

## Epidemiology and Symptomatology

Frey's syndrome commonly occurs after parotid surgery and the reported post-parotidectomy incidence is between 5 and 60%. Gustatory sweating has also been described after radical neck dissection, thoracocervical sympathectomies, and submandibular gland surgery. Bilateral gustatory sweating, which can affect the face, scalp, and neck, is seen in people with chronic diabetes and the incidence is increased with the development of neuropathies and nephropathies.

Frey's syndrome has been reported in 96% of post-parotidectomy patients when tested with a Minor's iodine test; however, only a minority of patients are symptomatic. In a retrospective series of 475 patients who underwent parotidectomy for pleomorphic adenoma, 13% reported subjective gustatory sweating (27). The development of Frey's syndrome after parotidectomy may be technique-dependent and reports show a wide range. Gustatory sweating is commonly associated with the autonomic dysfunction seen in diabetic neuropathy. Shaw et al. reported that 69% of patients with diabetic nephropathy and 36% of patients with diabetic neuropathy suffer from gustatory sweating (28).

## Clinical Diagnosis

A full history and physical should be part of the initial evaluation for gustatory sweating. Most patients with this complaint will have had a history of parotid surgery, facial trauma, or recurrent salivary gland infections. Comorbidities such as diabetes or neurological, cardiac, or autonomic problems should be elicited. Minor's sweat iodine test can be performed to demonstrate gustatory sweating. Care should be taken to distinguish focal hyperhidrosis from generalized sweating. Excessive sweating can have many different etiologies and requires a separate medical workup.

The diagnosis of hyperhidrosis and excessive gustatory sweating is often a subjective one. There is usually no clear-cut demarcation between normal physiological sweating and excessive sweat production. Symptoms are specific to individual circumstances; what is considered normal perspiration to some may be considered intolerable and socially crippling to others. Therapy must take into account patient's individual needs and circumstances.

### Clinical Evaluation

A complete physical should be performed, including careful evaluation of the head and neck. Cranial nerve examination should be performed. An examination looking for other autonomic dysfunction such as orthostatic hypotension should also be performed.

Minor's starch iodine test is easy to perform and can demarcate the area of pathological sweating. The iodine test involves painting the affected area with iodine and then lightly dusting the area with starch. Stimulation of sweating is done with food, usually lemon drops, and the area is inspected for sweating. Perspiration will darken the area by moistening the starch. Objective measurements of sweat production are generally only performed for research purposes. Gravimetric testing can generate a measure called the sweat rate, measured in milligrams per minute, which has been used for clinical trials in axillary hyperhidrosis *(29)*. Methods such as weighing absorbent dressings and gravimetric analysis have been used for quantitative analysis but because treatment approach is based on symptoms, these studies are generally not performed.

## Treatment Approach

There have been many proposed ways to avoid Frey's syndrome after parotidectomy. Most surgical methods involve creating obstacles between the parotid wound bed and the skin in order to block aberrant parasympathetic fibers from connecting to the skin. These methods include the use of local and regional flaps, autologous fascia, and cadaveric skin and fascia. Singha et al. reported a significant reduction in symptomatic gustatory sweating after laying AlloDerm graft onto the wound bed after parotidectomy. He reported a reduction from 80 to 20% in the incidence of gustatory sweating with this method *(30)*. Use of sternocleidomastoid muscle flaps to fill the parotid defect has also been tried with variable results. None of these methods have proven themselves in preventing Frey's syndrome and most methods required additional time under anesthesia and scars.

Surgical neurectomy of Jacobson's nerve has also been tried to reduce gustatory sweating with limited success. Although the procedure has good short-term benefits, there is a significant rate of relapse. Sectioning of the greater petrosal nerve has also been described with variable results *(31)*.

The treatment of gustatory sweating can be most cheaply and simply treated with topical antiperspirants that include aluminum chloride as an active ingredient. Glycopyrrolate cream is a local anticholinergic medication that can be applied topically to prevent excess perspiration *(32)*. The short duration of effect requires multiple applications of the cream.

Systemic anticholinergic medications have also been tried to decrease sweating. Glycopyrrolate and scopolamine have been discussed earlier in this chapter as a treatment for sialorrhea. These medications have significant side effects and a high rate of noncompliance.

BTX injection is being increasingly recognized as a first-line agent for the treatment of symptomatic Frey's syndrome. Almost all clinical series report close to a 100% improvement with intradermal injections. These reports also show a very high degree of safety in these injections and a long-lasting clinical response.

### Technical Aspects and Dosing

Minor's starch iodine test is typically used to demarcate the treatment area. Iodine is applied to the skin and neck. After drying, starch is lightly applied to the iodine. Lemon drops or other acidic food is then given to stimulate perspiration and the face is inspected for black discoloration that indicates active sweating. A grid is then drawn with 1- to 1.5-cm markings throughout the affected area. We use 2.5 U Botox in 0.1 cc bacteriostatic normal saline for each square centimeter of affected skin. Dosages vary based on report. We have results lasting 6–24 months, with an average of 12.1 *(32a)*. Restivo et al. reported using 5 U Dysport® per 2.25 cm$^2$ (1.5 × 1.5 cm grid) injected *(33)* and Drobik in his initial report used 0.5 U/cm$^2$

Botox. Each injection is administered intradermally. Massaging the area excessively is not desired because of potential diffusion to unwanted areas. The patient is instructed not to touch or press on the area for 6 hours after injection. Because individual responses to the toxin can vary considerably, a 2-week follow up visit is recommended and the Minor's iodine test repeated to see if there are any additional sites where BTX is needed.

*Adverse Reactions*

The most common side effect occurs from the diffusion of BTX into the underlying facial muscles and numbness in the skin. This can result in temporary facial asymmetry and weakness that can last for 3 to 4 months. If severe, orofacial function can be disrupted, resulting in drooling, inadvertent biting of the lips and inside of mouth, and speaking difficulties. Laccourreye reported transient upper lip asymmetry in 1 of 33 patients treated for postparotidectomy Frey's syndrome. Of 33 patients in his study, 2 also reported temporary numbness in the cheek *(34)*.

*Success*

BTX-A is a category 1 (efficacy studied by large-scale, randomized clinical trials) for treatment of axillary hyperhidrosis and category 2 (supported by convincing clinical evidence in controlled, nonrandomized studies) for gustatory sweating. Nauman et al. studied 45 patients with gustatory sweating after BTX injection and reported excellent results *(35)*. One to 2 U per 2 cm$^2$ skin area as determined by Minor's iodine test was injected intradermally. On a subjective rating scale, 50% of patients reported complete response and the remainder reported a significant response. All patients reported subjective improvement at 6 month follow-up. They reported no adverse effects. Dobik et al. published his follow-up of 19 patients treated over 3 years and reported a 100% success rate for an average of 17 months. There were no reported adverse effects *(36)*.

Although the physiological effects of BTX on acetylcholine release is 3 to 4 months in muscular denervation, the clinical improvement seen in the treatment of gustatory sweating appears to last much longer, 10 to 17 months on average. Laccourreye et al. performed a Kaplan-Meier actuarial life table method on 33 patients treated for Frey's syndrome after parotidectomy. In the 33 patients injected for the study, 100% reported improvement and 72% continued to have improvement 1 year after injection. Recurrent gustatory sweating was found in 27% 1 year after treatment, 67% after 2 years, and 92% after 3 years based on the actuarial estimate *(34)*. In a series of 15 patients, Bjerkhoel and Trobbe reported recurrence in gustatory sweating in 13.3% after 6 months *(37)*. Arad and Blitzer reported a series of seven patients with gustatory sweating after parotidectomy and diabetic neuropathy. They reported 100% success 2 weeks after treatment and the effects lasted for a mean of 12.3 months *(38)*.

*Conclusion*

The longevity of therapeutic effect on sweat glands has been a source of discussion. Although denervation effects generally last approximately 3 to 4 months, clinical improvement has been demonstrated 3 years after injection. Laskawi et al. proposed three possible mechanisms. The long duration of chemical denervation may partially or completely abolish sweat gland function. These autonomic nerve fibers have poor regenerative ability once chemically denervated. Also, post-surgical or posttraumatic local changes in the tissue may compromise axon regeneration potential *(36)*.

Based on the efficacy and minimum side affects reported by these studies, BTX is quickly becoming a first-line modality in the treatment of gustatory sweating.

# REFERENCES

1. Rossetto O, Seveso M, Caccin P, et al. Botulinum neurotoxins are metalloprotease specific for SNARE proteins involved in neuroexocytosis. In: Kreyden OP, Boni R, Burg G, eds. Hyperhidrosis and Botulinum Toxin in Dermatology. Basel: Karger; 2002, pp. 117–125.
2. Kontis Y, Johns ME. Anatomy and physiology of the salivary glands. In: Bailey BJ, ed. Head and Neck Surgery—Otolaryngology. 3rd ed. New York: Lippincott Williams & Wilkins; 2001, pp. 429–436.
3. Sullivan PB, Lambert B, Rose M, Ford-Adams M, Johnson A, Griffiths P. Prevalence and severity of feeding and nutritional problems in children with neurological impariement: Oxford Feeding Study. Dev Med Child Neurol 2000;42:613–617.
4. Harris SR, Purdy AH. Drooling and its management in cerebral palsy. Dev Med Child Neurol 1987;29:807–811.
5. Tahmassebi JF, Curzon ME. Prevalence of drooling in children with cerebral palsy attending special schools. Dev Med Chil Neurol 2003;45:613–617.
6. Hyson HC, Johnson A, Jog MS. Survey of sialorrhea in parkinsonian patients in southwestern Ontario. Can J Neurol Sci 2001;28:S46–S47.
7. Bhidayasiri R, Truong D. Expanding use of botulinum toxin. J Neurol Sci 2005;235:1–9.
8. Volonte MA, Porta M, Comi G. Clinical assessment of dysphagia in early phases of Parkinson's disease. Neurol Sci 2002;23:S121–S122.
9. Glickman S, Deaney CN. Treatment of relative sialorhoea with botulinum toxin type A: description and rationale for an injection procedure with case report. Eur J Neurol 2001;8:567–571.
10. Thomas-Stonell N, Greenberg J. Three treatment approaches and clinical factors in the reduction of drooling. Dysphagia 1988;3:73–78.
11. Reddihough D, Johnson H, Ferguson E. The role of a saliva control clinic in the management of drooling. J Paediatr Child Health 1992;28:395–397.
12. Mier RJ, Bachrach SJ, Lakin RC, Barker T, Childs J, Moran M. Treatment of sialorhea with glycopyrrolate: a double-blind, dose-ranging study. Arch Pediatr Adolesc Med 2000;154: 1214–1218.
13. Talmi YP, Finkelstein Y, Zohar Y. Reduction of salivary flow with transdermal scopolamine: a four year experience. Otolaryngol Head Neck Surg 1990;103:615–618.
14. Frederick FJ, Stewart IF. Effectiveness of transtympanic neurectomy in management of sialorrhea occurring in mentally retarded patients. J Otolaryngol 1982;11:289–292.
14a. Parisir SC, Blitzer A, Binder WA, Friedman WH. Tympanic neurectomy and chorda tympanectomy. Tran AAOO 1978;86:308–321.
15. Ethunandan M, Macpherson DW. Persistent drooling: treatment by bilateral sbmandibular duct transposition and simultaneous sublingual gland excision. An R Coll Surg Engl 1998;80: 279–282.
16. Shott SR, Myer CM, Cotton RT. Surgical management of sialorrhea. Otolaryngol Head Neck Surg 1989;101:47–50.
17. Mankarious LA, Bottrill IA, Huchzermyer PM, Bailey CM. Long-term follow up of submandibular duct rerouting for the treatment of sialorrhea in the pediatric population. Otolaryngol Head Neck Surg 1999;120:303–307.
18. Borg M, Hirst F. The role of radiation therapy in the management of sialorrhea. Int J Raol Oncol Biol Phys 1998;41:1113–1119.
19. Jongerius PH, van den Hoogen JA, Limbeek J, Gabreels FJ, van Hulst K, Rottevell JJ. Effect of botulinum toxin in the treatment of drooling: a controlled clinical trial. Pediatrics 2004;114: 620–627.
20. Brin MF, Lew MF, Adler CH, et al. Safety and efficacy of NeurobBloc (botulinum toxin type B) for type A-resistant cervical dystonia. Neurology 1999;53:1431–1438.

21. Comella CL, Jankovic J, Shannon KM, et al. Comparison of botulinum toxin serotypes A and B for the treatment of cervical dystonia. Neurology 2005;65:1423–1429.

22. Ellies M, Gottstein U, Rohrbach-Volland S, Arglebe C, Laskawa R. Reduction of salivary flow with botulinum toxin: extended report on 33 patients with drooling, salivary fistulas, and sialadenitis. Laryngoscope 2004;114:1856–1860.

23. Turk-Gonzales M, Odderson IR. Quantitative reduction of saliva production with botulinum toxin type B injection into the salivary glands. Neurorehabil Neural Repair 2005;19:58–61.

24. Frey L. Le syndrome du nerf auricuo-temporal. Rev Neurol 1923;2:97–114.

25. Arad A, Blitzer A. Botulinum toxin in the treatment of autonomic system disorders. Op Tech in Otolaryngol and Head and Neck Surg 2004;15:118–121.

26. Drobik C, Laskawi R. Frey's syndrome: treatment with botulinum toxin. Acta Otolaryngol (Stockh) 1995;115:459–461.

27. Laskawi R, Schott T, Schroder M. Recurrent pleomorphic adenomas of the arotid gland: Clinical evaluation and long term follow-up. Br J Oral Maxillofac Surg 1998;36:48–51.

28. Shaw JE, Parker R, Hollis S, Gokal R, Boulton AJM. Gustatory sweating in diabetes mellitus. Diab Med 1996;13:1033–1037.

29. Kreyden OP, Scheidegger EP. Anatomy of the sweat glands, pharmacology of botulinum toxin, and distinctive syndromes associated with hyperhidrosis. Clinics in Derm 2004;22:40–44.

30. Sinha UK, Saadat D, Doherty CM, Rice DH. Use of AlloDerm implant to prevent Frey syndrome after parotidectomy. Arch Facial Plast Surg 2003;5:109–112.

31. May M. Microanatomy and pathophysiology. In: May M, Schaitkin BM, eds. The Facial Nerve. 2nd ed. New York: Thieme; 2000, pp. 57–65.

32. Urman JD, Bobrove AM. Diabetic gustatory sweating successful treatment with topical glycopyrrolate: report of a case and review of the literature. Arch Intern Med 1999;159:877–878.

32a. Arad-Cohen A, Blitzer A. Botulinum toxin treatment for symptomatic Frey's syndrome Otolaryngol Head Neck Surg 2000;122:237–240.

33. Restivo DA, Lanza S, Patti F, et al. Improvement of diabetic autonomic gustatory sweating by botulinum toxin type A. Neurolog 2002;59:1971–1973.

34. Naumann M, Zellner M, Toyka KV, Reiners K. Treatment of gustatory sweating with botulinum toxin. Ann Neurol 1997;42:973–975.

35. Laskawi R, Drobik C, Schonebeck C. Up to date report of botulinum toxin type A treatment in patients with gustatory sweating (Frey's syndrome). Laryngoscope 1998;108:381–384.

36. Laccourreye O, Akl E, Gutierrez-Fonseca R, Garcia D, Brasnu D, Bonan B. Recurrent gustatory sweating (Frey Syndrome) after intracutaneous injection of botulinum toxin type A. Arch Otolaryngol Head Neck Surg 1999;125:282–286.

37. Bjerkhoel A, Trobbe O. Frey's syndrome: treatment with botulium toxin. J Laryngol Otol 1997;111:839–844.

38. Arad-Cohen A, Blitzer A. Botulinum toxin treatment for symptomatic Frey's syndrome. Otolaryngol Head and Neck Surg 2000;122:237–240.

# 10

# Cosmetic Applications

## Tara D. Miller and Isaac M. Neuhaus

### INTRODUCTION

The use of botulinum toxin (BTX) for facial enhancement is currently the most common cosmetic procedure performed in the United States *(1)*, with 2.8 million procedures performed in 2004 *(2)*. Although the only Food and Drug Administration (FDA)-approved cosmetic indication for BTX is "the temporary improvement in the appearance of moderate to severe glabellar lines associated with corrugator and/or procerus muscle activity in adult patients less than or equal to 65 years of age" *(3)*, the use of BTX has extended to other "off-label" indications, including crow's feet and horizontal forehead lines. This chapter reviews the pharmacology, safety profile, technique, and cosmetic indications for BTX.

### PHARMACOLOGY

Produced by the bacterium *Clostridium botulinum*, there are seven serotypes of BTX: A, B, C1, D, E, F, and G. Regardless of the type, all BTXs cause chemodenervation and paralysis of muscles by inhibiting the release of acetylcholine from the presynaptic motor neuron.

BTX type A (BTX-A) is currently the most commonly used serotype. Available as Botox® in the United States (Allergan Inc., Irvine, CA) and Dysport® in Europe (Ipsen Ltd., Maidenhead, UK), BTX-A inhibits release of acetylcholine by cleavage of synaptosome-associated protein-25, a presynaptic membrane protein required for fusion of neurotransmitter-containing vesicles. Because the onset of BTX-A's effect typically takes 3 to 7 days, patients must be informed at the time of treatment that improvement is not immediately noticed. For dosing purposes, 1 U Botox is equivalent to 3 to 5 U Dysport *(4)*.

BTX-B (Solstice Neurosciences, South San Francisco, CA) is the only other serotype of BTX that is commercially available. Its mechanism of action is cleavage of vesicle-associated membrane protein, also known as synaptobrevin *(5)*. BTX-B has a much more rapid onset of action.

Given the experience, safety, and FDA approval of Botox, it is the most widely used BTX preparation used by physicians. As such, all discussion in this chapter regarding BTX-A will refer to Botox.

### DILUTION AND DOSING

BTX-A is sold in a crystalline form, with each vial containing 100 U of vacuum-dried powder. Although the package insert recommends dilution with 0.9% normal saline, the authors prefer to reconstitute the product with preserved saline because the benzyl alcohol

From: *Therapeutic Uses of Botulinum Toxin*
Edited by: G. Cooper © Humana Press Inc., Totowa, NJ

preservative acts as an anesthetic and reduces the pain associated with injections *(6)*. For cosmetic purposes, 100-U vials are reconstituted with 1 to 5 mL saline. Although there are no well-controlled studies, smaller volumes with higher concentrations may allow for more precise placement of the toxin with less risk of diffusion to unintended areas *(7)*. Despite the package insert recommendations to use BTX-A within 4 hours, studies suggest that there is little loss of potency for upto 6 weeks following reconstitution *(8,9)*.

## CONTRAINDICATIONS

BTX-A is contraindicated in areas of active infection and in patients with known hypersensitivity to the drug. It should be administered with caution to patients with neuromuscular disorders, such as myasthenia gravis, or those with peripheral motor neuropathies. Caution should also be used in patients taking medicines that interfere with neuromuscular transmission because these can increase the effect of the toxin. Common examples of these agents include calcium channel blockers, penicillamine, quinine, or aminoglycoside antibiotics. BTX-A is pregnancy category C and is not recommended for pregnant or lactating women *(3)*.

## ADVERSE EVENTS

Adverse events with the cosmetic use of BTX-A are usually not serious and include transient pain, erythema, swelling at the injection site, headaches, nausea, and flu-like symptoms. Weakness of non-targeted muscles can occur within the first week and is generally transient but can persist for several months. Possible adverse events associated with each individual application are discussed in the "Clinical Applications" section. Serious adverse events associated with cosmetic use of BTX-A are quite low; medically therapeutic use is associated with a 33-fold increase in adverse events. This difference is likely a result of the higher doses used for these indications *(10)*.

## PATIENT EVALUATION

Before any cosmetic treatment with BTX-A, a detailed patient evaluation and history is required. Identifying specific patient desires, combined with a frank discussion of the abilities and limitations of BTX-A, are critical to achieving a satisfied patient outcome. For example, although a patient may have dynamic rhytids (lines in the face that are produced by muscular movement, such as wrinkles and furrows) that would benefit from BTX-A injection, he/she may be concerned with fat loss or uneven pigmentation. On the other hand, a patient may request BTX-A injections for an overall sagging appearance caused by cutaneous laxity or excess fat in the lower part of the face. Ideal treatment in this case would be facelift or liposuction, and the patient would be dissatisfied with the limited improvement that would be obtained with BTX-A. In addition to muscle contraction, facial rhytids can also be caused by gravity and sleeping positions. BTX-A treatments will not improve these non-dynamic wrinkles.

## GENERAL INJECTION GUIDELINES

A thorough understanding of facial anatomy is critical when treating a patient with BTX-A, rather than simply performing each procedure by rote. Having the patient frown, squint, raise their eyebrows, and so on is key to identifying the active muscle, revealing any variations in anatomy, and ensuring the proper placement of the toxin. After a complete discussion of the risks and benefits of the procedure, the patient should be sitting upright in a relaxed and comfortable position. A topical anesthetic or ice can be applied if needed *(11,12)*. The skin is then prepped with isopropyl alcohol. A thin, short needle allows for decreased pain and toxin conservation; the authors generally use a 30-gage 0.5-mm needle. Electromyography can be used to identify the intended muscle; however, an experienced physician will rarely need the device for superficial musculature of the face. The toxin is injected slowly into the belly of the muscle with the needle perpendicular to the skin. In the periocular and perioral areas where injections are more superficial, the needle should be directed toward the outer edges of the face, away from essential central structures, such as the eye *(13)*. Immediately after injection, pressure and/or cold compresses are applied to the area to reduce swelling and bruising. Patients should not massage the treatment area; however, some physicians recommend contracting the treated muscles for approximately 2 hours after the injection to expedite the toxin uptake. There is a theoretical risk of unwanted toxin diffusion with certain activities post-procedure but there are no controlled studies on the topic. A majority of physicians do not restrict activities, but some recommend avoidance of bending for 3 to 4 hours, exposure to heat for 2 hours, and flying for 2 hours after the treatment *(1)*.

## CLINICAL APPLICATIONS

### Glabellar Frown Lines

Contraction of the muscles in the glabellar complex (corrugator supercilii, procerus, and depressor supercilii) causes vertical frown lines. Treatment of this area is the most common site for BTX-A injection and the only FDA-approved cosmetic indication for BTX-A.

Twenty to 35 U of BTX-A are placed using a five-point injection method *(14–17)*. The authors typically start with the lower amount because our experience demonstrates that this effectively reduces muscle activity. Higher doses are used for male patients because of a larger muscle mass, with some studies demonstrating that 40 U may be the optimal dose for men *(18)*. However, doses exceeding 50 U show no difference in efficacy *(14)*. The patient should be seated upright and instructed to frown their brows; this helps identify the corrugators and ensure accurate placement (Fig. 1). Forty percent of the toxin is injected to each corrugator with two injections, one at the medial portion of the brow and the second at the mid-pupillary line (Fig. 2). To avoid adverse events resulting from diffusion, all injections should be placed at least 1 cm superior to the orbital rim. The remaining 20% of the toxin is placed midline in the procerus (Fig. 3). Maximum response occurs around 4 weeks after the injections and last approximately 12 to 16 weeks (Fig. 4; refs. *16–18*).

Complications can often be avoided with proper technique, placement, and dosage. Adverse events in this area include bruising, diplopia, lower lateral lid drooping, or upper eyelid ptosis *(19)*. If the toxin diffuses through the orbital septum into orbit, it can cause paralysis of the extraocular muscles resulting in diplopia. Diffusion can also affect the muscles responsible for elevating the upper eyelid, causing ptosis. Upper eyelid ptosis is most commonly seen within 2 to 14 days following treatment of the glabellar complex and can last up to 12 weeks *(20)*. Early studies reported a ptosis rate of 3 to 6% *(16,21)*; however, with improved injection techniques, the current rate is closer to 1% or less *(15,22)*. The use of α-adrenergic agonist eyedrops, apraclonidine hyprochloride 0.5% (Iopidine®, Alcon Labs,

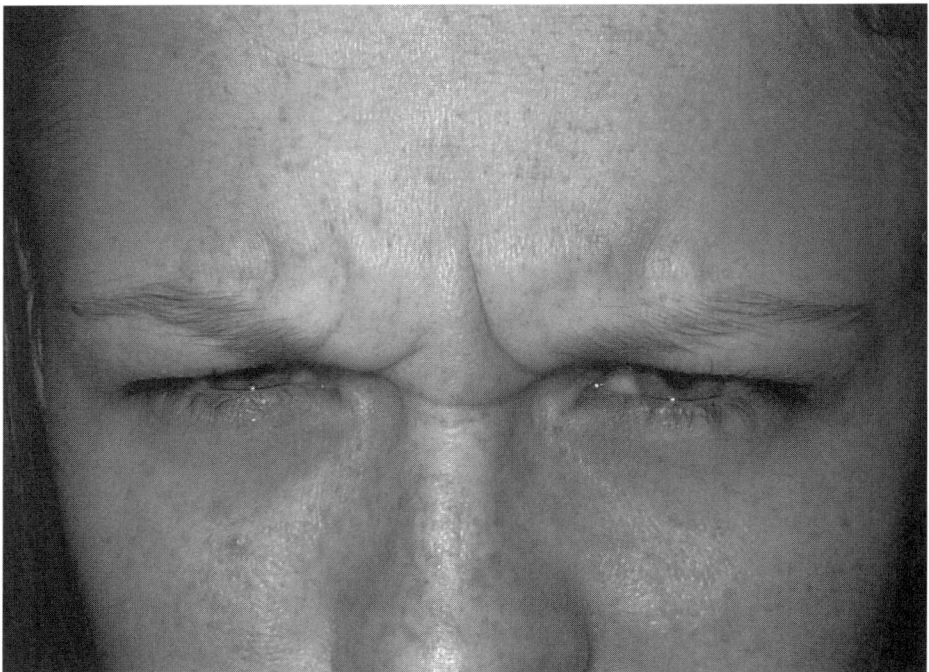

**Fig. 1.** Glabellar complex before treatment. The corrugator muscles become easily visible with furrowing of the brow.

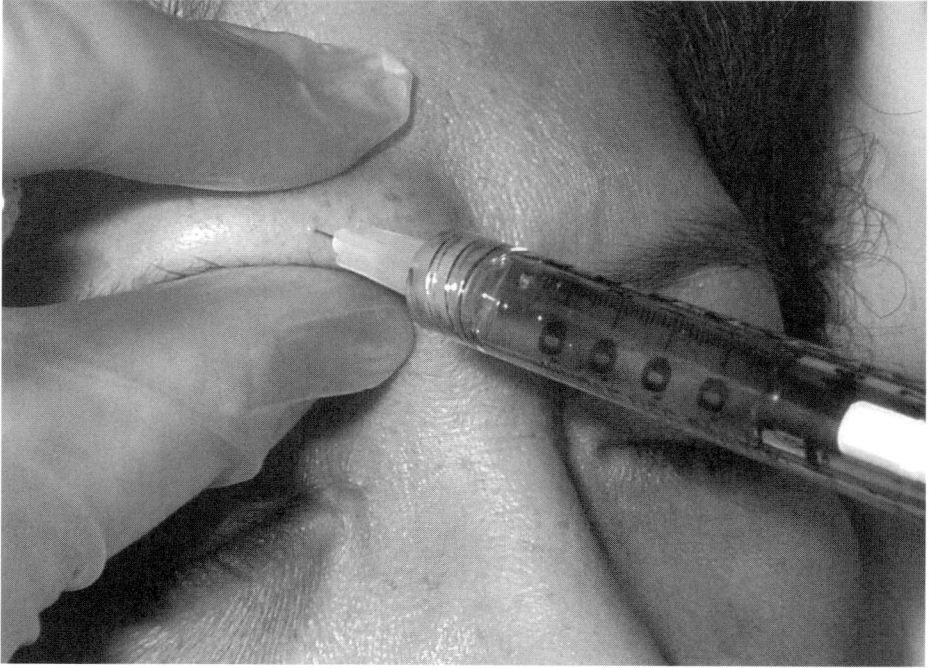

**Fig. 2.** Injection of botulinum toxin type A into the corrugator muscle. Note how the physician isolates the muscle by grasping it between the thumb and forefinger.

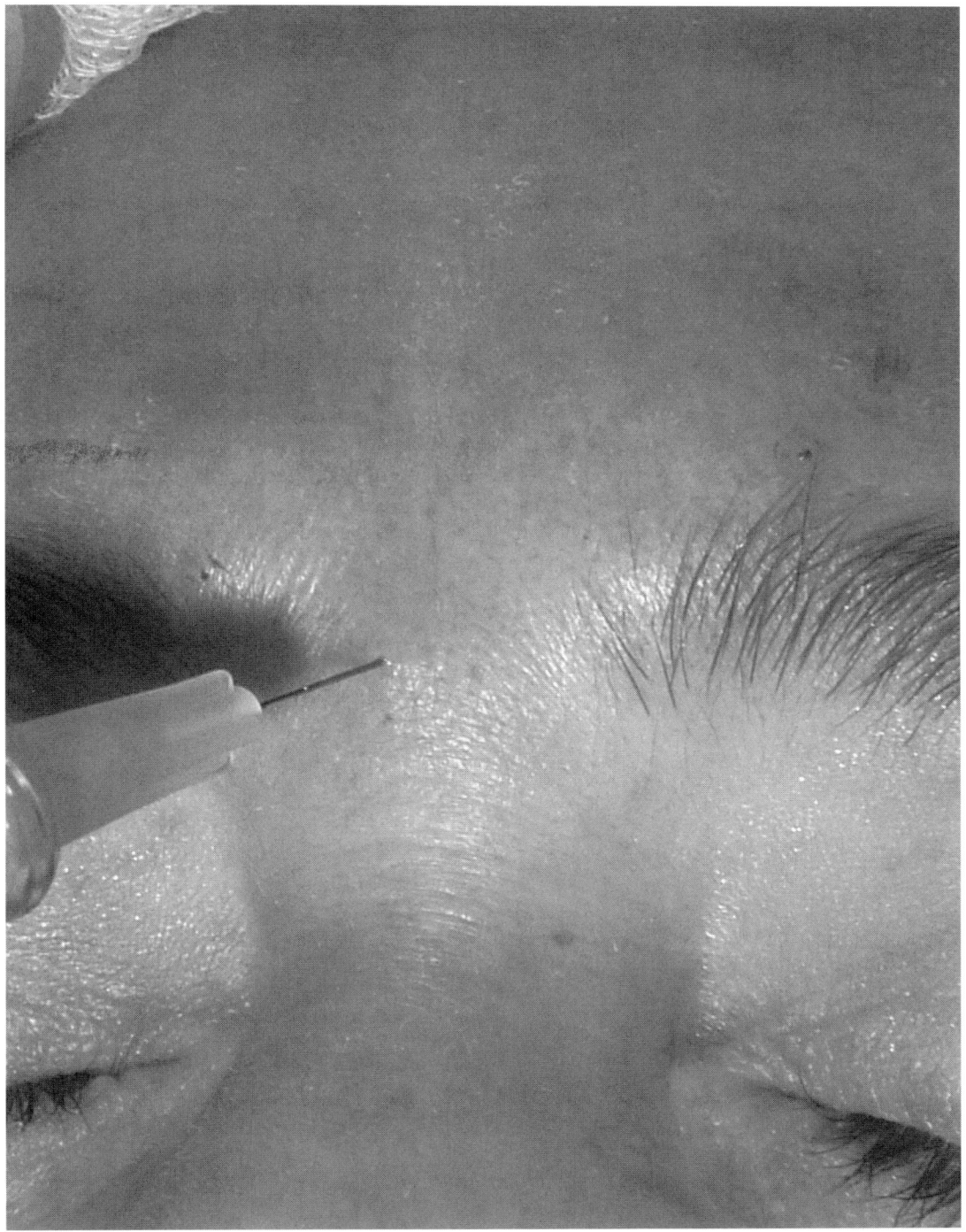

**Fig. 3.** Injection of botulinum toxin type A into the midline of the procerus muscle.

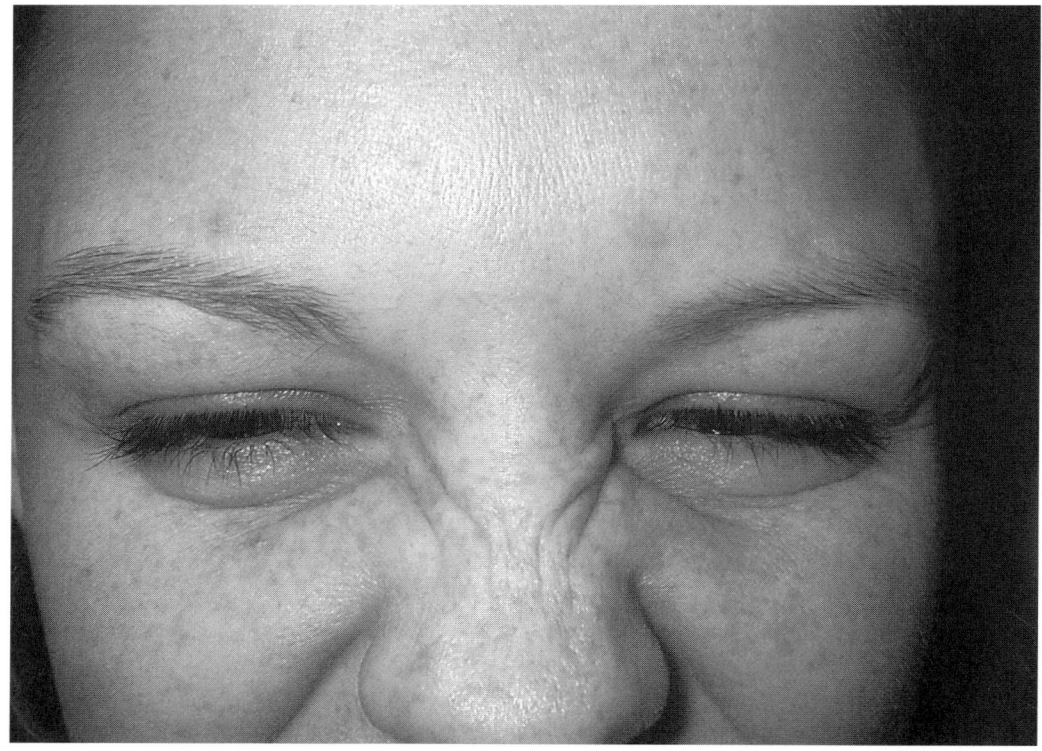

**Fig. 4.** Four weeks after botulinum toxin type A treatment of the glabellar complex.

Forth Worth, TX), or phenylephrine hydrochloride 2.5% (Neo-synephrine®, Sanofi, Winthrop Pharmaceuticals, New York, NY) can stimulate Müller's muscles in the lid, providing some relief of eyelid ptosis until the effects of BTX-A disappear *(19)*.

### Horizontal Forehead Lines

The frontalis muscle elevates the brow and its contraction causes horizontal forehead rhytids (Fig. 5). Treatment of this brow elevator results in a reduction of muscle activity and decreased forehead lines. Care must be taken when treating this area and injections are generally limited to the upper half to two-thirds of the frontalis. This placement avoids total paralysis of the frontalis, which can cause brow ptosis and heaviness. Physicians will often treat this area with the glabellar brow depressors to help decrease the occurrence of brow ptosis.

Ten to 20 U of BTX-A are placed in four to nine injections across the upper two-thirds of the forehead *(1,23,24)*. Slightly higher doses are sometimes required in men with larger muscles. Injections are placed along the rhytids, taking care to stay 2 to 3 cm above the orbital rim to avoid brow ptosis (Fig. 6; refs. *20* and *22*). This distance depends on the size of the patient's forehead; thus, some physicians recommend using the first horizontal line above the eyebrows as a landmark and only injecting above this line. Maximum response occurs at 2 to 4 weeks and the duration is often longer than seen when treating the glabellar complex (Fig. 7). Retreatment intervals range from 3 to 6 months *(1,25)*.

Another adverse event unique to treating the frontalis is raising the lateral eyebrow creating an elevated "quizzical" brow *(20)*. In general, if the upper lateral fibers are not treated,

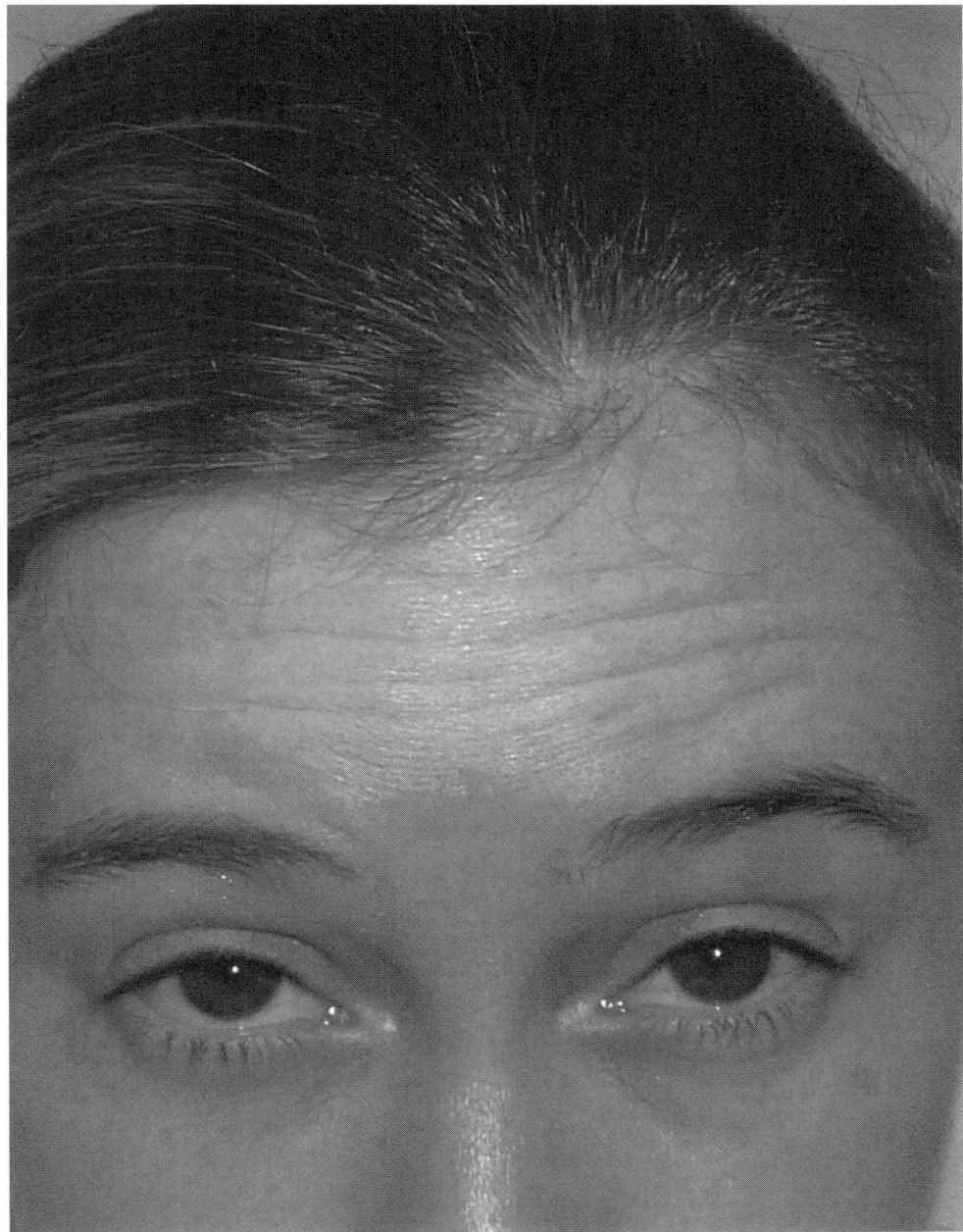

**Fig. 5.** Horizontal forehead rhytids, which are accentuated when the patient raises her eyebrows.

the unopposed muscle action will raise the lateral edge of the eyebrow. However, overtreatment of these fibers or inappropriate injections into the lower lateral fibers can cause significant ptosis that can partially cover the eye. As previously mentioned, mild ptosis can be improved with apraclonidine or phenylephrine eye drops.

Carruthers et al. performed a prospective blinded study comparing the safety and efficacy of BTX-A dosage in the treatment of horizontal forehead rhytids. Sixteen, 32, and 48 total

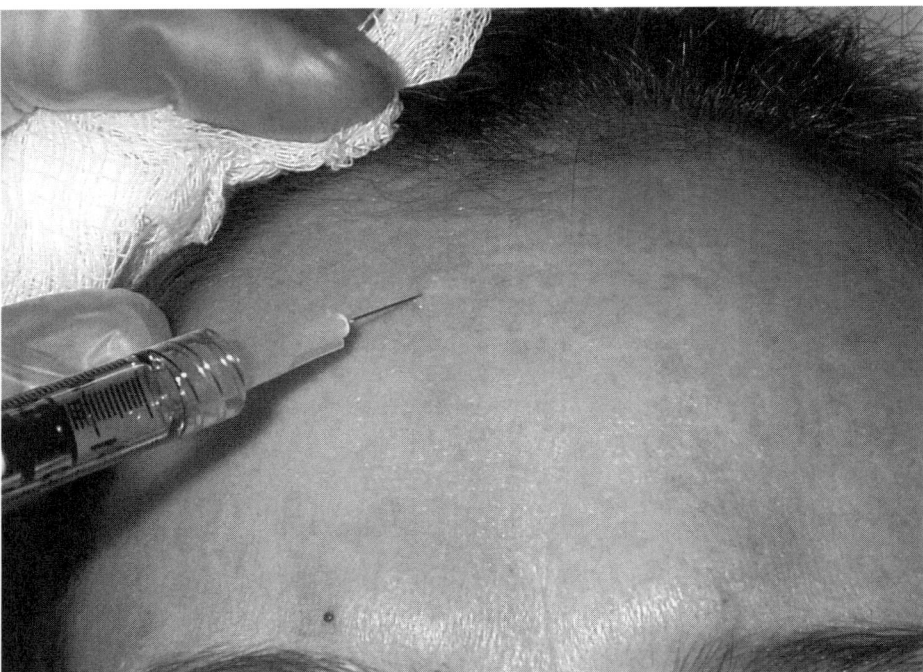

**Fig. 6.** For treatment of horizontal forehead wrinkles, botulinum toxin type A injections are placed into the frontalis muscle along the rhytids. Note that the injections are in the upper two-thirds of the forehead to avoid brow ptosis.

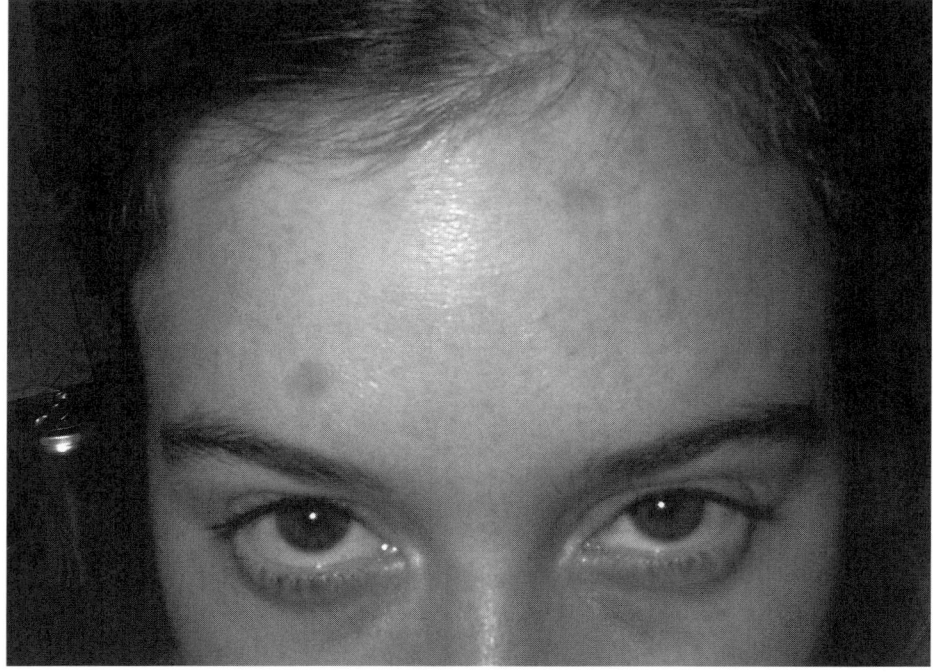

**Fig. 7.** Four weeks after treatment of horizontal forehead rhytids.

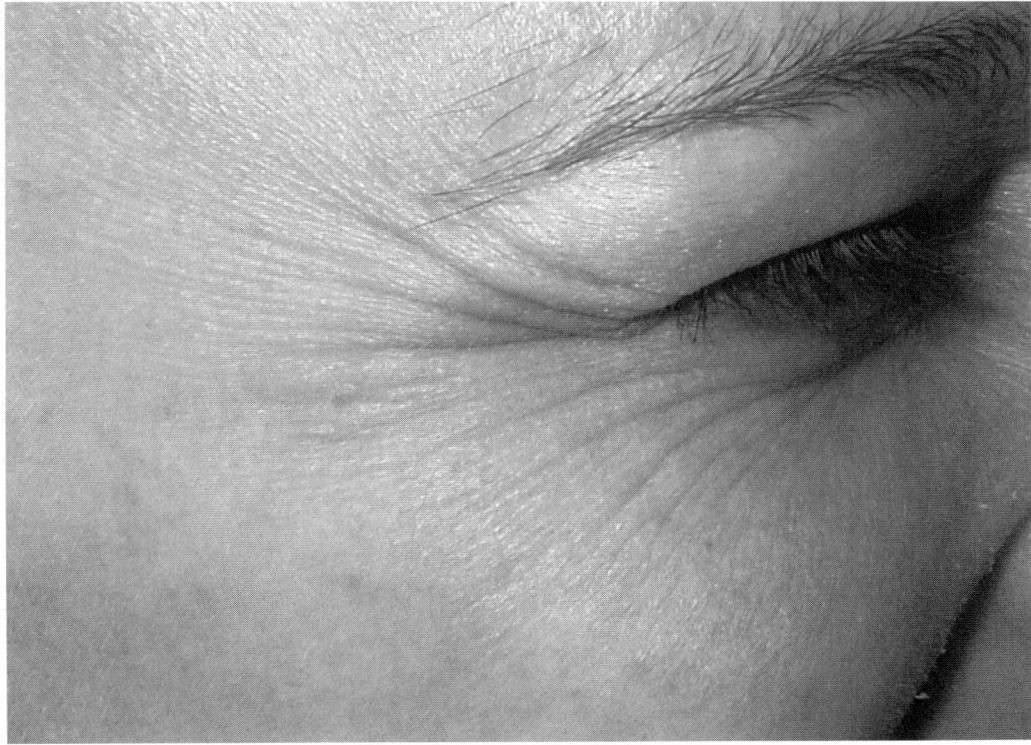

**Fig. 8.** Periocular rhytids (or "crow's feet") are easily identified when the patient squints the eyes.

units were administered over 8 injection sites into both brow depressors and elevators in 59 women, with 8, 16, and 24 U, respectively, into the frontalis muscle. A reduction in the severity of rhytids was noted in all three treatment groups, with the largest degree of response at the 48-U level. In addition, longer duration of response was associated with the higher doses of BTX-A, with some patients benefiting up to 24 weeks. However, although the percentage of adverse events was similar in all three groups, all six reports of eyebrow ptosis occurred in the 32- and 48-U groups *(25)*.

## Crow's Feet

Crow's feet are periocular rhytids that radiate outward from the lateral canthus. These dynamic wrinkles are caused by contraction of the orbicularis oculi. However, natural aging and sun exposure add a static component. The primary function of the orbicularis oculi is the involuntary and voluntary closure of the eyelids to protect the globe. Thus, similar to the treatment of horizontal forehead wrinkles, the goal is to relax and not to immobilize the muscle. A close evaluation of the patient is also imperative before injection. For example, a patient with excessive lower eyelid skin or fat pads would not only be at increased risk for adverse events from BTX-A injections, but would also likely derive greater benefit from a blepharoplasty.

The authors routinely have the patient squint to identify the exact location of the rhytids, and then 8 to 12 U are used on each side (Fig. 8). Injections are placed approximately 1 cm

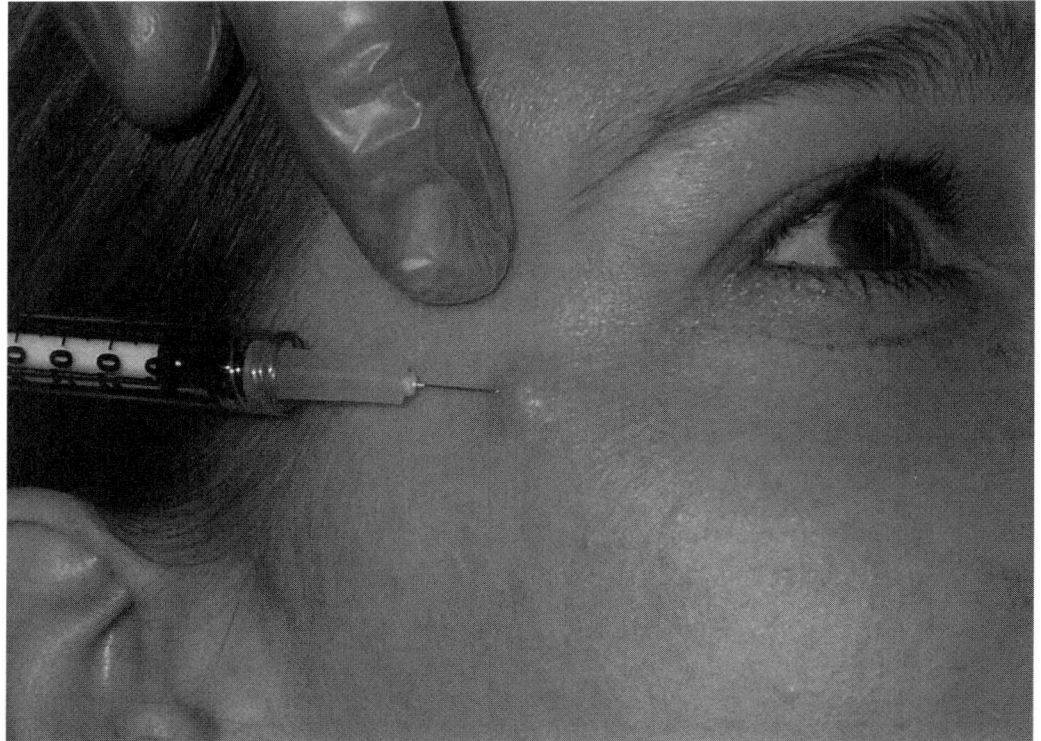

**Fig. 9.** Botulinum toxin type A is placed into the obicularis oculi, approximately 1 cm lateral to the orbital rim. Note the superficial bleb that is raised with injection.

lateral to the orbital rim. A superficial bleb is raised with a series of three injections on each side, followed by gentle massage to diffuse the toxin (Fig. 9). Care is taken to avoid any superficial veins that are frequently present in this location. In some patients, the orbicularis oculi may extend more than 3 cm laterally; in this case, an additional injection can be placed 1 cm distal to conventional injection points *(9)*. An additional 2 to 4 U can be placed into the lower eyelid to minimize infraorbital rhytids and widen the eye. The dose is often divided between two injection sites, one at the midpupillary line and the second halfway between the midpupillary and the lateral canthus *(26)*. The maximum response is seen approximately 4 weeks after the injection and the average duration is between 4 and 6 months (Fig. 10; refs. *27–29)*.

Lowe et al. performed a double-blind, randomized, placebo-controlled dose–response trial comparing placebo with 3, 6, 12, and 18 U BTX-A for the treatment of crow's feet *(28)*. Improved efficacy and longer duration was achieved with higher doses, but no difference was seen between the 12- and 18-U dosing. This prompted the authors to recommend 12 U per side as the most appropriate dose *(28)*.

Potential adverse events in this area include bruising, ectropion, upper lid ptosis, asymmetrical smile, strabismus, and dry eyes *(20)*. The increased risk of bruising results from the many periocular superficial veins. Using proper lighting and stretching the skin can help the physician visualize these small veins. Ice and/or pressure immediately after the injections can also help. Limiting the number of injections can further decrease the incidence of bruising. If the patient has lower lid retraction at baseline or if a snap test reveals lower lid laxity, a high

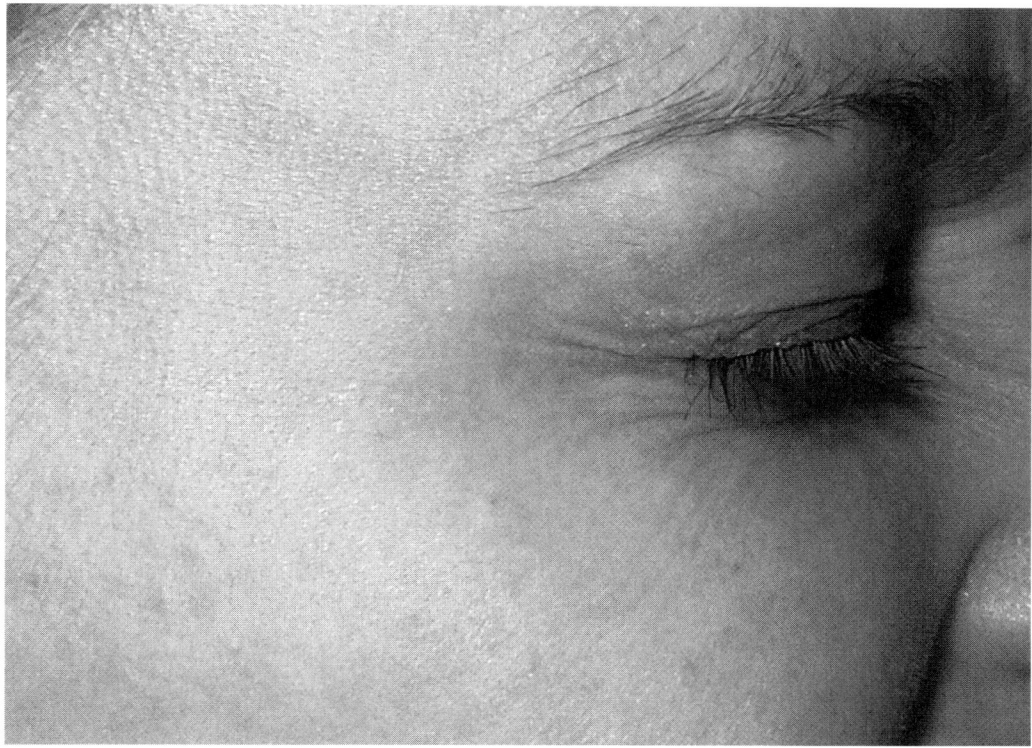

**Fig. 10.** Two weeks after treatment of periocular rhytids.

risk of ectropion is associated with BTX-A treatment *(1)*. The lower portion of the orbicularis oculi should not be injected in these patients. Strasbismus is caused by the diffusion of toxin into the ocular muscles, such as the lateral rectus. Tear formation can also be affected if diffusion around lacrimal glands occurs. Lip ptosis, a more distal adverse event, results from diffusion of the toxin into the zygomaticus major, which inserts near lateral aspect of orbicularis oculi and the levator labii superioris muscle *(30)*. Weakening of these muscles causes an asymmetric smile. Although these complications can often be avoided with proper injection technique, they appear to be more common in patients who have had previous facial plastic surgery and/or vision correction surgery such as laser-assisted *in situ* keratomileusis *(1,31)*.

### *"Bunny" Lines*

Bunny lines are rhytids on the sides of the nose that result from contracting the transverse portion of the nasalis muscle, which runs from the maxilla diagonally across the bridge of the nose. These wrinkles radiate downward and should be distinguished from the transverse lines across the nasal bridge, which are caused by procerus contraction.

For treatment of bunny lines, a total of one to three injections are placed into the nasalis. Some authors recommend a single superficial injection into the midline of the muscle while some prefer injecting each side, placing the toxin into the lateral wall of nose anterior to the nasofacial groove. Still others combine the methods for a total of three sites. The recommended total starting dose is between 2 and 6 U, divided evenly if more than one injection is placed. A recent study of 250 patients with nasal rhytids injected 3 U to each side of the nose with 40% of the patients having satisfactory treatment *(32)*. The authors went back and treated the persistent wrinkles (at the nasal root and between the eyes) for complete satisfaction. No complications were reported.

The adverse event unique to this area is drooping of the upper lip. Placing an injection into the nasofacial groove or a vigorous downward massage can affect the levator labii alaeque nasi and the levator labii superioris. As with other sites, injections should be kept superficial to avoid bruising, but in this area particular caution should be undertaken to avoid the angular vein. Of note, treatment may be less effective in patients who have undergone rhinoplasty *(1)*.

### Perioral Lines

Perioral rhytids radiate vertically outward from the vermillion border. They primarily result from the purse string-like contraction of the orbicularis oris muscle. Although predominately associated with smokers, these wrinkles also result from photodamage, expression, and aging. In addition to softening the rhytids, BTX-A injection also gives the appearance of fuller lips as weakening of the muscles results in slight eversion *(33,34)*. Injections can weaken the orbicularis oris muscle and reduce rhytids. Care must be taken to avoid weakness, which can interfere with speech and mouth function.

Injections are placed into the muscle adjacent to each visible crease either along or just above (<5 mm) the vermillion border. If the lines are not apparent, have the patient pucker the lips, and then mark the areas of muscle contraction adjacent to the rhytids. Usually 1 to 4 U are placed per lip with no more than 2 U per lip quadrant *(34,35)*. The average total dosing is 5 to 6 U spread over six to eight injection sites.

Potential adverse events resulting from the treatment of perioral lines are both cosmetic and functional. Even small doses of BTA in this area can decrease the patient's ability to purse his or her lips, making it difficult to whistle, use a straw, or play a musical instrument. Patients may also have speech difficulties, specifically with pronouncing "b" and "p" sounds. Treatment of the lower lip is more likely to affect function, thus some authors recommend treatment of the upper lip only *(1)*. The midline of the upper lip should be avoided during treatment to prevent flattening of cupid's bow. One should also not inject into the corners of mouth because weakening of these muscles can cause drooling and/or drooping as well as an asymmetrical smile *(20)*. Injections placed too far above the vermillion border can cause the upper lip to invert or evert *(33)*.

### Mental Crease and Dimpled Chin

The mental crease is the groove between the lower lip and prominence of the chin. It is accentuated by the contraction of the mentalis muscle during expression. The mentalis muscle runs from mandible across the chin and inserts below the upper lip. Contraction in addition to loss of dermal collagen and subcutaneous fat also causes wrinkling and dimpling of the chin giving a *peau d'orange* appearance.

To soften the mental crease, 3 to 5 U BTX-A is placed into each mentalis band just lateral to midline on both sides and anterior to the bony mentum *(33)*. To treat the dimpled chin, one injection is typically placed midline into the mass of muscle on the prominence of the chin. The starting dose is usually 5 to 6 total units but can be increased to 12 U depending on response *(1,35)*.

Adverse events in this area most commonly involve inadvertent weakening of the orbicularis ori or the depressor labii, which result in lower lip incompetence and drooling *(20)*. Conservative dosing regimens, proper placement of injection low on the chin, and avoidance of injection into the mental crease can help avoid complications.

## Mouth Frown

Contraction of the depressor anguli oris (DAO) pulls down the lateral corners of the mouth, producing a permanent frown. Weakening this muscle allows for the upward pull of zygomaticus major and minor to elevate the corners of the mouth. The DAO extends superiorly from the lateral surface of the mandible to insert into the modiolus at the angle of the mouth and lays directly over the depressor labii inferioris. Some authors recommend injecting 2 to 3 U BTX-A directly into each DAO, while others place 3 to 5 U at the level of the mandible to avoid inadvertent asymmetrical weakening of the depressor labii inferioris *(33,35)*. In addition to an asymmetrical appearance, other adverse events include flaccid cheeks, mouth incompetence/drooling, and difficulty with speech *(20)*.

## Platysmal Bands

The platysmal is a large sheet arising from the pectoralis and deltoid fascia, crossing the clavicle, and extending along the sides of the neck. The anterior fibers spread widely to insert into the mandible or interdigitate with the opposite platysma and the muscles of the lower part of the face. Platysmal bands occur with age as the cervical skin loses its elasticity, submental fat descends, and the platysma separates to form two vertical bands *(33)*.

Patient selection and education is critical because BTX-A will not correct skin laxity or fat deposits, and injections can worsen the appearance of platysmal banding in patients who have jowl formation. These patients would have greater benefit with a traditional rhytidectomy rather than BTX-A injection. BTX-A has the best results in patients with obvious banding and good skin elasticity *(36,37)*. Injections can also be used as an adjuvant therapy to liposuction of the neck or as post-surgical treatment for residual bands after a rhytidectomy.

Contraction of the platysma allows the bands to "pop out" of the neck and they are easily grasped with the physician's non-dominant hand. Injections are placed along the band into the belly of the muscle approximately 1 cm apart. Anywhere from 2 to 12 injection sites per band are placed for a 10- to 40-U total starting dose *(1)*. Excessive or misplaced toxin, such as injecting into the strap muscles of the neck, can result in dysphagia, dysphonia, and neck weakness *(20)*.

## Horizontal Neck Lines

Horizontal or "necklace" lines are indentations in the skin caused by the attachment of the superficial musculoaponeurotic system in the neck. Treatment usually consists of deep intradermal injections of 1 to 2 U at 1-cm intervals along the horizontal lines for a total of 10 to 20 U *(33)*.

The most common adverse event is bruising. This area is especially prone to bruising because of deep venous perforators, which can easily bleed. A gentle massage immediately after injection can diminish bruising. The deglutition muscles are also located in this area and are cholinergic; thus diffusion of toxin could potentially cause difficulty swallowing.

## SUMMARY

BTX-A is a safe and effective treatment for dynamic rhytids of the upper, middle, and lower face. A thorough understanding of facial anatomy combined with appropriate patient selection, dosage, and injection technique maximizes clinical benefit while minimizing adverse events.

## REFERENCES

1. Carruthers J, Fagien S, Matarasso S, and the Botox Consensus Group. Consensus recommendations on the use of botulinum toxin type A in facial aesthetics. Plast Reconstruct Surg 2004;114: 1S–22S.
2. The American Society for Aesthetic Plastic Surgery. 11.9 Million Cosmetic Procedures In 2004. Available from: http://surgery.org/press/news-release.php?iid=395. Accessed 1/13/06.
3. PDR (package insert;Allergan Botox Cosmetic). Available from: http://www.botox.com/site/professionals/prescribing_info/botox_cosmetic.asp. Accessed 1/3/2006.
4. Wohlfarth K, Kampe K, Bigalke H. Pharmacokinetic properties of different formulations of botulinum neurotoxin type A. Mov Disord 2004;19:S65–S67.
5. Flynn TC. Myobloc. Dermatol Clin 2004;22:207–211.
6. Alam M, Dover JS, Arndt KA. Pain associated with injection of botulinum toxin A exotoxin reconstituted using isotonic sodium chloride with and without preservative: A double-blind, randomized controlled trial. Arch Dermatol 2002;38:510–514.
7. Carruthers A, Carruthers J. Botulinum toxin type A: history and current cosmetic uses of the upper face. Semin Cutan Med Surg 2001;20:71–84.
8. Klein AW. Dilution and storage of botulinum toxin. Dermatol Surg 1998;24:1179–1180.
9. Hexsel DM, De Almeida AT, Rutowitsch M, et al. Multicenter, double-blind study of the efficacy of injections with botulinum toxin type A reconstituted up to six consecutive weeks before application. Dermatol Surg 2003;29:523–529.
10. Cote TR, Aparna KM, Polder JA, Walton MK, Braun MM. Botulinum toxin type A injections: adverse events reported to the US Food and Drug Administration in therapeutic and cosmetic cases. JAAD 2005;53:407–415.
11. Sarifakioglu N, Sarifakioglu E. Evaluating the effects of ice application on the pain felt during botulinum toxin type-A injections. Ann Plast Surg 2004;53:543–546.
12. Lowe PL, Patnaik R, Lowe NJ. Single-center, double-blind, randomized study to evaluate the efficacy of 4% lidocaine cream versus vehicle cream during botulinum toxin type A treatments. Dermatol Surg 2005;31:1651–1654.
13. Hexsel D, Dal'Forno T. Type A botulinum toxin in the upper aspect of the face. Clin Dermatol 2003;21:488–497.
14. Hankins CL, Strimling R, Rogers GS. Botulinum A toxin for glabellar wrinkles. Dose and response. Dermatol Surg 1998;24:1181–1183.
15. Carruthers JD, Lowe NJ, Menter MA, et al. Double-blind, placebo-controlled study of the safety and efficacy of botulinum toxin type A for patients with glabellar lines. Plast Reconstr Surg 2003;112:1089–1098.
16. Carruthers JA, Lowe NJ, Menter MA, et al. A multicenter, double-blind, randomized, placebo-controlled study of the efficacy and safety of botulinum toxin type A in the treatment of glabellar lines. J Am Acad Dermatol 2002;46:840–849.
17. Carruthers A, Carruthers J, Said S. Dose-ranging study of botulinum toxin type a in the treatment of glabellar rhytids in females. Dermatol Surg 2005;31:414–422.
18. Carruthers A, Carruthers J. Prospective, double-blind, randomized, parallel-group, dose-ranging study of botulinum toxin type A in men with glabellar rhytids. Dermatol Surg 2005;31:1297–1303.
19. Klein AW. Contraindications and complications with the use of botulinum toxin. Clin Dermatol 2004;22:66–75.
20. Klein AW. Complications and adverse reactions with the use of botulinum toxin. Dermatol Surg 2003;29:549–556.

21. Frampton JE, Easthope SE. Botulinum toxin A (Botox Cosmetic): a review of its use in the treatment of glabellar frown lines. Am J Clin Dermatol 2003;4:709–725.
22. Flynn TC. Periocular botulinum toxin. Clin Dermatol 2003;21:498–504.
23. Klein AW. Botox for the eyes and eyebrows. Dermatol Clin 2004;22:145–149.
24. Connor MS, Karlis V, Ghali GE. Management of the aging forehead: a review. Oral Surg Oral Med Oral Pathol Oral Radiol Endod 2003;95:642–648.
25. Carruthers A, Carruthers J, Cohen J. A prospective, double-blind, randomized, parallel-group, dose-ranging study of botulinum toxin type A in female subjects with horizontal forehead rhytides. Dermatol Surg 2003;29:461–467.
26. Flynn TC, Carruthers JA, Carruthers JA, Clark RE. Botulinum A toxin (Botox) in the lower eyelid: dose-finding study. Dermatol Surg 2003;29:943–951.
27. Lowe NJ, Lask G, Yamauchi P, et al. Bilateral, double-blind, randomized comparison of 3 doses of botulinum toxin type A and placebo in patients with crow's feet. J Am Acad Dermatol 2002; 47:834–840.
28. Lowe NJ, Ascher B, Heckmann M, et al. Double-blind, randomized, placebo-controlled, dose-response study of the safety and efficacy of botulinum toxin type A in subjects with crow's feet. Dermatol Surg 2005;31:257–262.
29. Levy JL, Servant JJ, Jouve E. Botulinum toxin A: a 9-month clinical and 3D in vivo profilometric crow's feet wrinkle formation study. J Cosmet Laser Ther 2004;6:16–20.
30. Matarasso SL, Matarasso A. Treatment guidelines for botulinum toxin type A for the periocular region and a report on partial upper lip ptosis following injections to the lateral canthal rhytids. Plas Reconstr Surg 2001;108:208–214.
31. Speigel JH. treatment of periorbital rhytids with botulinum toxin type A maximizing safety and results. Arch Facial Plast Surg 2005;7:198–202.
32. Tamura BM, Odo MY, Chang B, Cuce LC, Flynn TC. Treatment of nasal wrinkles with botulinum toxin. Dermatol Surg 2005;31:271–275.
33. Carruthers J, Carruthers A. Aesthetic botulinum A toxin in the mid and lower face and neck. Dermatol Surg 2003;29:468–476.
34. Semchyshyn N, Sengelmann RD. Botulinum toxin A treatment of perioral rhytides. Dermatol Surg 2003;29:490–495.
35. Atamoros FP. Botulinum toxin in the lower one third of the face. Clin Dermatol 2003;21:505–512.
36. Kane MA. Nonsurgical treatment of platysmal bands with injection of botulinum toxin A. Plast Reconstr Surg 1999;103:656–663.
37. Matarasso A, Matarasso SL, Brandt FS, Bellman B. Botulinum A exotoxin for the management of platysma bands. Plast Reconstr Surg 1999;103:645–652.

## Joely Kaufman and Leslie Baumann

## INTRODUCTION

Hyperhidrosis is defined as the overproduction of sweat, in excess of what can be evaporated and what is typically needed for normal, physiological thermoregulation (1,2). Hyperhidrosis can be primary or secondary. Primary hyperhidrosis is by definition idiopathic in nature. Secondary hyperhidrosis can be generalized or localized. There are many causes of secondary hyperhidrosis and each patient should be evaluated with a complete history of these causes a diagnosis of primary hyperhidrosis is given. Secondary causes of hyperhidrosis are generally related to systemic conditions, the most common being endocrine abnormalities. Other common causes of secondary hyperhidrosis include febrile illness, neurological disorders, spinal cord injury, and diabetes. Table 1 gives a complete list of additional causes. In this chapter, we focus our attention on primary idiopathic hyperhidrosis. In most cases, primary hyperhidrosis is seen in its localized form, yet cases of generalized primary hyperhidrosis are also reported. Primary localized hyperhidrosis most commonly occurs symmetrically in the axillae, palms, and/or soles and is usually absent during sleep (2–4).

Primary hyperhidrosis is thought to occur as a result of overactivity of the sympathetic nervous system, yet proof of this causality remains to be demonstrated. Onset of the disorder is usually around the time of puberty. The prevalence of localized hyperhidrosis is generally estimated to be around 0.6 to 1% (5). This prevalence rate may be significantly underestimated because only a small percentage of patients actually seek medical care for their condition. A national survey done in 2004, using the validated hyperhidrosis disease severity scale (HDSS), reported the incidence of hyperhidrosis to be 2.8%, with an equal proportion of men and women affected. The average age of individuals with hyperhidrosis was 40 years. Of those affected, only 38% reported that they had discussed the condition with a health care professional. Women were more likely to consult for care than men (3). Hyperhidrosis, although not life threatening, can be extremely disabling. The excess sweating can be socially and professionally distressing. The stress associated with the sweating frequently leads to additional anxiety and a subsequent increase in sweating, which only exacerbates the condition. Patients suffering from hyperhidrosis report a decrease in their quality of life, as measured on self-assessment scores. The negative impact on quality-of-life scores for patients with hyperhidrosis has been reported by validated questionnaires, and has been found to be similar to the impact of other well-documented diseases, such as psoriasis (6). Of affected patients,

From: *Therapeutic Uses of Botulinum Toxin*
Edited by: G. Cooper © Humana Press Inc., Totowa, NJ

**Table 1**
**Causes of Hyperhidrosis**

1. Idiopathic
2. Physiological
3. Febrile illness
4. Endocrine and metabolic disorders
5. Drugs, toxins, and substance abuse
6. Cardiovascular disorders
7. Respiratory failure
8. Hodgkin's disease
9. Intrathoracic neoplasms or lesions
10. Carcinoid tumor
11. Gustatory sweating
12. Olfactory sweating
13. Spinal cord injuries
14. Compensatory hyperhidrosis
15. Familial dysautonomia (Riley-Day syndrome)
16. Cold-induced hyperhidrosis
17. Hypothalamic lesions
18. Nail-Patella syndrome
19. Cutaneous diseases

Adapted from ref. *22*.

32% report that their sweating is barely tolerable and frequently interferes with daily activities *(3)*. In addition to the emotional implications, excessive sweating can also cause medical complications in the skin, such as maceration and secondary infection of the compromised skin barrier.

Localized primary hyperhidrosis is a disorder of sweating. It is still considered to be idiopathic in nature because no clear etiology has been found. Some have proposed an autosomal-dominant inheritance pattern; one study showed 15 of 18 patients with hyperhidrosis had a family member who was also affected *(7,8)*. Sweating is an important physiological mechanism that assists with thermoregulation and skin hydration. Humans have three different types of glands that carry out this function, and it has become a recent debate whether hyperhidrosis is solely a disorder of eccrine glands. Several investigators have looked at the possibility of some contribution from apoeccrine glands because the hyperhidrosis disease onset is usually around the time of apocrine gland maturation, during puberty *(9)*. It remains to be determined how much of a role, if any, the apoeccrine glands play in hyperhidrosis. Eccrine glands are small (0.05–1 mm in diameter) and are located deep in the middle dermis. There are approximately two million eccrine glands in the human skin *(10)*. The eccrine secretory coil is surrounded by myoepithelial cells. The duct then connects directly to the skin surface. The resultant product is a watery, hypotonic solution that is produced continuously in copious amounts. The nerve supply to the eccrine glands is via the sympathetic nervous system, yet uses acetylcholine (ACh) as the neurotransmitter, which binds to the muscarinic receptor on the eccrine gland to initiate the sweating response *(9,11,12)*. The exact type of muscarinic receptor has not been identified. Eccrine glands can also respond to adrenergic stimuli, yet this stimulation plays only a minor role in the sweating response. Eccrine glands are found in all areas of the body except for the labia minora, lips, and external auditory canal. In the axilla, it is generally accepted that the majority of the hyperhidrosis is from the hair bearing areas of the axilla, which is also where the apocrine and apoeccrine glands are located. However, hyperhidrosis of the palms is clearly not related to apocrine or apoeccrine glands because neither of these glands are found on the palm *(9,11,12)*. Apocrine glands are also present at birth, but do not become clinically active until puberty. They are found primarily in the axilla, vermillion border of the lips, breasts, and perineum. They are never found on the palms. The gland is much larger than the eccrine gland and the apocrine duct does not open directly to the skin surface like the eccrine duct does. The apocrine duct instead empties its contents into the hair follicle between the sebaceous gland and the skin surface. Apocrine sweat is milky, viscous, and produced in an intermittent fashion *(13)*. Apoeccrine glands are thought to evolve from eccrine glands and are first seen in the skin at around age eight. They have only been found in the axilla and become more numerous as puberty evolves. They are situated in the deep dermis, similar to apocrine glands, yet their ducts connect directly with the skin surface, similar to the eccrine duct. The sweat produced from the apoeccrine gland is watery, thin, and produced in a continuous fashion, similar to eccrine gland *(14,15)*. In vitro, the apoeccrine gland is more responsive to stimulation than either the eccrine or the apocrine glands *(14,15)*.

Several researchers have looked at the morphology of the glands themselves in the search for the cause of hyperhidrosis. The eccrine glands of patients with hyperhidrosis are anatomically normal, yet demonstrate the morphology of a chronically activated gland *(16)*.

This active phenotype displays an overall increase in the linear dimensions of the gland of up to eight times greater than normal. The secretory cells themselves were also found to be larger than normal cells. In addition, there is devesiculation of granular cells, distended basal infoldings and canaliculi between non-granular cells, and a contracted myoepithelium. All of these findings are consistent with a morphologically normal, yet hyperactive eccrine gland. Apocrine gland morphology from hyperhidrosis patients also demonstrates this altered chronically active appearance. The glands are also anatomically normal, yet enlarged, more coiled, and have a greater luminal diameter *(17)*. Again, this may imply that in axillary hyperhidrosis there is some involvement of the apocrine as well as the eccrine glands.

## DIAGNOSIS

Hyperhidrosis is primarily diagnosed by patient history, HDSS, and observation of sweat in the affected area. There are no quantitative measures required for diagnosis. For study purposes, sweat production can be quantitatively measured via gravimetric measures and/or other methodologies. The use of a starch iodine test, which will be described in detail later in this chapter, is not a quantitative measure of sweat production, but rather a general measure of the area of involvement of sweating. This measurement helps to outline areas for treatment. Before initiating therapy, a complete history and physical exam should be completed with each patient. A search for a secondary cause can be ruled out with a thorough history that includes age of onset, precipitation factors, drug and psychosocial history, medical and surgical history, associated signs and symptoms, and family history. The younger the patient is at age of presentation, the more likely a secondary cause will be found. Laboratory tests should be ordered when the history or physical examination indicate the possibility of a secondary cause, but are not indicated in routine screening.

## TREATMENT ALGORITHM

Although treatments are available, they usually provide little benefit and adequate treatment is often frustrating to both physician and patient alike. Patients should generally start with the least invasive from of therapy and progress to more complicated therapies as these other therapies fail. Approved therapies include topical medications, iontopheresis, systemic medications, botulinum toxin type A (BTX-A), and surgery. Topical therapies consist of aluminum chloride hexahydrate preparations that patients must apply consistently to achieve mild improvement of their condition. The most popular of these agents is a 20% solution (Drysol®), which is applied at night to the affected area and washed off in the morning. The mechanism of action of this group of topical agents is suggested to be related to plugging of the acrosyringium. The reduction in sweating is temporary and may be associated with irritation of the skin in the application areas. Antiperspirants containing aluminum chloride hexahydrate are also available. The use of tanning agents has been described in the treatment of hyperhidrosis, but this is generally not well accepted because of unwanted side effects *(18)*. Other treatments include iontophersesis, which involves the introduction of electric current to the skin causing a blockage of the acrosyringium. This process was first described for the treatment of arthritis by Pivatti in 1740. In 1936, Ichihashi described its use in treating hyperhidrosis *(19)*. This procedure can be used for palmar or plantar hyperhidrosis, but is physically difficult for axillary hyperhidrosis. The patient places their hands into basins of tap water attached to an electric current. The area to be treated receives the anode current, while the opposite side receives the cathode current. Most iontopheresis systems employ an average direct current of 15 mA at a voltage of 20 to 40 V. Recommended treatment times of 10 to 30 minutes daily are used until the desired anhidrotic effect is attained. Maintenance therapy consists of twice weekly treatments *(20)*. Again, these treatments are time consuming, temporary, and have variable outcomes. The incidence of irritation is lower than in the topical therapies, but not absent. Treatment is sometimes associated with a stinging or burning sensation when the skin barrier is disrupted, as is frequently seen with severe hyperhidrosis patients. Iontopheresis is typically done with tap water; however, successful reports with various additives such as poldine methylsulfate, glycopyrronium bromide, and BTX have been documented *(21–23)*.

Alternative treatments have been reported, including hypnosis, biofeedback, and acupuncture, all again with variable success rates *(18,24)*. Systemic anticholinergic agents are riddled with side effects that preclude their widespread use in most instances. These side effects include dry mouth, dry eyes, constipation, urinary retention, and blurry vision. Surgical excision of the glands can be done for axillary hyperhidrosis, but it is generally painful and results in severe scarring. Liposuction of the glandular tissue has also been reported for axillary hyperhidrosis and results in a better cosmetic outcome with similar success rates. However, relapse rates tend to be high as well as the need for retreatment for residual sweating *(25,26)*. Surgical therapy is available via ablation of the sympathetic nerves, yet should be reserved for only the most refractory cases. Although this procedure is now done via laparoscopy, there are still side effects not only from the surgery itself, but also with regard to compensatory sweating. With transthoracic videothoracoscopy, the intra-operative time is generally less than 60 minutes. Isolation and ablation of few nerve ganglia has resulted in fewer side effects than traditional sympathectomies. In one study, the mean interval between hospital discharge and return to work was 12 days, making it a fairly quick recovery *(27)*. In this same retrospective study, 87% of patients suffered from compensatory sweating. Most patients reported this as mild to moderate, and tolerable.

**Table 2**
**Injection Equivalents**

| *Botox* | *Reloxin/Dysport* | *BTX-B/Myobloc* |
|---|---|---|
| Axilla | 50 U | |
| Palms | 60–100 U | |
| Soles | 60–100 U | |

Severe compensatory sweating generally occurs in 2 to 8% of patients postoperatively *(28–30)*. Other side effects include pneumothorax and Horner's syndrome. The success rates of thorascopic sympathectomy differs by area, with most surgeons reporting a success rate in the 90th percentile with respect to palmar hyperhidrosis, but much lower success rates with axillary and palmar involvement. With this relative lack of a simple, low-risk, effective therapy for such a debilitating disease, the introduction of BTX has rapidly found a place in the treatment armamentarium.

BTX is a toxin made from bacteria that block the release of Ach from the presynaptic nerve terminal. In doing so, any nerve that uses Ach as its transmitter can be affected, including sympathetic nerves. In the treatment of hyperhidrosis, BTX-A blocks the release of ACh from the presynaptic nerve terminal, thereby resulting in a decrease in stimulation of the eccrine gland, and hence decreased sweat production *(31,32)*. Since its introduction, numerous reports of BTX-A use for hyperhidrosis have clearly shown its clinical effectiveness. In addition to its quantitative reduction in sweat production, several studies have also shown improvement in the quality-of-life index ratings of patients after treatment with BTX-A. These qualitative improvements are perhaps even more significant than the quantitative measures *(33–35)*.

BTX-A is approved for use by the Food and Drug Administration for axillary hyperhidrosis. Treatment in this area is associated with mild side effects related to the injection procedure. At the recommended doses, there are very few other side effects reported, such as dry mouth, dry eyes, and indigestion. In addition to treatment of the axilla, BTX-A is also being used off-label for treatment of hyperhidrosis of the palms and soles, as well as for some of the less common areas of involvement. Currently, only Botox® (Allergan Inc., Irvine, CA) is approved in the United States for treatment of hyperhidrosis, but there are reports of other formulations of BTX-A and BTX-B (Reloxin® and Dysport®, respectively) also being used successfully. For purposes of simplicity, when we refer to BTX-A and the unit dosing, we will be referring to Botox. (*See* Table 2 for doses of other forms of BTX).

In addition to the published studies on treatment of axillary hyperhidrosis, there are also several studies on the use of BTX-A for the treatment of palmar hyperhidrosis. Because this area is more sensitive to pain and contains more fine motor musculature, the palms and soles have become a more delicate treatment area. Double-blind, placebo-controlled studies have indicated that the treatment is effective at reducing sweating from these areas. One study demonstrated improvements in sweating by gravimetric measure, iodine starch, and patient and physician ratings. The results were statistically significant in all areas of assessment. They also noted no significant difference in grip strength between treated and untreated hands *(36–39)*. There are, however, several reports of reduced grip strength, pinch strength, and muscular activity after BTX-A treatment *(38,39)*. It seems that depth of injection may play a role in the frequency of occurrence of side effects. Injections in

**Table 3**
**Hyperhidrosis Disease Severity Scale**

Which of the following best describes the impact of your sweating on your daily activities?
1. Never noticeable, never interferes.
2. Tolerable, sometimes interferes.
3. Barely tolerable, frequently interferes.
4. Intolerable and always interferes.

studies in which no changes in grip strength were noted were done intradermally, as opposed to subcutaneously, with a wheal at the area of injection. Zaiac et al. reported use of a specialized needle to try to control the depth of injection during treatment. In their series of 10 patients, none of the patients reported muscle weakness *(40)*. One study looked at muscle action potentials before and after injection of BTX-A and found that even with intradermal injection the compound muscle potentials for the abductor pollicis brevis and abductor digiti minimi were decreased post-injection by as much as 64%. This value returned to normal at 37 weeks. It seems that, despite careful administration of BTX-A intradermally, there is still diffusion of the toxin and its associated side effects. Patients should be warned of the likelihood of experiencing some motor weakness of the hand that normally returns to baseline after approximately 6 months. The palmar eccrine glands are located at the junction between the dermis and the subcutaneous tissues, and ideally, this is where the BTX-A should be placed. Because of the diffusion capabilities of the toxin, placement in the dermis will also result in improvement with possibly fewer side effects. The pain associated with injections of the palms and soles are often too much for the patient to tolerate without some form of anesthesia. Topical anesthesia, nerve blocks, cooling, and vibration are just some of the techniques used to make the injections more tolerable. Treatment of plantar hyperhidrosis is even more difficult because sensory nerves supplying these areas are situated deep in the dermis, making nerve blocks difficult. One study showed the successful use of BTX-A injection via a Dermojet® (Akra, Pau, France) in treatment of plantar hyperhidrosis *(41)*. The Dermojet injection technique is not recommended for use in palmar hyperhydrosis because the nerves and vessels are located more superficially and injection with the Dermojet does not allow for consistent superficial placement of the toxin.

## BTX INJECTION PROCEDURE

Before BTX treatment for any patient, a complete history, including previous treatments, medications, and family history is taken. Patients are also given the simple HDSS four-point scale to determine the severity of their hyperhidrosis (Table 3). In general, a score of three or four on this scale indicates need for some kind of treatment. Most patients at our facility have already tried and failed topical treatments, iontopheresis, and oral treatments. Before any surgical therapy, patients should be considered for BTX treatment (Table 4).

### Axilla

For the first treatment of hyperhidrosis with BTX, the physician should set aside approximately 45 minutes for initial evaluation, delineation of the treatment area, injection, and observation. Each successive treatment may not require as much time because some of the steps will not need to be repeated.

**Table 4**
**Treatment Steps: Axilla**

1.  HDSS severity score determination (score of 3 or 4 needed).
2.  Patient consent.
3.  Starch iodine-outlining procedure.
4.  Topical anesthesia application for at least 30 minutes.
5.  Marking of sites to be injected: placed approximately 2 cm apart in staggered fashion.
6.  Mix Botox®: 4 cc 0.9% sterile saline per 100-unit vial.
7.  Draw up Botox into 4 1-cc syringes with 25-gage needle, then replace with 30-gage needle.
8.  Count injection sites and determine volume to be injected per site.
9.  Injection of each site: 3-mm depth with bleb.
10. 30 Minutes in office observation.

The area of involvement of hyperhidrosis is generally the hair-bearing areas in the axilla. Although some patients will have sweating outside of this area, injections in the hair-bearing areas can be used as a general guideline if no form of outlining is going to be done. Patients who do not have an outlining procedure done before the first treatment should be seen for follow-up to touch up remaining hyperhidrotic areas. Whenever possible, it is best to outline the area of involvement using the starch iodine test before the patient's first treatment. If the first set of injections results in successful cessation of sweating, a photograph of the original starch iodine test can be used for future treatments to avoid performing this messy procedure with each visit.

The Minor's starch iodine test is done using iodine or betadine swabs (Figs. 1 and 2). Before initiating this test, patients should be questioned about iodine allergy. The area to be outlined is cleansed thoroughly, dried, and then brushed with the iodine or betadine swabs. The starch powder (potato starch) is then lightly sprinkled over the area. The color change of the iodine from orange/red to black is indicative of areas of active sweating. These areas can then be outlined with a surgical marking pen. The skin is cleaned of all the iodine and photos should be taken at this time for use in follow-up procedures.

After outlining the area to be treated with a marking pen, topical anesthetic can be applied to the area. Topical anesthesia containing lidocaine, such as ElaMax 5% cream is generally sufficient for treatment of the axilla. Other anesthesia options include the use of vibration and cooling. In our practice, if a patient cannot tolerate the procedure with topical anesthesia alone, a Zimmer cooler or ice is applied to each site immediately before each injection. The accepted diffusion rate from the point of injection of BTX-A in the axilla is approximately 2 cm. Hence each injection should be placed 2 cm apart to completely cover the entire area. These sites can be mapped out before injection using a marking pen to facilitate even placement of the product. The injections should be placed in the superficial dermis, approximately 2 to 3 mm deep. The 100-U Botox vial is diluted with 4 cc 0.9% sterile normal saline and gently mixed. This gives a concentration of 2.5 U per 0.1 cc Botox. Most studies indicate that the ideal total treatment of the axillae should consist of 100 U BTX-A (50 U per axilla). Studies using higher doses to increase the efficacy or duration of the response have been conflicting *(42,43)*. The actual amount of BTX-A injected per site will vary depending on the number of injection sites needed. Each patient's anatomy and outlining procedure will determine the number of injection sites needed to treat the entire area of involvement. What is most important is the total dosage used and that care is taken to treat the entire area in a complete and uniform manner. When first beginning to treat patients for

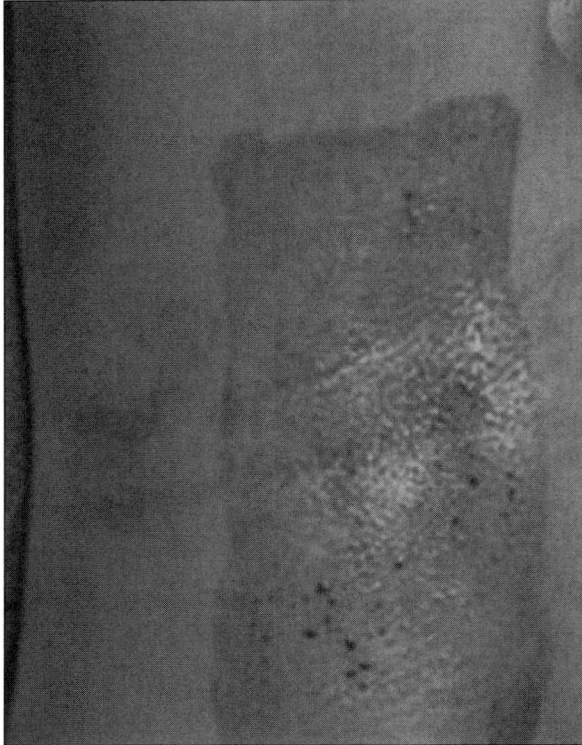

**Fig. 1.** Application of iodine to area to be tested.

hyperhidrosis, the easiest way to ensure consistent results is to map the area and the exact sites to be injected. Again, each injection site should be approximately 1.5 to 2 cm apart and should be done in a staggered fashion to avoid any skip areas. One technique published by Lam uses a grid pattern, injecting the BTX into the center of each square *(44)*. Follow-up should be done 10 to 14 days after injection on patients who receive the grid-pattern injection as their initial treatment to determine any sites of residual sweating. Patients who have been treated successfully previously do not need this visit. If these sites are present, outlining should be done again with the starch iodine test and the area should be retreated. Treatment with 100 U Botox should produce an anhidrotic effect for at least 5 months for the majority of patients *(45)*. The range of duration of action has been reported by one study to be between 17 and 57 weeks *(46)*.

Successful treatment of axillary hyperhidrosis has also been reported using BTX-B (Myobloc®; ref. *47*). The dose used was 2500 U per axilla. Myobloc is very successful at ameliorating hyperhidrosis at this dose; however, side effects noted include dry eyes, dry mouth, and indigestion *(47)*. The mean duration of action of BTX-B at this dose was 5 months, similar to the duration of action of BTX-A treatment. Others have reported effectiveness using lower doses, including one study with 250 U BTX-B *(48)*. The duration of action at this dose is much less than that of higher doses, but no side effects related to BTX were noted.

Other forms of BTX-A are also used in other countries for hyperhidrosis. Reloxin/Dysport has been shown to be effective at doses of 100 to 250 U per axilla *(49–51)*.

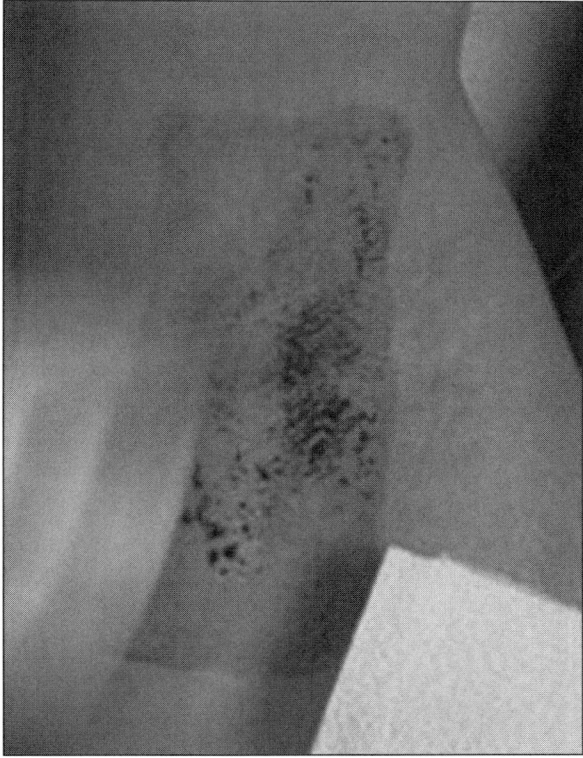

**Fig. 2.** Shows black areas corresponding to areas of sweating.

## Palms

Treatment of hyperhidrosis for the palms and soles is more complicated because of the anatomy of these areas and the additional pain associated with injections in these areas. The nerves and muscles, especially in the palms, lie closer to the surface of the skin and are hence more vulnerable to injury and side effects as a result of their physical location. In addition, topical anesthetics do not seem to function as well on these areas where the epidermis is thicker. Muscular weakness is also a major factor in treatment of the palms, and all patients should be advised to this likely yet transient side effect. Topical anesthetics are many times not adequate for pain control during treatment. Additional techniques, such as cooling and vibration, may also be used to maintain pain control, but many times peripheral nerve blockade is required. The physician must be familiar with the anatomy of the sensory nerves of the wrist and palm, including the median nerve, ulnar nerve, superficial radial nerve, and the lateral cutaneous nerve of the forearm. When doing peripheral nerve blocks, the patient must be alert and able to provide feedback to prevent nerve injury. A separate consent form should be used when performing peripheral nerve blocks. The area around the nerve should be infiltrated with the anesthesia, but never the nerve itself. If the patient feels pain in the distribution of the nerve, then the nerve itself has been infiltrated, and the needle should be withdrawn until the pain dissipates, before injection *(52–54)*. Nerve blocks should be performed approximately 30 minutes before injection of BTX.

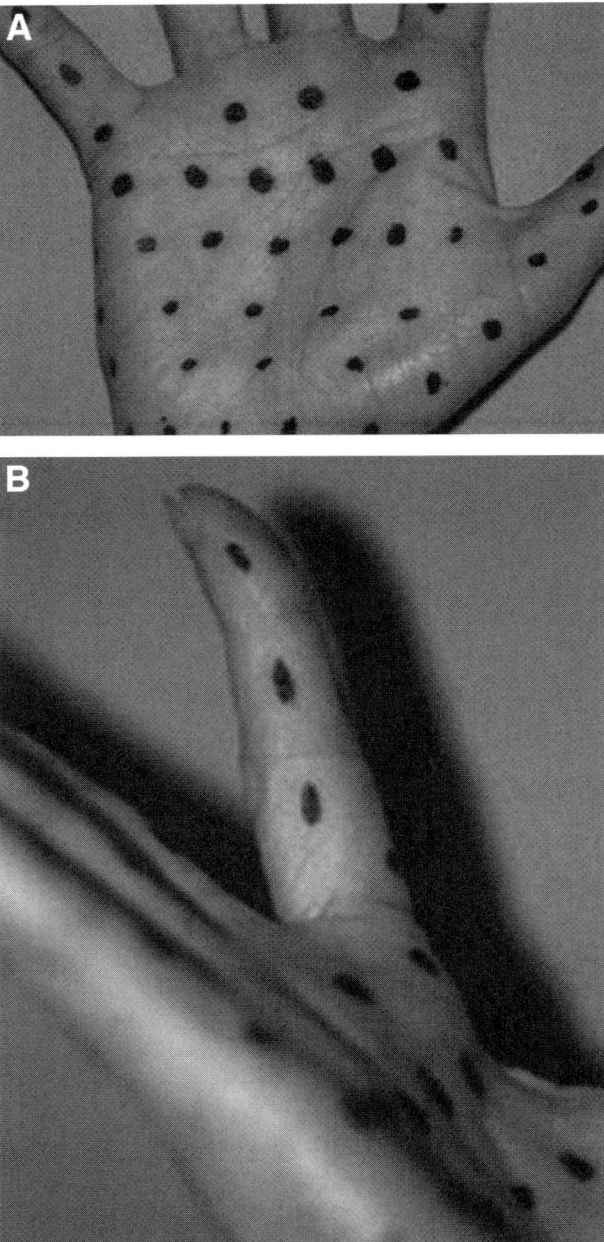

**Fig. 3.** Injection sites on fingers and hand for palmar hyperhidrosis.

The median nerve supplies most of the sensory innervation to the palm and many times blockade of this nerve alone is sufficient for pain control during treatment. The median nerve is positioned between the palmaris longus tendon and the flexor carpi radialis tendon. These tendons can be easily located with the wrist in the fully flexed position. To locate the palmaris longus tendon, the patient should put the thumb and the last two fingers together. Injections should be made between these two tendons, or radial to the palmaris longus tendon, and just proximal to the wrist crease. Approximately 2 to 4 cc 2% lidocaine should be injected at each site while withdrawing the needle. Again, care should be taken to withdraw the needle if any pain in the distribution of the nerve is felt.

The cutaneous branch of the ulnar nerve can be blocked at its location near the ulnar styloid process. This injection should be placed radial to the flexor carpi ulnaris tendon. This tendon can be located on the ulnar side of the wrist during wrist flexion. Again, 2 to 4 cc 2% lidocaine should be injected during withdrawal of the needle. Usually, blockade of the median nerve and the cutaneous branch of the ulnar nerve gives sufficient pain control to allow for full treatment of the palm. However, the superficial branch of the radial nerve, which supplies sensory innervation to the thumb, can also be blocked. This injection is done in a subcutaneous manner on the lateral aspect of the wrist. Again, 2 to 4 cc 2% lidocaine can be used in this area. Patients should be instructed that their hands may feel clumsy and they will not be able to drive for 3 hours following the procedure. Nerve blocks have been associated with paresthesias. In our practice, we have switched to using topical anesthetics and spraying Frigiderm on the skin immediately before injection *(47)*.

Although the iodine starch test is not necessary in all patients, it can help delineate what unique areas need to be treated, such as higher on the wrist and between the fingers. Some hyperhidrotic areas will extend onto the lateral aspects of the palm and fingers, and these areas need to be identified and treated if present.

The iodine starch test is performed before nerve block and BTX injections. A surgical marker is used to mark the areas that need to be treated. If the patient elects not to have a nerve block performed, the palms should be covered with topical lidocaine and placed in plastic bags to aid in penetration of the anesthetic. Application of a cooling device, such as ice packs, ice, or a Zimmer™ cooler, can also aid in pain control. These devices should be used on each specific site, immediately before each injection.

Botox 100-U vial should be diluted with 4 cc 0.9% sterile saline and gently mixed. Each palm will typically require between 60 and 100 U Botox. A 30-gage needle is used on a 1-cc syringe with needle-locking capabilities, such as the leur lock syringe, to prevent the needle from falling off during the injection process. Injection points on the palm should be placed slightly closer together than those of the axilla because diffusion of BTX seems to be less prevalent on the palms. Care should also be taken to inject the sides of the fingers because sweating commonly occurs in this location also (Fig. 3). After injection, the patient should be told not to move the hands for at least 30 minutes and should not drive or operate other machinery for 3 hours if a nerve block was performed. For new patients, follow-up should be done within 2 weeks to assess for additional hyperhidrotic areas. These areas, if identified, can be treated with as little as 2 U per 1-cm area involved. Full retreatment should not be performed before 3 months.

### Soles

Topical mapping of the affected areas should be done before injection. As with the palms, BTX treatment of the soles can be painful and many times requires peripheral nerve blocks for pain control during treatment. Because of the deep placement of the nerves in the feet, a thorough understanding of the anatomy of this area is required. Again, as with the palms, the patient must be alert in order to give feedback regarding nerve pain to prevent inadvertent damage to the nerve. The posterior tibial nerve and the sural nerve supply sensory innervation to the soles. The patient should be placed in the prone position allowing for comfortable access to these nerve branches. For the posterior tibial nerve, the posterior tibial artery should be palpated and marked. The injection should be placed posterior to the posterior tibial artery, midway between the medial malleolus and the Achilles tendon. The needle is inserted to the bone and approximately 3 to 5 mL 2% lidocaine should be injected while withdrawing the needle. The sural nerve can be anesthetized in the area between the Achilles tendon and the lateral malleolus in a similar fashion. After nerve blockade of the soles, patient should not drive for 2 to 3 hours.

After mapping of the hyperhidrotic areas, marks should be placed 1 to 2 cm apart where injections will be placed. The 100-U vial of Botox should be diluted with 4 cc 0.9% sterile saline. The soles are mapped with the starch iodine test and injection points are drawn with a surgical marker. Again, similar to the palms, 100 U BTX-A are used per sole. If a patient suffers from both palmar and plantar hyperhidrosis, the palms are always treated first because several patients have cessation of sweating of the soles after treatment of the palms.

## CONCLUSION

BTX is an excellent choice for treatment of hyperhidrosis. Several well-controlled studies have been published demonstrating the success of BTX-A in the treatment of hyperhidrosis. Side effects, including dry eyes, dry mouth, and indigestion, may be seen using very high doses and if retreatment is done before 3 months. These side effects are more commonly seen with BTX-B than BTX-A. Other side effects include parasthesias from peripheral nerve blocks. Separate consent forms should always be obtained when administering nerve blocks. Temporary weakness of the small muscles in the hands is frequently encountered when treating the palms and patients should be advised of this side effect. If additional treatment is needed at the 2-week follow-up, it should be done only in specific areas, not full retreatment. In addition, we recommend careful mapping of affected areas before treatment, for at least the first visit. To determine patients who would likely benefit from treatment with BTX, the HDSS questionnaire is used in our practice. Gravimetric measurements provide little in determining the effect of the condition on a patient's daily activities. Successful treatment results depend on careful injection technique as well as satisfactory pain control for the patient.

## REFERENCES

1. Stolman LP. Treatment of hyperhidrosis. Dermatol Clin 1998;16:863–869.
2. Atkins JL, Butler PE. Hyperhidrosis: a review of current management. Plast Reconstr Surg 2002;110:222–228.
3. Strutton DR, Kowalski JW, Glaser DA, Stang PE. US prevalence of hyperhidrosis and impact on individuals with axillary hyperhidrosis: results from a national survey. J Amer Acad Derm 2004;51:241–248.
4. Hashmonai M, Kopelman D, Assalia A. The treatment of primary palmar hyperhidrosis: a review. Surg Today 2000;30:211–218.
5. Adar R, Kurchin A, Zweig A, Mozes M. Palmar hyperhidrosis and its surgical treatment: a report of 100 cases. Ann Surg 1977;186:34–41.
6. Cina CS, Clase CM. The illness intrusiveness rating scale: a measure severity in individuals with hyperhidrosis. Qual Life Res 1999;8:693–698.
7. Hurley HJ, Shelly WB. Axillary hyperhidrosis. Clinical features and local surgical management. Br J Dermatol 1966;78:127–40.
8. Hurley HJ. Diseases of the eccrine sweat glands. Philidelphia: W.B. Saunders; 1992.

9. Lonsdale-Eccles A, Leonard N, Lawrence C. Axillary hyperhidrosis: eccrine or apocrine? Clin and Exp Dermatol 2003;28:2–7.

10. Bisbal J, de Cacho C, Casalots J. Surgical treatment of axillary hyperhidrosis. Ann Plast Surg 1987;18:429–436.

11. Sato K, Kang WH, Saga K, et al. Biology of sweat glands and their disorders. I. Normal sweat gland function. J Am Acad Dermatol 1989;20:537–561.

12. Chalmers TM, Keele CA. The nervous and chemical control of sweating. Br J Dermatol 1952;64: 43–54.

13. Urmacher CD. In: Histology for Pathologists, 1st ed. New York: Raven Press; 1992.

14. Sato K, Sato F. Sweat secretion by human axillary apoeccrine sweat gland in vitro. Am J Physiol 1987;252:R181–R187.

15. Sato K, Leidal R, Sato F. Morphology and development of an apoeccrine sweat gland in human axillae. Am J Physiol 1987;252:R166–R180.

16. Bovell DL, Clunes MT, Elder HY, Milsom J, et al. Ultrastructure of the hyperhidrotic eccrine sweat gland. Br J Dermatol 2001;145:298–301.

17. Clunes MT, Holdsworth R, Bovell DI. A morphological study of hyperhidrotis and normal human apocrine sweat glands. Br J Surg 2002;89:31.

18. White JW Jr. Treatment of primary hyperhidrosis. Mayo Clin Proc 1986;61:951–956.

19. Ichihashi T. Effect of drugs on the sweat glands by cataphoresis and an effective method for suppression of local sweating. Observation on the effect of diaphoretics and adiaphoretics. J Oriental Med 1936;25:101–102.

20. Kreyden O. Iontopheresis for palmoplantar hyperhidrosis. J Cosm Dermatol 2004;3:211–214.

21. Moran KT, Brady MP. Surgical management of primary hyperhidrosis. Br J Surg 1991;78:279–283.

22. Leung A, Chan P, Choi M. Hyperhidrosis. Int J Dermatol 1999;38:561–567.

23. Kavanagh GM, Oh C, Shams K. Botox delivery by iontopheresis. Br J Dermatol 2005;151: 1093–1095.

24. Duller P, Gentry WD. Use of biofeedback in treating chronic hyperhidrosis: a preliminary report. Br J Dermatol 1980;103:143–146.

25. Lillis PJ, Coleman WP. Liposuction for treatment of axillary hyperhidrosis. Dermatol Clin 1990; 8:479–482.

26. Lee M, Ryman W. Liposuction for axillary hyperhidrosis. Australas J Dermatol 2005;46:76–79.

27. Dumont P, Denoyer A, Robin P. Long-term results of thoracoscopic sympathectomy for hyperhidrosis. Ann Thoracic Surg 2004;78:1801–1807.

28. Lin TS, Wang NP, Huang LC. Pitfalls and complication avoidance associated with transthoracic endoscopic sympathectomy for primary hyperhidrosis (analysis of 2200 cases). Int J Surg Investig 2001;2:377–385.

29. Zacherl J, Huber ER, Imhof M, et al. Long-term results of 630 thoracoscopic sympathicotomies for primary hyperhydrosis: the Vienna experience. Eur J Surg Suppl 1998;580:43–46.

30. Drott C, Gothberg G, Claes G. Endoscopic transthoracic sympathectomy: an efficient and safe method for the treatment of hyperhidrosis. J Am Acad Deratol 1995;33:78–81.

31. Pearce LB, First ER, MacCallum RD, Gupta A. Pharmacologic characterization of botulinum toxin for basic science and medicine. Toxicon 1997;35:1373–1412.

32. Naumann M. Evidence-based medicine: botulinum toxin in focal hyperhidrosis. J Neurol 2001;248:31–33.

33. Campanati A, Penna L, Guzzo T, et al. Quality-of-life assessment in patients with hyperhidrosis before and after treatment with botulinum toxin: results of an open label study. Clin Therap 2002;25:298–308.

34. Swartling C, Naver H, Lindberg M. Botulinum A toxin improves quality of life in severe primary focal hyperhidrosis. Eur J Neurol 2001;8:247–252.

35. Naumann MK, Hamm H, Lowe NJ. Effect of botulinum toxin type A on quality of life measures in patients with excessive axillary sweating: a randomized controlled trial. Br J Dermatol 2002;147:1218–1226.

36. Lowe N, Yanauchi P, Lask G, et al. Efficacy and safety of botulinum toxin A in the treatment of palmar hyperhidrosis: a double blind, randomized, placebo-controlled study. Dermatol Surg 2002;28:822–827.

37. Shelley WB, Talanin NY, Shelley ED. Botulinum toxin therapy for palmar hyperhidrosis. J Am Acad Dermatol 1998;38:227–229.

38. Schnider P, Binder M, Auff E, et al. Double-blind trial of botulinum toxin A for the treatment of focal hyperhidrosis of the palms. Br J Dermatol 1997;136:548–552.

39. Saadia D, Voustianiouk A, Wang AK, Kaufmann H. Botulinum toxin type A in primary palmar hyperhidrosis: randomized, single-blind, two-dose study. Neurology 2001;57:2095–2099.

40. Zaiac M, Weiss E, Elgart G. Botulinum toxin therapy for palmar hyperhidrosis with ADG needle. Dermatol Surg 2000;26:230.

41. Vadoud-Seyedi J. Treatment of plantar hyperhidrosis with botulinum toxin A. Int J Dermatol 2004;43:969–971.

42. Heckmann M, Plewig G. Low-dose efficacy of botulinum toxin A for axillary hyperhidrosis. Arch Dermatol 2005;141:1255–1259.

43. Karamfilov T, Konrad H, Karte K, Wollina U. Lower relapse rate of Botulinum Toxin A therapy for axillary hyperhidrosis by dose increase. Arch Dermatol 2000;136:487–490.

44. Lam D. Use of a grid to simplify botulinum toxin injection for axillary hyperhidrosis. Plas Reconst Surg 2003;112:1741–1742.

45. Odderson IR. Long term quantitative benefits of botulinum toxin type A in the treatment of axillary hyperhidrosis. Dermatol Surg 2002;28:480–483.

46. Lowe PL, Cerdan-Sanz S, Lowe N. Botulinum toxin type A in the treatment of bilateral primary axillary hyperhidrosis: efficacy and duration with repeated treatments. Dermatol Surg 2003; 29:545–548.

47. Baumann L, Slezinger A, Halem M, Vujevich J, et al. Pilot study of the safety and efficacy of Myobloc for treatment of axillary hyperhidrosis. Int J Dermatol 2005;44:418–424.

48. Hecht M, Birklein F, Winterholler M. Successful treatment of axillary hyperhidrosis with very low doses of botulinum toxin B: a pilot study. Arch Dermatol Res 2004;295:318–319.

49. Heckmann M, Teichmann B, Pause BM, Plewig G. Amelioration of body odor after intracutaneous axillary injection of botulinum toxin type A. Arch Dermatol 2003;139:57–59.

50. Heckmann M, Ceballos-Baumann AO, Plewig G. Botulinum toxin A for axillary hyperhidrosis. N Engl J Med 2001;344:488–493.

51. Galadari I, Alkaabi J. Botulinum toxin in the treatment of axillary hyperhidrosis. Skinmed 2003;2:209–211.

52. Hayton MJ, Stanley JK, Lowe NJ. A review of peripheral nerve blockade as local anesthesia of palmar hyperhidrosis. Br J Dermatol 2003;149:447–451.

53. Fujita M, Mann T, Mann O, Berg D. Surgical pearl: use of nerve blocks for botulinum toxin treatment of palmar–plantar hyperhidrosis. J Am Acad Dermatol 2001;45:587–589.

54. Trindade De Almeida AR, Kadung BV, Martins De Oliveira EM. Improving botulinum toxin therapy for palmar hyperhidrosis: wrist block and technical considerations. Dermatol Surg 2001;27:34–36.

## SUGGESTED FURTHER READING

Fujita M, Mann T, Mann O, Berg D. Surgical pearl: use of nerve blocks for botulinum toxin treatment of palmar-plantar hyperhidrosis. J Am Acad Dermatol 2001;45:587–589.

Leung AKC, Chan PYH, Choi MCK. Hyperhidrosis. Int J Dermatol 1999;38:561–567.

Lonsdale-Eccles A, Leonard N, Lawrence C. Axillary hyperhidrosis: eccrine or apocrine? Clin and Exp Dermatol 2003;28:2–7.

Naumann MK, Hamm H, Lowe N. Effect of botulinum toxin on quality of life measures in patients with excessive axillary sweating: a randomized controlled trial. Br J Dermatol 2002;147: 1218–1226.

# 12

# Urological Applications

## David E. Rapp and Gregory T. Bales

## INTRODUCTION

Botulism was first described in the early 19th century as a life-threatening, paralytic illness associated with sausage intake *(1)*. The botulinum toxin (BTX) was subsequently isolated in 1897 by van Ermengem and has been since identified as the most potent biological toxin known to exist *(2)*. In the last decades, BTX has emerged as a powerful therapy in the treatment of a variety of medical disorders. Certainly, the introduction of BTX within the field of urology has transformed the treatment of urological disorders. It can be argued that in no other medical specialty does BTX offer the promise for treatment of such a wide range of disorders.

BTXs are polypeptides produced by the facultative anaerobe *Clostridium botulinum*. Currently, seven toxin subtypes have been identified, designated as subtypes A, B, C, D, E, F, and G. Research has demonstrated that the parental form of BTXs are comprised of both a heavy- and light-chain component *(1)*. The heavy and light chains are connected through a disulfide bond interaction. Toxin action is thought to involve four steps *(1,3)*. The first step involves recognition and binding of the toxin with the presynaptic neuronal membrane, which is mediated by the toxin heavy chain. The toxin is then internalized and heavy- and light-chain separation occurs through cleavage of the disulfide bond. The light chain is then translocated into the cytosol, following which neurotransmitter release is inhibited through the action of the light chain. The specific mechanism of inhibition is thought to occur through toxin interaction and cleavage of specific vesical and target membrane proteins. Owing to the different toxin subtypes that are known to exist, and their corresponding light chains, different vesical and membrane proteins are targeted by the specific toxin subtypes (Table 1). Although the majority of early research focused on the toxin-induced somatic blockade of acetylcholine release, it is now clear that inhibition occurs in other neuronal populations as well (e.g., autonomic and sensory).

Currently, three commercial preparations of BTX are available for medical therapeutics. BTX type A (BTX-A) is available as Botox® (Allergan, Inc., Irvine, Ca) and Dysport® (Ipsen, Inc., Berkshire, United Kingdom). BTX-B is available as Myobloc® and Neurobloc® in the United States and Europe, respectively. Distinct differences exist between these available preparations (Table 1). In addition, in vitro data suggest that biochemical differences also exist between the various subtypes. For example, BTX-D is shown to effect an earlier inhibition of parasympathetic, as compared to somatic, neurotransmission *(4)*. In other investigations,

From: *Therapeutic Uses of Botulinum Toxin*
Edited by: G. Cooper © Humana Press Inc., Totowa, NJ

**Table 1**
**Protein Target and Commercial Preparations of Botulinum Toxin Subtypes**

| BTX subtype | Protein target | Commercial preparation | Molecular weight (kDa) | Preparation units | Formulation |
|---|---|---|---|---|---|
| BTX-A | SNAP-25 | Botox | 900 | 100 | Vacuum dried |
|  |  | Dysport | 900 | 500 | Lyophilized |
| BTX-B | VAMP | Myobloc | 700 | 2500/5000/10,000 | Solution |
| BTX-C | SNAP-25 | NA |  |  |  |
| BTX-D | VAMP | NA |  |  |  |
| BTX-E | SNAP-25 | NA |  |  |  |
| BTX-F | VAMP | NA |  |  |  |
| BTX-G | VAMP | NA |  |  |  |

Source: ref. *3.*
BTX, botulinum toxin; SNAP-25, synaptosomal-associated protein-25; VAMP, vesical-associated membrane protein.

BTX-A has shown the greatest potency for inhibition of sensory neurotransmission *(5)*. Finally, animal models demonstrate that Dysport and Myobloc preparations may be associated with a greater degree of diffusion and, for this reason, a higher incidence of systemic effects *(6)*. The clinical manifestations of these differences, if any, remain unknown. Despite the importance of research to better define the subtype differences, the vast majority of clinical urological research has used BTX-A. For this reason, this chapter focuses on BTX-A unless otherwise indicated.

This chapter reviews the use of BTX in the treatment of the broad group of urological disorders known as lower urinary tract (LUT) dysfunction. A brief overview of the diagnosis and evaluation of LUT dysfunction is provided. Further, a summary of the rationale behind and clinical experience with BTX is given for each urological disorder for which sufficient clinical experience exists. Finally, a broad discussion focuses on the clinical issues relevant to BTX administration, such as side effects and administration protocol.

## DIAGNOSIS AND EVALUATION OF LUT DYSFUNCTION

As discussed previously, clinical experience has been reported using BTX in the treatment of a wide range of urological disorders. A basic discussion of the pathophysiology underlying each disorder, and the rationale for BTX injection as a treatment modality, is given in the following sections. In general, these disorders are classified under the broad category of LUT dysfunction. This section provides a brief overview of the diagnosis and evaluation of patients with LUT dysfunction.

In the context of this text, the LUT is comprised of all portions of the urinary system excluding the kidneys and ureters. The majority of LUT dysfunction can be classified as disorders of urine storage versus elimination (micturition), and disorders of the bladder versus urinary tract outlet. An abbreviated table demonstrating examples of this classification is shown in Table 2, and focuses on those disorders discussed in this chapter. The different anatomical targets/injection sites corresponding to the various types of LUT dysfunction are shown in Fig. 1.

Despite the breadth of pathologies underlying the various types of LUT dysfunction, patients often present with a common constellation of symptoms. These symptoms most often include urgency, frequency, incontinence, or pain. Because of the broad differential that must be considered, patients presenting with these symptoms should undergo a broad work-up. The complete

**Table 2**
**Classification of Lower Urinary Tract Dysfunction**

| Anatomic dysfunction | Physiological dysfunction | |
| --- | --- | --- |
| | *Storage* | *Elimination* |
| Bladder | DO | Hypocontractility |
| | Sensory dysfuction | |
| Outlet | | BPH |
| | | DSD |

DO, detrusor overactivity; DH, detrusor hypocontractility; BPH, Benign prostatic hypertrophy; DSD, detrusor-sphincter dyssnergia.

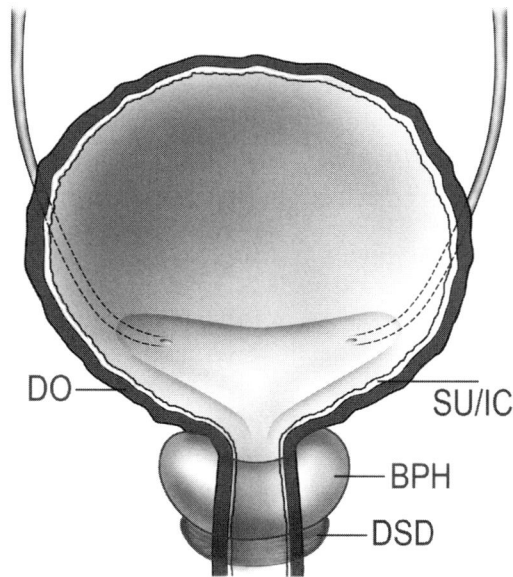

**Fig. 1.** Potential targets of botulinum toxin injection classified by urological disorder. DO, detrusor overactivity; IC, interstitial cystitis; SU, sensory urgency; BPH, benign prostatic hypertrophy; DSD, detrusor-sphincter dyssynergia.

algorithm for work-up of LUT dysfunction is beyond the scope of this chapter. However, an abbreviated description of important components to this diagnostic investigation is given.

### History and Physical Examination

A complete history and physical examination are crucial to the evaluation of LUT dysfunction. History should include a complete past medical history to evaluate for medical disease, surgical history, medications, and drug and alcohol intake that may contribute to urinary symptoms. In addition, a focused evaluation of urinary symptoms should be performed. For example, specific voiding symptoms should be detailed in an attempt to differentiate stress, urge, total, and mixed incontinence subtypes when applicable. The presence of frequency, urgency, and painful symptoms should also be addressed. Physical examination should include a routine survey, with specific focus on findings associated with neurological disease or previous surgery that may affect bladder function. Examples include spinal or lumbar abnormalities suggestive of spinal dysraphism. A female or male pelvic examination should be performed in all patients. Specific to female patients, this examination must include both a speculum and bimanual examination to evaluate for prolapse. Additionally, the Q-tip test may be used to evaluate for urethral hypermobility, in which a Q-tip is inserted into the urethra and mobility is assessed during valsalva *(7)*. The male pelvic examination should include a full external genitalia and perineal exam, in addition to digital rectal examination.

## Validated Questionnaires and Voiding Diary

The subjective nature of LUT dysfunction often makes assessment and follow-up difficult. As a result, clinicians and investigators often use validated questionnaires to assess both disease severity and related quality of life (QOL). These questionnaires not only aid the physician in the diagnosis of LUT dysfunction, but also allow them to use follow-up scores to assess treatment response and the need for further intervention. Designed by Shumaker et al., the incontinence impact questionnaire (IIQ) consists of 30 questions directed at four QOL areas (physical activity, social relationships, travel, and emotional health; ref. *8*). The same investigators designed the complementary urogenital distress inventory (UDI), created to assess the severity of incontinence-related symptoms *(8, 9)*. Short forms of both questionnaires (IIQ-7 and UDI-6) are available to make administration easier in the context of an office visit *(8)*. Additional study has been conducted using these questionnaires and both questionnaires have demonstrated significant correlation with other objective outcomes, such as pad test, volume of urine loss, and frequency severity *(10–12)*. A voiding diary is another simple method by which patients may document the severity of urinary symptoms. Data obtained via voiding diary may include volume voided, frequency of urination, time and number of incontinence episodes, and amount and type of fluid intake.

## The Pad Test

The pad test is another objective measure that may be used to identify the degree of urinary incontinence. A simple pad test may be performed by having a patient change incontinence pads every 6 hours and compare the wet weight with that of a dry, unused pad. Generally, each gram of wet weight difference corresponds to a urine loss of 1 mL. Conversely, pads can be examined for incontinence degree following administration of pyridium, which results in orange discoloration of urine. Many authors continue to advocate the use of pad tests as a diagnostic tool, given data suggesting that validated questionnaires may not demonstrate excellent validity in certain clinical situations *(13,14)*.

## Routine Urological Assessment

Routine urological assessment should include urinalysis and urine culture. Both of these studies are mandatory because urinary tract infection is a common cause of frequency, urgency, or incontinence. Serum creatinine should be used to evaluate renal function. Assessment of micturition is essential in the diagnostic work-up. Accordingly, uroflow offers a noninvasive method by which the urine flow rate is measured and can help to identify patients with outlet obstruction and/or detrusor hypocontractility. Further, measurement of postvoid residual (PVR) urine volume is essential to determine voiding ability and bladder capacity. PVR may be measured through noninvasive methods such as office sonography or via bladder catheterization following voiding.

## *Urodynamics*

Urodynamics is instrumental in the diagnosis of LUT dysfunction. In general, urodynamics consists of filling cystometry and voiding cystometry, in which pressure and flow parameters are measured during bladder filling and emptying. Accordingly, a physiological assessment of bladder function can be made. Detrusor spasticity during filling, poor bladder compliance, low bladder capacity, detrusor hypocontractility, and outlet obstruction are all examples of diagnoses that are made through urodynamic evaluation. Each of these pathologies may contribute to the urinary symptoms seen in patients with LUT dysfunction and are important to the subsequent discussion of outcomes following BTX injection. Most authors believe that urodynamic evaluation is mandatory before proceeding with more invasive surgical management, including BTX injection.

## *Cystourethroscopy*

Cystourethroscopy (CU) is not indicated in all patients with frequency, urgency, and incontinence. Hematuria on urinalysis should prompt CU. In addition, CU may be useful in patients with a history of previous pelvic, bladder, or urethral surgery to rule out the presence of scars, sutures, or other explainable etiologies of patient symptoms. In particular, male patients with a history of prostatectomy should undergo CU to rule out the possibility of stricture formation. Given that CU is performed in conjunction with BTX injection, we prefer to perform both in the same setting. In the advent of unexpected findings such as those listed previously, BTX injection is aborted.

# CLINICAL APPLICATION OF BTX IN THE TREATMENT OF LUT DYSFUNCTION

## *Detrusor–Sphincter Dyssynergia and Related Disorders*

### *Background*

The first reported urological application of BTX injection was in the treatment of detrusor–sphincter dyssynergia (DSD). Fundamental to the normal physiology of micturition is the coordinated relaxation of the external sphincter during bladder contraction and emptying. DSD is the contraction of the urinary sphincter simultaneously with voluntary or uninhibited involuntary contraction of the detrusor muscle. This phenomenon results in a functional bladder outflow obstruction, which can increase intravesical pressures and result in secondary bladder and renal damage.

Because of this risk, clean intermittent catheterization (CIC) has become central to the treatment of DSD in an effort to decrease bladder filling pressures. However, a portion of patients will be unable to perform catheterization or will continue to have deleterious bladder pressures despite catheterization. Following CIC failure, other alternatives are described that include sphincterotomy, transurethral prostatectomy, dorsal rhizotomy, and urethral stent placement *(15)*. Although these methods have demonstrated reasonable efficacy, their permanency makes them less desirable. BTX exists as an alternative that may produce a chemical dennervation of a transient nature, thereby allowing for assessment of clinical benefit, as well as for the undesired effect of incontinence, before permanent sphincter disruption. For example, the finding by Smith et al. of worsening or *de novo* stress incontinence in 4% of injected patients allows these patients the option of pursuing other treatment options following toxin reversal *(16)*.

Subsequent to initial experience in the treatment of DSD, the application of BTX was expanded to include other related pathologies. As opposed to the sphincteric obstruction seen in DSD, a number of neurogenic patients have difficulty voiding because of detrusor hypoactivity. The application of sphincteric BTX injection has been applied to these patients as well, in an attempt to decrease sphincteric resistance such that it may be overcome despite a dysfunctional detrusor muscle. In a similar fashion, BTX injection has now been used in cases of overt urinary retention.

*Clinical Investigation (Table 3)*

In 1988, Dykstra and colleagues utilized external urethral sphincter injection of BTX in 11 patients with DSD resultant from spinal cord injury *(17)*. Evidence of sphincter chemodenervation was seen using electromyography (EMG), which corresponded to subjective and objective improvement in most patients. Objective improvement was seen in parameters including PVR, urethal pressure profile, and incidence of autonomic dysreflexia. Toxin effects lasted an average of 50 days.

Subsequent to this initial report, a number of small studies have confirmed the efficacy of sphincter chemodenervation in the treatment of DSD. Schurch et al. used BTX sphincter injection in the treatment of 24 patients with DSD *(19)*. These authors demonstrated an 88% response rate, with objective improvements in maximum urethral pressure and mean urethral sphincter pressure. In addition, complete disappearance of DSD was seen in one-third of the patients. Additional studies have demonstrated similar subjective and objective improvement in outcome parameters following BTX injection (Table 3).

As discussed previously, the indications for urethral/sphincter injection of BTX have expanded to include a variety of related disorders. Kuo evaluated the use of sphincteric injection of BTX (50 U) in 20 patients with detrusor hypocontractility *(21)*. Seven (35%) of these patients voided with straining, while the remaining patients required indwelling or clean intermittent catheterization. Following injection, 11 of 13 patients in retention were able to void using valsalva alone. An overall decrease in PVR, mean urethral closing pressure (UCP), and increased QOL scores were demonstrated. This experience expands the use of BTX to patients whose primary disorder relates to bladder hypocontractility, in contrast to those patients suffering from primary DSD.

Kuo presented an expanded cohort of 103 patients with LUT dysfunction of multiple etiologies *(22)*. LUT dysfunction was defined as severely difficult urination, large residual volumes, or chronic urinary retention. Underlying etiologies included DSD, dysfunctional voiding, nonrelaxing urethral sphincter, cauda equina lesion, peripheral neuropathy, and detrusor underactivity. Following urethral injection of BTX (50 or 100 U), 85% of patients demonstrated subjective improvement. In addition, 87% of those patients requiring CIC or indwelling catheterization were able to discontinue these interventions 4 weeks post-operatively. These outcomes were accompanied by decreased voiding pressures, UCP, and PVR in the vast majority of patients.

Additionally, Phelan et al. investigated the efficacy of sphincteric injection of BTX in an expanded cohort that included patients with pelvic floor spasticity *(23)*. In this investigation, 21 patients with DSD, pelvic floor spasticity, or detrusor hypocontractility were treated with sphincteric toxin injection (80 or 100 U). Following injection, 17 of 19 patients requiring CIC pre-operatively were able to void spontaneously. Only one patient was considered a treatment failure, with the remaining patient electing to continue CIC secondary to a lack of home social support.

**Table 3**
**Clinical Outcomes in Patients Undergoing Urethral Injection of BTX-A in the Treatment of Detrusor-Sphincter Dyssynergia and Related Disorders**

| Reference | Diagnosis pt. (no.) | Dose (U) | Subjective outcome | Objective outcome | Effect duration[a] months (range) |
|---|---|---|---|---|---|
| 17 | DSD | 11 | 20–240[b,c] | Decreased AD Imp PVR, UPP | 2 |
| 18 | DSD | 5 | 140–240[c] | Decreased AD Imp PVR, UPP | 3 |
| 19 | DSD | 24 | 100/250[c,d] | No Δ AD Imp UP, DSD | 2–3/9–12 |
| 20 | DSD | 5 | 100 | Decreased AD, 40% able to dc cath Imp VP, no Δ PVR | 3 (3–5) |
| 3 | DSD | 16 | 100[c] | Imp UDI, bladder perception scores Imp freq, urg, leaks, PVR | 3–6 |
| 16 | DSD+ | 68 | 100–200 | Imp cath req (60 to 12%) Imp VP, PVR | 6 |
| 21 | DSD+ | 20 | 50 | 55% voiding by valsalva alone, imp QOL Imp VP, UCP, PVR | 3 |
| 22 | DSD+ | 103 | 50–100 | Sx improvement (85%), 87% able to discontinue catheterization Imp VP, UCP, PVR | 4 (2–6) |
| 23 | DSD+ | 21 | 80–100 | 17 of 19 patients able to discontinue CIC Imp VP, PVR | NA |
| 24 | DSD+ | 17 | 150 | Dec cath freq Imp VP, no Δ PVR | 2–5 |

BTX-A, botulinum toxin type A; DSD, detrusor-sphinter dyssynergia; DSD+, DSD and related disorders (e.g., hypocontractility); AD, autonomic dysreflexia; PVR, post void residual; UPP, urethral pressure profile; VP, voiding pressure; Freq, frequency; Urg, uregency; UDI, urinary distress inventory; CIC, clean intermittent catheterization; QOL, quality of life; UCP, urethral closing pressure; Imp, improved.

[a]Duration in some investigations limited by short-term study follow-up.
[b]Three different protocols using Botox or Dysport.
[c]Protocol using repeat injections.
[d]Three different protocols used.

*Section Conclusion*

These data suggest that BTX injection is efficacious in the treatment of DSD, detrusor hypocontractility, and related disorders. Despite the variety of injection doses and protocols reported, sphincter injection induces durable improvements to PVR, UCP, and bladder pressures. Subjective improvements are associated in the majority of studies, including decreased CIC requirements, improved incontinence episodes, and decreased autonomic dysreflexia. Long-term study of functional bladder and upper tract outcomes is needed. Furthermore, additional investigations, including randomized and controlled trials with larger number of patients need to be undertaken. Nonetheless, sphincteric toxin injections would appear to offer a reversible surgical option that may protect patients from urinary tract damage and allow clinicians to assess response in anticipation of repeat toxin injection or more permanent surgical options.

## Neurogenic and Idiopathic Detrusor Overactivity

### Background

To date, one of the most widespread urological applications of BTX has been in the treatment of detrusor overactivity (DO). DO is implicated as a major pathology underlying urge urinary incontinence and urgency–frequency syndromes. In a general sense, the constellation of symptoms including urgency, frequency, and incontinence is referred to as overactive bladder (OAB). It is currently believed that OAB symptoms may result from a variety of underlying pathologies. One of these, DO, is defined as the presence of uninhibited bladder contractions during bladder filling, as demonstrated on urodynamic evaluation. When seen in association with symptoms of urgency or incontinence, a diagnosis of DO is confirmed.

In a portion of patients with DO, neurogenic dysfunction can be identified as the underlying pathology and is therefore classified as neurogenic DO (NDO). Examples of neurological impairment include spinal cord lesions, stroke, multiple sclerosis, Parkinson's disease, and dementia. In other cases, no demonstrable neurological impairment can be identified. Accordingly, the disorder is classified as non-neurogenic or idiopathic DO (IDO). Other defects, such as detrusor myocyte hyperactivity, have been suggested as possible etiologies in these patients who have no underlying neurological dysfunction (25). However, the exact etiology of IDO is currently unknown.

Finally, symptoms of frequency, urgency, and incontinence may occur in the absence of demonstrable DO despite these patients having equally severe urinary symptoms. In contrast to the motor overactivity characteristic of DO, it is possible in these cases that an underlying sensory neuron dysfunction exists. Although this theory is not definitively proven, many of these patients are diagnosed with sensory urgency (SU) and urgency–frequency syndrome. The role of BTX in the treatment of bladder sensory dysfunction is discussed later.

Anticholinergic therapy is currently the first-line treatment for patients with DO. Despite the success seen using anticholinergic therapy, a significant number of patients fail to respond to treatment (26,27). Further, anticholinergic side effects are significant and result in the discontinuation of therapy in a substantial number of patients (27). Invasive surgical intervention (e.g., sacral nerve stimulation, bladder augmentation) may be offered to a subset of treatment failures. However, it is clear that other less invasive therapies are needed in the treatment of these disorders. Accordingly, BTX injection emerged as a potential treatment option that could theoretically decrease bladder spasticity through a partial inhibition of the detrusor muscle.

### Clinical Investigation, NDO (Table 4)

Stohrer et al. reported the first use of BTX in the treatment of NDO (28). The expanded results of the abstract were reported 1 year later (30). The authors treated 21 patients suffering from NDO resultant from spinal cord injury with 200 to 300 U BTX. At 6-week follow-up 17 of 19 (89%) patients were completely continent. In addition, urodynamic evaluation revealed increased mean reflex volume (MRV), increased maximum bladder capacity (MBC), and decreased detrusor voiding pressures. Of the 11 responders available for 36-week follow-up, all demonstrated continued improvement over baseline. Minor incontinence episodes were reported in four of these responders.

In the largest analysis to date, Reitz et al. report the results of a European multi-center, retrospective analysis of 200 patients receiving BTX injection of the detrusor muscle in the treatment of neurogenic incontinence owing to spinal cord injury/disease *(32)*. Urodynamic evaluation at 12 weeks following injection revealed decreased mean cystometric bladder capacity and MRV, and increased mean bladder compliance. Continued urodynamic improvement was seen at 36-week follow-up. A significant reduction/cessation of anticholinergic medications was possible in the majority of patients.

Additional experience was reported by Schulte-Baukloh and associates, who injected 20 children failing anticholinergic therapy and CIC in the treatment of NDO *(33)*. Significant improvement in reflex volume, uninhibited detrusor contractions, maximal detrusor pressure, bladder capacity, and compliance was demonstrated 4 weeks following injection. Continued improvement was seen through 3-month follow-up, however, at 6-month follow-up most end points failed to demonstrate statistically significant improvement over baseline values.

Schurch et al. recently reported the results of the first multi-center, placebo-controlled trial using BTX in the treatment of NDO of spinal cord origin *(31)*. Fifty-nine patients with NDO requiring CIC were randomized to receive BTX (200 or 300 U) or placebo (saline). Patients were followed over a 24-week period with subjective and urodynamic evaluation. A statistically significant reduction in the primary study end point, incontinence episodes, was established in both treatment arms and persisted through the study conclusion. In addition, improvement in urodynamic outcomes was seen in both study groups throughout the study. Improvement in the mean QOL total scores was also observed. In contrast, no statistically significant difference in subjective or objective end points over baseline was demonstrated for the placebo arm.

*Clinical Investigation, IDO/OAB (Table 4)*

Far fewer data exists to investigate the role of BTX in the treatment of IDO or in a generalized OAB population. At the University of Chicago, we evaluated the clinical outcomes of BTX injection in 35 patients with refractory symptoms of frequency, urgency, and/or urge incontinence, who had failed treatment with anticholinergic medication *(36)*. Using our reported technique (*see* "Injection Technique"), 300 U BTX was injected throughout the trigone, bladder base, and lateral walls. Patients were evaluated at 3 weeks and 6 months after treatment by completion of the IIQ-7 and UDI-6, as well as questions assessing global response to the treatment.

After 3 weeks, statistically significant reductions in the mean IIQ-7 and mean UDI-6 scores were demonstrated. Overall, 60% (21 of 35) of patients reported complete (34%) or slight (26%) improvement of voiding symptoms after 3 weeks. Among initial responders followed for 6 months, continued, though diminished, improvements to the mean IIQ-7 and UDI-6 symptom scores were seen.

In their analysis of 110 patients undergoing BTX injection in the treatment of urological disorders, Smith et al. report 42 patients receiving intravesical toxin injection. Of these patients, 17 (40%) were enrolled for treatment of IDO *(16)*. Intravesical injection of BTX resulted in a decreased number of patients requiring pad use, decreased micturition frequency per 24-hour period, and increased cystometric capacity. Although no specific subset analysis is presented in this report, the authors state that similar response ratios were seen when comparing the nonneurogenic and neurogenic cohorts.

Rajkumar et al. conducted a prospective evaluation of 15 women with IDO receiving a single dose of 300 U BTX-A via intradetrusor injection *(35)*. In this analysis, symptomatic and urodynamics were evaluated at baseline, 6 weeks, and every 4 weeks thereafter until return to baseline values were reached. Symptomatic improvement was seen in 14 of 15 patients. In

**Table 4**
**Clinical Outcomes in Patients Undergoing Bladder Injection of BTX-A in the Treatment of Detrusor Overactivity**

| Reference | Diagnosis pt. (no.) | Dose (U) | Subjective outcome | Objective outcome | Effect duration[a] months (range) |
|---|---|---|---|---|---|
| 29 | NDO | 15 | 300 TS | 87% cont, 13% minor leakage Improved MDP, MBC | 7 (4–12) |
| 30 | NDO | 21 | 2–300 TS | 89% cont at 6 wk Improved MBC, MRV, DVP | 9 |
| 31 | NDO | 59 | 2–300 TS | Improved cont Improved MBC, MRV, MDP | 24 wk |
| 32 | NDO | 200 | 300 TS | Improved cont, reduced AC Improved MBC, MRV, DVP | 9 |
| 33 | NDO | 20 | 300 (max) TS | Improved cont Improved MBC, MRV, MDP | 6 |
| 34 | NDO | 10 | 3–400 NA | Improved cont Improved MRV, MBC, MDP | 3+ |
| 35 | IDO | 15 | 300 TS | Improved freq, urg, BFLUTS/KHQ score Improved MBC, DO, VFD | 6 (2–12) |
| 3 | IDO/OAB | 18 | 300 T | Improved leakage, freq, urg, IIQ, UDI NA | 3–6 |
| 36 | IDO/OAB | 35 | 300 T | Improved leakage, freq, urg, IIQ, UDI NA | 6 |
| 16 | Mixed | 42 | 1–300 T | Pad use in 93% → 12% Improved MBC | 3–6 |
| 37 | Mixed | 22 | 300 TS | Improved freq, urg, pad use Improved MBC, compliance, MDP | 5 (1–7) |
| 38 | Mixed | 75 | 2–300 TS | Improved freq, urg, pad use Improved MBC, MDP | 4 |

T, trigone; TS, trigone-sparing, NDO, neurogenic detrusor overactivity; IDO, idiopathic detrusor overactivity; OAB, overactive bladder; AC, anticholinergics; Cont, continent; Freq, frequency; Urg, urgency; IIQ, incontinence impact questionnaire; UDI, urinary distress inventory; BFLUTS, Bristol female lower urinary tract questionnaire; KHQ, King's health questionnaire; MDP, maximum detrusor pressure; MBC, maximum bladder capacity; MRV, mean reflex volume; DVP, detrusor voiding pressure; VFD, volume at first desire.

[a]Duration in some investigations limited by short-term study follow-up.

addition, improvement in volume at first desire to void, MBC, and absence of DO was seen in 13, 10, and 6 patients, respectively. This data providing urodynamic response rates is particularly important because most studies express objective response as mean improvement to specific urodynamic parameters, which makes counseling patients on the likelihood of response difficult.

*Clinical Investigation of DO, Comparative Study*

Owing to the more recent application of BTX injection in the treatment of IDO, very few studies exist to compare toxin efficacy between NDO and IDO cohorts. Kessler and colleagues conducted a prospective analysis of 22 patients with NDO or IDO in an attempt to compare treatment response following BTX injection *(37)*. Subjective improvement, as measured by bladder diary and patient satisfaction survey, and urodynamic outcomes were assessed. Both cohorts demonstrated a statistically significant improvement in subjective (median daytime frequency, nocturia, and pad use) as well as objective (MBC and mean bladder compliance) parameters. No significant difference in clinical and urodynamic outcomes was observed between NDO and IDO cohorts.

Popat et al. performed a prospective evaluation of 44 patients receiving BTX injection in the treatment of neurogenic (300 U) or idiopathic (200 U) DO *(38)*. At both 4 and 16 weeks following therapy, significant improvements in urodynamic and LUT symptom parameters were observed in both groups. Comparison of percent change in clinical parameters revealed a greater improvement in urinary frequency in the NDO cohort. However, all other parameters revealed no statistically significant difference between the cohorts, leading the authors to conclude that patients with refractory IDO and NDO respond similarly to toxin injection despite differing disease etiology and injection dose.

Comparative investigation has also sought to determine the efficacy of BTX injection in comparison to other agents used in the treatment algorithm of DO. Giannantoni et al. compared the efficacy of BTX injection versus intravesical instillation of resiniferatoxin *(39)*. A total of 25 patients were randomized to receive BTX injection of 300 U or 0.6 µM resiniferatoxin in the treatment of NDO. Both cohorts demonstrated significant improvement in catheterization frequency and incontinence episodes, volume at first detrusor contraction, and MBC at 6, 12, and 18 months following treatment. However, BTX injection demonstrated superior results with respect to these clinical and urodynamic outcomes.

*Section Conclusion*

Intradetrusor BTX injections offers a viable option in patients with DO/OAB failing medical therapy. Durable improvements in objective parameters such as MBC, MRV, and detrusor voiding pressure are consistently seen in reported study. Further, subjective improvement is consistent with respect to improved urgency and incontinence. Toxin effects seem to begin within several weeks and last approximately 6 months. Continued investigation is needed to better define the optimal injection protocol and dose.

### Sensory Disorders/Interstitial Cystitis/Pelvic Pain Disorders

*Background and Laboratory Investigation*

The inhibitory effect of BTX on the motor end plate with resultant muscle relaxation provided the rationale behind the first urological applications in the treatment of detrusor muscle and external sphincter spasticity. However, a large amount of in vitro data suggests that BTX also has an inhibitory effect on the afferent innervation of the bladder. Concurrently, a significant amount of basic science research has suggested a large role of sensory neurons in the pathophysiology of the subset of OAB thought to suffer from sensory neuron dysfunction (SU and urgency–frequency syndrome) (discussed previously; refs. *40* and *41*). Further, research supports that neuronal actions may act as possible mediators of interstitial cystitis (IC) *(42)*. The etiology of IC, a debilitating condition most commonly associated with bladder and pelvic pain, is poorly understood. Despite this limitation, significant research suggests that this disorder resembles a non-traumatic, non-infectious inflammation that may result, in part, from neuron-induced inflammation *(43)*. Combined, these data tend to support the extended application of BTX in patients with sensory bladder dysfunction and IC.

An inhibitory action of BTX-A on pain sensation has been supported by several experiments. BTX-A has been shown to inhibit the calcium-dependent release of the nociceptive neurotransmitter, substance P, from rat dorsal root ganglion neurons in primary culture *(5)*. In this experiment, BTX subtypes A, B, C, and F were used, with BTX-A demonstrating the greatest potency for inhibition of the sensory neurons. Inhibition of substance P by BTX subtypes correlated with cleavage of their respective BTX substrate proteins (e.g., synaptosomal-associated protein-25 for BTX-A). This finding suggests that inhibition may occur through a similar mechanism as that observed during inhibition of motor neurons at the neuromuscular junction. Finally, investigation of the temporal effects of BTX-A demonstrated that onset of inhibition required 4 hours and was maintained throughout the experiment duration of 15 hours.

Pre-treatment with BTX-A decreases formalin-induced pain in rat hindpaw that is associated with a decrease in neurotransmitter release from primary afferent terminals *(44)*. These authors also demonstrated the inhibition of formalin-induced glutamate release. This finding is particularly noteworthy because glutamate release may be an important mediator of sensory neuron activity through purinergic signaling mechanisms.

Recently, research has focused on BTX-A-induced inhibition of bladder sensation. Vemulakonda et al. reported a significant decrease in the level of *c-fos* expression following intravesical BTX-A instillation in a rat model of chronic bladder inflammation *(45)*. The *c-fos* gene, and resultant protein, are associated with the cellular stress response and are thought to be important mediators of inflammation. In addition, Chuang and colleages demonstrated that BTX-A application increases bladder tissue calcitonin gene-related peptide (CGRP) immunoreactivity in an acetic acid-induced bladder pain model *(46)*. CGRP is a sensory neurotransmitter that is widely used as a measure of sensory neuron activity. The sensory afferent axons of the bladder are the only structures within the bladder that contains high levels of CGRP, suggesting a role for this peptide in bladder sensation *(47)*. Consistent with this hypothesis, CGRP is released from isolated sensory neurons by agonists that cause pain in human and animal models *(48)*. The data reported by Chuang et al. indirectly suggest that BTX may decrease CGRP release, thereby inhibiting sensory neuron signaling.

Based on this background, we developed a rat model to determine the effect of BTX-A on basal and chemically evoked release of CGRP from an isolated bladder preparation *(49)*. Using this model, retained sensory afferent innervation to the bladder was chemically stimulated and the effect of BTX-A on both basal and stimulated sensory neuron activity was measured. BTX-A application resulted in a 19% reduction in basal release of CGRP; however, this difference did not achieve statistical significance. BTX-A application significantly reduced chemically stimulated CGRP by 62% versus control ($p < 0.005$).

This in vitro data using animal models has been reinforced by recent investigation utilizing human tissue. Apostolidis and associates investigated the possible effect of BTX-A on expression of the sensory receptors, TRPV1 and P2X$_3$, in bladder biopsy specimens obtained from patients with both NDO and IDO undergoing BTX-A injection *(50)*. Expressed primarily by sensory neurons, previous experiments have suggested a role for these receptors in bladder sensory signal transduction and, further, that increased expression of these receptors is present in patients suffering from NDO *(51,52)*. These authors found that decreased levels of both receptors were present at 4 and 16 weeks following injection and that decreased receptor expression correlated with both symptomatic and urodynamic improvements at these time-points.

*Clinical Investigation*

To date, there are no published reports specifically evaluating the effect of BTX on SU. Zermann and associates demonstrated decreased frequency and increased bladder capacity in the majority of patients undergoing BTX injection in the treatment of urgency–frequency syndrome *(53)*. More recently, Flynn et al. investigated the effect of BTX in seven patients with severe urge urinary incontinence *(54)*. The authors sought to evaluate outcomes in a cohort of subjects with urge incontinence resulting from IDO. Accordingly, evidence of stress urinary incontinence and underlying neurological disorder were used as exclusion criteria. Despite the use of pre-operative urodynamic evaluation, the presence of DO was not used as a specific inclusion criterion and no discussion of this patient parameter is made. Accordingly, it may be possible that a percentage of the included patients suffered incontinence resulting from underlying SU as opposed to DO. This study demonstrated a significant reduction in incontinence episodes, 24-hour pad weight, subjective symptom scores, and urodynamic outcomes.

Similarly, our investigation of a broad group of patients suffering from symptoms of OAB likely included patients having underlying sensory dysfunction. In this investigation (detailed previously), we sought to evaluate subjective outcomes in a broad group of patients with symptoms of frequency, urgency, and incontinence. Pre-operative urodynamic evaluation was not included in the study protocol. Accordingly, it is likely that this cohort included not only patients with NDO and IDO, but also those with sensory disorder. In this study, a 60% response rate was seen. Despite these outcomes, it is evident that further investigation focused on bladder disorders of sensory origin is needed.

Other investigation has evaluated the effect of BTX injection in the treatment of IC and has demonstrated contrasting results. Rackley et al. report the use of intravesical injection versus instillation of BTX (200 U) in the treatment of 10 patients with IC. Instillation of BTX was performed using 200 U diluted in 60 mL saline *(3)*. Retrospective analysis of patient outcomes revealed that neither group experienced a statistically significant change in objective or subjective outcome measures. Smith et al. presented the results of a multi-institutional case series examining the efficacy of intravesical Botox or Dysport injection in 13 patients with refractory IC *(55)*. Of these patients, 69% reported subjective improvement in disease symptoms following treatment, lasting a mean of almost 4 months.

## Benign Prostatic Hypertrophy

*Background and Clinical Investigation*

Interest in BTX injection for the treatment of benign prostatic hypertrophy (BPH) was based on animal models demonstrating that intraprostatic toxin injection resulted in denervation and gland atrophy *(56)*. In addition, the localization of muscarinic receptors on prostatic epithelial cells and the parasympathetic actions of neurons associated with the prostate suggest that BTX may block some of these functions *(57)*. Whether this blockade results in local relaxation, glandular atrophy, or some other clinically applicable effect remains undefined.

Only two reported studies have investigated the role of BTX injection in the treatment of BPH. Maria et al. conducted a randomized, placebo-controlled study in the treatment of 30 patients with voiding dysfunction resulting from BPH *(56)*. Inclusion criteria included an American Urological Association (AUA) symptom score of at least 8, mean peak flow rate less than 16 mL per second, and an enlarged prostate gland on DRE. Of note, patients did not undergo routine pre-operative urodynamic study to confirm outlet obstruction. Patients were randomized to receive intraprostatic injection of BTX-A (200 U) or saline and assessment of outcomes was performed at 1 and 2 months following injection. At 1 month, improved AUA symptom score, PVR, and peak urinary flow rate were seen following BTX but not saline injection. In addition, a decrease in prostate volume and PSA by 54 and 42% were observed, respectively. Further improvements in all parameters were observed in the treatment arm at 2 months.

Kuo and colleagues performed intraprostatic injection of BTX in 10 patients with BPH who were poor candidates for surgery because of comorbid disease *(57)*. All patients underwent pre-operative urodynamic evaluation, confirming high voiding pressures in combination with a low urinary flow rate. A total of 200 U BTX was injected into the prostate transitional zone at 10 sites. At 3 months, improved voiding detrusor pressure, maximal flow rate, PVR, and total prostate volume were seen. Subjective improvement was seen in all patients, with 80% reporting excellent results. Interestingly, compared with the overall reduction in prostate volume, the transitional zone index remained unchanged following injection.

Despite the promising findings observed in these investigations, several questions remain. The observed reduction in prostate volume is particularly noteworthy and suggests that local neuronal innervation may directly or indirectly regulate prostate growth. Conversely, it is possible that BTX may have a toxic effect on prostatic tissue. In addition, it remains possible that the clinical benefit observed may result not secondary to decreased prostate size, but rather from sphincter relaxation or a combination of the two actions. Such information is of significant clinical relevance. If the clinical effects observed result from a reduction in prostate size, it may confer a heightened treatment response to patients with larger prostate size. Further, it may be advantageous to continue α-adrenergic blockade following BTX injection to concomittently induce sphincteric relaxation. A notable limitation to BTX application in the treatment of BPH is the clinical utility of this therapy. Because of the high cost of BTX and the efficacy of current surgical therapy (e.g., transurethral resection of prostate), BTX injection should currently remain a treatment choice only in patients who are poor surgical candidates. Certainly, additional long-term investigation is needed to better define the efficacy and mechanism of BTX action in the treatment of BPH.

## BTX-B in the Treatment of Urological Disorders

Far less investigation has focused on the use of BTX-B in the treatment of urological disorders. BTX-A has been the predominant subtype used in urological disorders, presumptively owing to a greater experience with this subtype in other disorders and its greater potency. However, toxin resistance may develop and be an underlying cause for treatment failure. The development of anti-toxin antibodies is known to occur and has been proposed to potentially underlie the development of resistance *(58)*. This data served as one rationale for the investigation of BTX-B in the treatment of urological disorders. Owing to the different molecular target of subtypes A and B, it is possible that antibody development to type A may not confer resistance against type B. However, in vitro study in patients treated with BTX-A has demonstrated the development of antibodies that are cross-reactive to subtype B despite never receiving BTX-B injection *(59)*. Based on this data, the role of BTX-B in the primary treatment of bladder overactivity and/or its role in BTX-A treatment failures has been the focus of recent research.

The first urological application of BTX-B was reported by Dykstra et al. in 2003. In this case report, the authors treated one patient with DO resulting from multiple sclerosis *(60)*. Treatment consisted of two separate intradetrusor injections of 5000 and 7500 U BTX-B. An immediate treatment response was demonstrated and the patient was able to discontinue CIC. A second injection was performed following symptom recurrence and resulted in similar outcomes. The authors report that treatment duration appears to last 4 months.

Based on these results, Dystra et al. expanded their experience to 15 patients with OAB. This investigation was performed as a dose-escalation study, using intradetrusor injection of BTX-B (range 2500 to 15,000 U; ref. *61*). A treatment response rate of 93% (14 of 15) was observed, defined as decreased frequency, urgency, and absence of incontinence. A decrease in frequency (by a mean of 5.27 episodes per day) was seen following treatment and the response degree was not dose-dependent. In contrast, duration of response demonstrated a significant correlation with injection dose. Using the 10,000- and 15,000-U doses, a response duration of approximately 3 months was seen.

Simultaneous case reports by Reitz et al. and Pistolesi et al. described the first urological applications of BTX-B in patients resistant to BTX-A *(58,62)*. In total, three patients who failed to demonstrate subjective and objective improvement to intradetrusor injection of BTX-A were accrued. Resistance to BTX-A was established through the extensor digitorum brevis test, in which electrophysiological testing of muscle action potentials demonstrated no response following injection of BTX-A *(63)*. Following injection of BTX-B, subjective and urodynamic improvement was observed in all patients and appeared to last 6 months.

Recently, Ghei et al. published the first prospective randomized crossover study of BTX-B injection for refractory DO *(64)*. Twenty patients with urodynamic evidence of DO were randomized to receive intradetrusor injection of BTX-B (5000 U) or placebo. A crossover injection was then performed at 6 weeks without washout. Significant differences were found between the two treatment arms and in comparison to baseline with respect to the primary study outcome, average voided volume, and weekly incontinence and frequency. Improvement in several subjective domains on QOL assessment was also seen. However, the duration of effect was reported as approximately 6 weeks.

*Section Conclusions*

The results of these combined investigations suggest that BTX-B may have a role in the treatment of urological disorders. However, significant issues remain. Foremost, the short duration of action seen by Ghei (6 weeks) would suggest that BTX-A, which generally achieves durable responses of at least 6 months, may be a more useful therapy in the generalized patient population. Accordingly, the utility of BTX-B may be limited to those patients resistant to BTX-A or those experiencing an adverse response to BTX-A injection. The question then becomes, in what patient is BTX-B injection appropriate? It is unclear whether all patients failing to respond to BTX-A should be viewed as candidates for BTX-B. Other experts believe that only patients initially responding to BTX-A and then developing suspected resistance should be considered *(65)*. In addition, it is unclear what criteria should be used to demonstrate BTX-A resistance. Most would argue that treatment failure following BTX-A is not sufficient to demonstrate resistance. However, is treatment failure after prior response sufficient to demonstrate resistance or are more invasive diagnostics, such as electrophysiological testing, necessary in all patients before considering BTX-B injection? Although the literature regarding the urological application of BTX-B suggests that it offers promise as a treatment modality, a significant amount of research is needed to better elucidate these issues.

## CLINICAL ISSUES RELATED TO BTX INJECTION

### Injection Duration

As discussed previously, the action of BTX is thought to result from toxin-induced inhibition of neurotransmitter release. This information is of particular importance because the specific mechanism and duration of the local toxin effects may provide data relevant to the anticipated clinical response. Histological evidence suggests that toxin injection is followed by a chemical denervation, which is followed by re-sprouting of axons *(66,67)*. In contrast, the muscular integrity is not altered following intradetrusor injection *(68)*. Axonal re-sprouting is variable, accruing over weeks to months *(66,67)*. However, Haferkamp et al. found that only three of seven biopsy specimens demonstrated axonal sprouting at 9 months following injection *(68)*. Despite this finding, symptom benefit has been generally shown to subside by this time point, suggesting that axonal sprouting may not relate to duration of effect.

Contrasting histological data suggests that the local action of intradetrusor BTX injection may affect a functional inhibition that is not associated with neuronal death. Apostolidis and associates demonstrated through immunohistochemistry evaluation that neuronal density within bladder biopsy specimens was not significantly reduced at 4 and 16 weeks following toxin injection *(50)*. Bladder neuronal density was measured through the use of the pan-neuronal marker PGP9.5-IR. This effect was observed despite a reduced expression of the sensory neuron receptors TRPV1 and $P2X_3$, and a corresponding clinical benefit seen in the patients. Again, this data is particularly important because the time required for neuronal recovery after functional inhibition versus that required for neuronal regeneration following cell death may relate to durability of clinical effect.

Combined, these data underscore the need for further research to better define the exact mechanism of toxin-induced neuronal inhibition and how these structural effects relate to duration of clinical response. Further, it is possible that the duration of both structural and clinical effects may relate to other factors, such as differing toxin subtypes (e.g., A versus B) and/or different neuronal population targets (e.g., somatic versus autonomic).

Irrespective of these factors, the clinical benefit of intradetrusor BTX injection appears to last at least 6 months. Shurch and colleagues reported a duration of at least 9 months in their initial experience. Subsequent to this study, most authors have reported a duration range of 6 to 9 months (Table 4). The duration and efficacy of repeat injections is discussed subsequently. Certainly, the duration of treatment effect may be affected by injection protocol and dose. Further study is needed to better define the protocol and dose resulting in optimal treatment efficacy and duration, while minimizing side effect profile. However, we believe that it is appropriate to counsel patients that the treatment effect may last approximately 6 months.

In contrast to intradetrusor injection, it appears that the clinical effect of sphincteric injection may have a shorter duration. Treatment duration following sphincteric injection varies in the reported studies to date. In general, a response duration of 1 to 5 months is seen (Table 3).

Although no direct, single-study comparisons of intradetrusor and sphincteric injection are reported, some conclusions may be drawn from those authors with reported experience using both techniques. Schurch et al. report that the duration of detrusor paresis was at least 9 months, as compared with 3 to 4 months observed with a single sphincter injection *(30)*. In contrast, Smith et al. report that a treatment response of at least 6 months was seen in patients undergoing both urethral and bladder injection of BTX *(16)*. Further study is needed to determine whether treatment duration truly differs between the urethral and bladder injection techniques. Based on available data, it appears appropriate to counsel patients that injection duration will likely last approximately 3 months or more.

### Treatment Onset

It is difficult to define the exact onset of treatment response given the available literature. Foremost, most investigations define treatment onset based on subjective response. As such, it is often difficult for patients to define a specific time when clinical improvement began. Larger studies are then subject to significant interpatient variation and recall bias. In contrast, objective outcomes, as demonstrated by urodynamic evaluation, are often not performed until 4 to 6 weeks following therapy. For these reasons, most reported studies do not include data regarding treatment onset.

Smith et al. reported that maximal efficacy was seen between 7 and 30 days following intradetrusor and sphincteric injection of BTX *(16)*. Time to maximal efficacy was defined using patient interview conducted via telephone consultation or during clinic visit. In our investigation of 35 patients undergoing bladder injection of BTX for treatment of OAB, patient questionnaires included specific items assessing time to first and time to maximal symptom improvement *(36)*. Among those patients reporting slight or complete symptom improvement after 3 weeks, patients first noted an improvement to their symptoms at a range of 1 to 14 days (mean 5.3) postoperatively and described reaching the maximal symptom improvement at 2 to 20 days (mean 8.3) postoperatively.

### Repeat Injection

There is one investigation to date specifically designed to evaluate the efficacy of BTX in patients undergoing repeat injection. Grosse and colleagues reported 66 patients undergoing repeat BTX injection (Botox, 300 U; Dysport, 750 U) in the treatment of neurogenic urinary tract dysfunction *(69)*. All patients underwent one repeat injection, with a portion undergoing as many as six repeat injections. The interval between injections was approximately 10 months through the fourth injection. No difference was seen when comparing the difference between these intervals (injection 1 to 2, 2 to 3, 3 to 4). Major improvement of subjective satisfaction was seen in 71% of patients undergoing repeat injection and was comparable to the 74% rate observed following the initial injection. Major satisfaction percent increased to 96 and 89% in those undergoing a second and third repeat injection, respectively. This finding is not surprising as only one-half and one-fourth of patients underwent these injections, respectively, and were presumptively those who exhibited a significant response to the initial injections. Urodynamic improvement in cystometric capacity and reflex volume were seen through the measured endpoint of the third injection, although comparison was only conducted with baseline values.

Repeat injection is also reported in other studies. Smith et al. reported 27 patients undergoing repeat injection at intervals of 6 months or longer *(16)*. All patients receiving a second injection revealed improved symptoms. The authors comment that repeat injections usually lasted longer than the initial injection, with some patients having a durable response greater than 1 year. However, no specific data regarding repeat injection is provided in this report.

Based on these data, it appears that the efficacy of BTX injection continues in the majority of patients undergoing repeat injection. Undoubtedly, however, a small percentage of patients will fail repeat injection. As discussed previously, multiple toxin injection may cause resistance and associated treatment failure. Currently, it is unclear which patients are likely to respond to repeat injection, which criteria should be used to time re-injection, and the role that BTX-B will play in this treatment algorithm.

### Side Effects

Side effects and adverse events following BTX injection are rare. Hematuria and postoperative pain are the most common symptoms observed. Given the paralytic nature of BTX, systemic effects are of significant theoretical concern. However, systemic absorption of BTX is minimal because of the high molecular weight. Del Popolo reported muscular weakness in 8% (5 of 61) of patients undergoing intravesical BTX injection *(70)*. All patients experienced symptom resolution within 4 weeks of injection. Dykstra et al. also reported upper extremity weakness in three patients undergoing urethral toxin injection, which resolved by postoperative week 3 *(18)*. Two other authors report a longer lasting duration of associated muscle weakness. Wyndaele et al. reported upper extremity weakness in two patients following intravesical injection of BTX (300 U Botox, 1000 U Dysport), persisting in these cases for 90 days *(71)*. Gross and colleages describe four patients suffering from transient muscle weakness in the trunk and/or extremities (range 2 weeks to 2 months). Although these reports are of concern, no incidence of extremity weakness has been described in the numerous other series reported in the literature. Further, no severe systemic complication (e.g., respiratory muscle weakness/paralysis) has been reported.

Because of the mechanism of action underlying BTX therapy, urinary retention is an obvious surgical concern during intravesical injection. Despite being shown to increase PVR, early reports of intravesical BTX injection did not demonstrate a significant rate of postoperative urinary retention. However, urinary retention has been reported with increasing frequency in more recent, large-scale investigations. In assessing this risk, it is important to stratify patients based on underlying pathology. For example, a large percentage of patients with NDO may require CIC at baseline and, for this reason, urinary retention is not a significant clinical concern. However, in those patients with NDO not requiring CIC, *de novo* urinary retention is certainly an undesired outcome. In contrast, patients with IDO are unlikely to require pre-operative catheterization and the postoperative development of urinary retention represents a debilitating outcome.

Following intravesical BTX injection, Rajkumar et al. report an increased PVR in an IDO cohort *(35)*. However, no incidence of urinary retention requiring catheterization was reported. In a mixed population, Smith et al. report that several patients needed to strain during urination and an increased residual not requiring catheterization was seen in one patient *(16)*. Kessler et al. reported *de novo* CIC in nine patients (four IDO, five NDO) owing to a PVR greater than 150 mL *(37)*. Finally, Popat and colleagues report *de novo* CIC in 69% of NDO patients as compared with 19% of those with IDO *(38)*. Despite these reports, no incidence of urinary retention is reported in the majority of investigation. When occurring, urinary retention is transient, although specific duration is variable. However, based on these data, we feel that it is appropriate to counsel all patients regarding this risk and that temporary catheterization may be required postoperatively. Patients who find this possible outcome unsatisfactory are counseled against toxin injection.

Certainly dose and injection technique may be directly related to incidence of adverse events. However, in the only direct comparison of two treatment doses, no reported difference in adverse events was noted between intradetrusor injection of 200 versus 300 U Botox *(31)*. Variable toxin preparations may also have differing side effect profiles. Grosse et al. report that muscular weakness was observed exclusively in patients receiving Dysport (versus Botox) and that systemic dispersion may be higher for this preparation *(69)*. However, the authors concluded that available literature and unreported personal experience would suggest that a similar side effect profile may be seen with both preparations.

## PROTOCOL FOR BTX INJECTION

Despite the initial success achieved via endoscopic injection of BTX in the treatment of voiding dysfunction, further improvement is necessary. Perhaps the most important immediate obstacle to the more successful widespread utilization of BTX in the treatment of urological disorders is the lack of a standardized technique for BTX administration. Published studies to date have utilized varying doses, injection volumes, and injection site/numbers. Foremost, this variation makes systematic assessment of the efficacy of BTX difficult. Further, it remains difficult to provide urologists seeking to incorporate BTX administration into their treatment armamentarium with a standardized protocol for administration. This section addresses the generalized injection principals and the common protocols used to date.

### Injection Dose

Published experience has utilized a total injection dose of 100 to 300 U (Botox) and 500 to 1000 U (Dysport). Because of the lack of significant literature regarding Dysport dosing, the following discussion will center on the Botox preparation. In one of the first published investigations of intravesical BTX injection for DO, Schurch and colleagues reported the use of varying doses, ranging from 200 to 300 U *(30)*. The authors reported that the administration dose was based on a previous titration study demonstrating that this range was most likely to result in a complete blockade of acetylcholine at the detrusor level. Although a dose–response comparison was not formally conducted, the two patients failing to respond to treatment both received 200 U. As a result, the authors concluded that 300 U may be the optimal dose for DO.

More recently, Schurch and associates reported the first direct comparison of two doses *(31)*. In this prospective, multi-center investigation, patients with incontinence resulting from NDO were randomized to receive intravesical injection of 200 or 300 U of BTX-A. Significant improvement was seen in both groups with respect to subjective and objective outcomes. In this analysis, no clear dose difference in the clinical outcomes was demonstrated between the two groups. However, the authors caution that this outcome may have been affected by the small study sample size. As a result, they caution that additional, long-term investigation is needed to better define potential dose–response differences with respect to not only clinical efficacy, but also the effect that a higher dose may have on treatment duration.

The majority of remaining investigations of intravesical injection of BTX have utilized a 300-U dose. Several studies reported using 100- and 200-U doses *(16,30)*. In these studies, improvement similar to investigation using 300 U is seen with respect to both subjective and objective outcomes, including decreased incontinence episodes, increased mean cystometric capacity, and decreased mean voiding pressures. Nonetheless, definitive conclusions regarding the optimal dose remain difficult in the absence of further study directly focused on dose–response outcomes.

In addition, dose modification based on specific patient parameters has been reported in an attempt to reduce the risk of clinically significant PVR and/or urinary retention. Rackley et al. report the use of a 100-U trial dose in patients with DO combined with urodynamic evidence of borderline contractility *(3)*. These authors also use this trial dose in patients of advanced age, given evidence demonstrating advanced age to predict for hypocontractile bladder conditions. Smith and colleagues report the use of a greater number of injections (and resultant dose) in patients with NDO as compared with those with IDO or IC *(16)*. This approach may be particularly effective in this subset of patients, who perform CIC but remain incontinent as a result of DO. Accordingly, detrusor hypocontractility may actually be a desired effect in these patients.

## Injection Volume

Published investigation to date has generally used an injection volume of 0.1 mL to 0.5 mL per injection site. More recently, protocol modifications have been proposed using a larger injection volume (0.5–1.0 mL; ref. *15*). Kim et al. demonstrated that larger dilution volumes resulted in increased gastrocnemius muscle relaxation in an animal model *(72)*. Theoretically, it is possible that larger dilution volumes will result in greater suburothelial diffusion, thereby allowing for toxin action on a larger surface area of muscle. However, no evidence has been presented to suggest that increased dilution volume used during intravesical injection BTX will result in superior clinical outcomes. In contrast, larger volumes may have the deleterious effect of increasing the potential for serosal extravasation. Further, as BTX administration is more frequently performed in the outpatient clinical setting, larger volumes may also result in increased patient discomfort and analgesic requirements.

## Injection Distribution

In general, the entire volume of toxin is injected, divided among 20 to 40 evenly distributed intramural injection sites. These sites include the bladder base and posterolateral walls of the bladder (Fig. 2). Because the wall of the bladder dome is the thinnest bladder region and lies in an intraperitoneal position, this area should be avoided to prevent inadvertent bowel injury.

Central to the issue of optimal injection site is the question of whether the trigone should be included in the injection distribution site. In the early experience investigating the use of BTX-A in NDO, Schurch et al. report a trigone-sparing injection distribution *(30)*. These investigators reported that the decision to avoid the trigone was multifactorial, including a desire to avoid inducing reflux to the upper tracts. Further, it was felt that injection of the trigone, containing dense innervation from both adrendergic, cholinergic, and non-cholinergic excitatory pathways, might complicate the efficacy analysis of a cholinergic blockade. Finally, these authors felt that trigonal injection might include the suburothelial sensory plexus, resulting in possible impairment of the sensory nerve endings. Subsequent investigations have predominantly utilized trigone-sparing injections *(27,30)*. Whether these protocols were adapted based on similar concerns, simply a lack of other protocols to define trigonal inclusion, or for other reasons is unclear.

Given the concerns raised by Schurch et al., it was indeed reasonable for early investigators to spare the trigone in the absence of persuasive evidence to support trigonal inclusion. However, a significant amount of subsequent basic and clinical research (discussed previously)

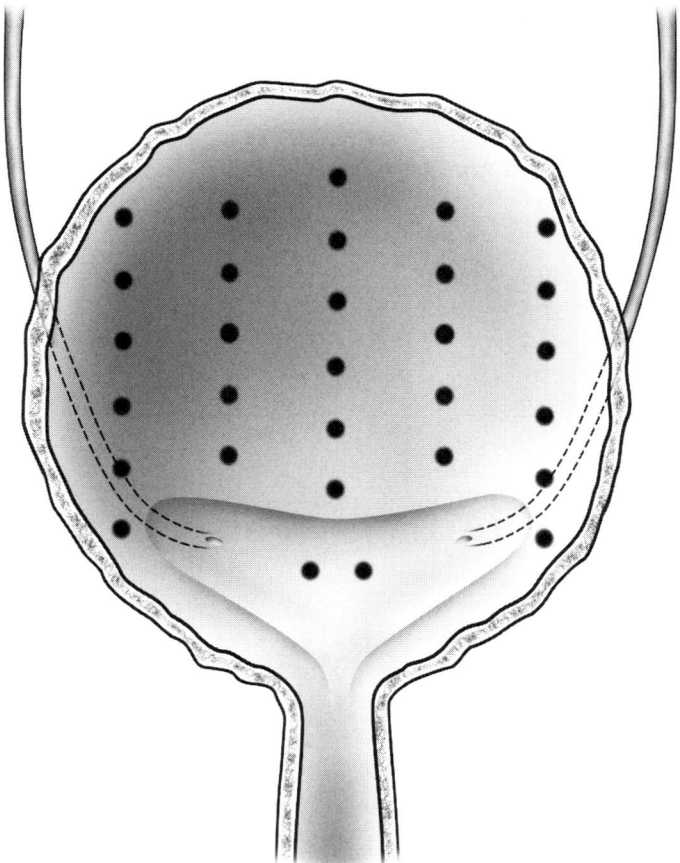

**Fig. 2.** Botulinum toxin injection sites, University of Chicago protocol. Reprinted from ref. *36*, © 2004, with permission from Elsevier.

has suggested that sensory neuron dysfunction may actually contribute to the pathophysiology of DO, SU, and IC. Given the recently defined inhibitory effect of BTX on sensory neuron activity, it is possible that trigonal BTX injection might have therapeutic benefit in this patient population.

Two recent studies report successful outcomes utilizing a BTX injection with trigonal inclusion *(3,16)*. However, no direct comparison was made with patients receiving trigone-sparing injections. Although routine postoperative voiding cystourethrogram was not performed to rule out the possibility of iatrogenic reflux, neither study reported postoperative urinary tract infection based on urinalysis and symptom presentation.

At the University of Chicago, we conducted a pilot study to assess the subjective benefit of trigonal-inclusion during BTX injection. A total of 40 patients with OAB refractory to anticholinergic treatment received trigone or trigone-sparing injections of BTX-A (300 U). A statistically significant improvement in UDI and IIQ symptom scores was seen at 3-week and 6-month follow-up in both groups. However, no difference between the treatment arms was found. In our experience, patients undergoing trigonal injection received 30 evenly distributed injections (10 U per injection site), with two injections being placed in the trigonal region (Fig. 2). Care is taken to avoid injection in proximity to the ureteral orifices. Despite these findings, further investigation is needed to determine whether trigonal injection is associated with improved urodynamic outcomes or may be more appropriately used in patients with isolated sensory and/or pain complaints.

## Bladder Injection Technique

We routinely perform BTX injection in the outpatient setting under intravenous sedation. Other authors describe the use of local anesthesia, reporting minimal associated discomfort or complications. Rackley et al. report The Cleveland Clinic Foundation injection protocol, in which 100 mL 2% lidocaine solution is instilled into the bladder to provide local anesthesia *(3)*. A 15- to 20-minute dwell time is allowed. In addition, lidocaine-enhanced electromotive drug administration has been reported to decrease post-injection pain scores compared with lidocaine instillation alone *(73)*. As more experience with BTX administration under local anesthesia is accrued, this technique may be used to allow for cost reduction, avoidance of anesthetic risks, and injection in the clinic setting. All patients receive peri-operative antibiotics and discontinuation of antiplatelet medications is not necessary because minimal bleeding is induced by the small-gage injection needle.

Intravesical injection of BTX is performed by first diluting the toxin to the desired concentration. Botox is preserved in a vacuum-dried formulation, with each vile containing 100 U. At our institution, each vile of Botox is diluted using 1 mL preservative-free saline, yielding 10 U per 0.1 ml for injection at each site. The entire dilution is then drawn into a 1-mL syringe. A total of three vials are used, providing three 1-mL syringes with 100 U Botox per syringe. Because excessive movement can decrease the potency of the toxin through disruption of its disulfide bonds, care is taken to avoid shaking during toxin preparation *(74)*.

BTX injection is performed with the patient in the dorsal lithotomy position. Injections are performed using a rigid 21 F cystoscope and a collagen injection needle inserted through the endoscopic working port. Following entry into the bladder with the cystocope, the needle tip is visualized under direct vision (Fig. 3). As the needle sheath volume approximates 0.5 mL, priming is required. Accordingly, 0.5 mL BTX is injected into the needle before insertion into the detrusor muscle. Visual confirmation of a sufficient priming dose is provided by observing for cessation of air bubble flow from the needle tip.

The bladder wall is then injected with BTX, divided among evenly distributed intramural injection sites. The injection needle allows the surgeon to control for a precise injection depth. In male patients, a longer injection needle may be used when necessary. Twenty to 30 evenly distributed intradetrusor injections are generally administered based on the specific protocol used. Our injection technique involves the creation of a submucosal bleb, allowing for action on the underlying detrusor muscle. This technique allows for visual confirmation of the insertion depth and diffusion along the suburothelial space. Other authors attempt direct needle insertion and toxin injection within the detrusor muscle itself. When using this technique, care must be taken to avoid the risk of inserting the needle through the bladder serosa, with resultant toxin extravasation and risk to neighboring pelvic structures. As a result of sheath priming, the final 0.5 mL of toxin are injected by flushing the sheath with a fourth 1-mL syringe containing 0.5 mL saline.

## Urethral Injection Technique

A variety of reported protocols are available for BTX injection of the external urinary sphincter. Foremost, BTX injection can be performed via a cystoscopic or, in the female

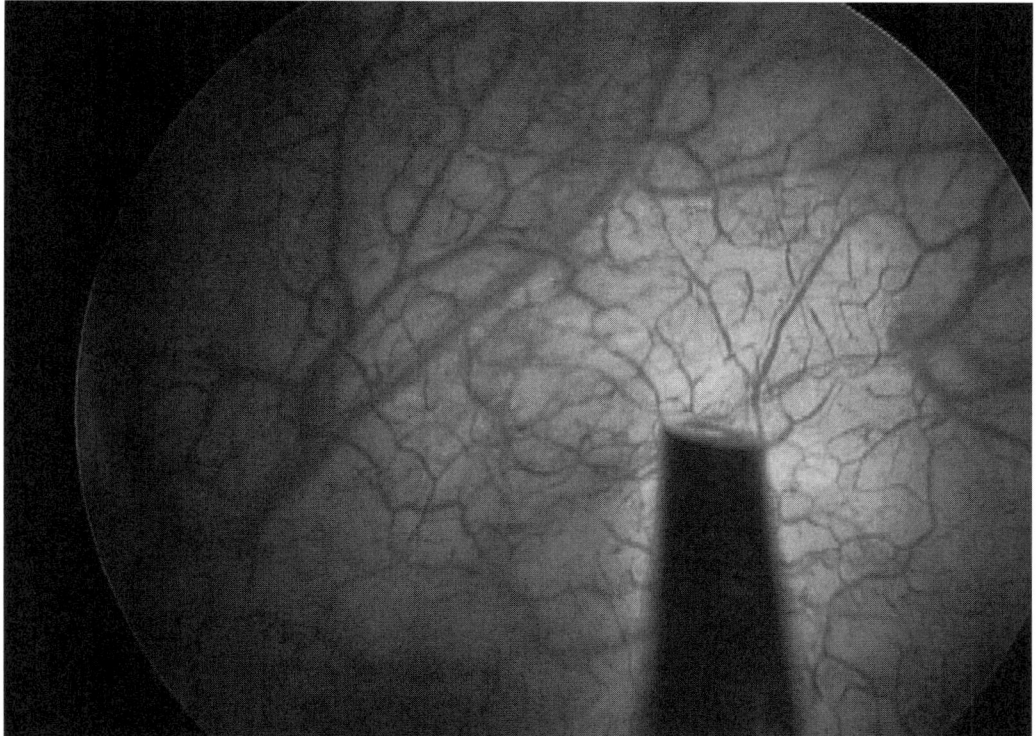

**Fig. 3.** Cystoscopic injection of botulinum toxin performed under direct vision.

patient, a transurethral approach. Under both approaches, the toxin is prepared as described for the bladder injection technique. The cystoscopic approach is performed using standard cystoscopic equipment and a collagen injection needle. Urethroscopy is initiated and, under direct vision, the external sphincter is localized and injected. Using the transurethral approach, a fine-gauge spinal needle is inserted periurethrally with the patient in the lithotomy or "frog-leg" position. The spinal needle is advanced directly into the sphincter muscle and injection is initiated.

Under both techniques, sphincter localization can be performed with or without the use of EMG. When using EMG, an EMG needle is inserted periurethrally and neurodiagnostic testing is used to confirm sphincter localization. More recently, a greater number of authors have reported toxin injection without EMG localization *(3,23)*. In these cases, patient participation (when using local anesthesia) can be used to assist with sphincteric localization. Accordingly, the sphincter may be visualized under cystoscopic guidance during voluntary sphincter contraction or valsalva. Alternatively, the crede maneuver may also aid in cystoscopic visualization of the sphincter when sedation is used.

Injection distribution also varies depending on the reported protocol. The majority of reported techniques utilize sphincteric injection at the 3-, 6-, 9-, and 12-o'clock or 3-, 6-, and 9-o'clock positions *(23,74)*. The Cleveland Clinic Foundation injection protocol for intraurethral injection uses a 2- and 10-o'clock distribution pattern *(3)*. In general, a complete and evenly distributed injection pattern is desired to ensure pharmacological sphincterotomy.

## CONCLUSION

The introduction of BTX injection offers a promising treatment for a variety of LUT dysfunction. Certainly, significant clinical experience supports a positive subjective response following injection in the treatment of DO and DSD. These outcomes are accompanied by data demonstrating improvement in many objective parameters of LUT function. Growing experience suggests that BTX application may be useful in a greater number of urological disorders, such as detrusor hypocontractility, IC, sensory disorders, and BPH. More basic science research is needed to better define the effects of BTX on the somatic, autonomic, and sensory innervation to the bladder. Further, better definition of the optimal protocol for BTX injection is needed. Despite these issues, BTX injection exists as a powerful treatment modality that provides urologists with an additional tool to treat urological disease.

## REFERENCES

1. White SR. Botulism. In: Ford MD, ed. Clinical Toxicology. Philadelphia: WB Saunders Co; 2001, p. 934.
2. van Ermengem E. Ueber einen neuen anaeroben Bacillus and seine Beziehungen zum Botulisms. Ztsch Hyg Infekt 1897;26:1–56.
3. Rackley RR, Frenkl TL, Abdelmalak JB. Botulinum toxin: the promise of therapy for complex voiding dysfunction. Cont Urol Feb 2005;38–52.
4. Carpenter FG. Motor responses of the urinary bladder and skeletal muscle in botulinum intoxicated rats. J Physiol 1967;188:1–11.
5. Welch MJ, Purkiss JR, Foster KA. Sensitivity of embryonic rat dorsal root ganglia neurons to Clostridium botulinum neurotoxins. Toxicon 2000;38:245–25.
6. Roger Aoki K. Botulinum neurotoxin serotypes A and B preparations have different safety margins in preclinical models of muscle weakening efficacy and systemic safety. Toxicon 2002;40:923–928.
7. Sirls LT, Choe JM. The incontinence history and physical examination. In: O'Donnell PD, ed. Urinary Incontinence. St Louis: Mosby-Year Book, Inc.; 1997, pp. 54–63.
8. Shumaker SA, Wyman JF, Uebersax JS, et al. Health-related quality of life measures for women with urinary incontinence: the Incontinence Impact Questionnaire and the Urogential Distress Inventory. Qual Life Res 1994;3:291–306.
9. Uebersax JS, Wyman JF, Shumaker SA, et al. Short forms to assess life quality and symptom distress for urinary incontinence in women: the Incontinence Impact Questionnaire and the Urogential Distress Inventory. Neurourol Urodyn 1995;14:131–139.
10. Abrams P, Blaivas JG, Stanton SL, et al. The standardization of terminology of lower urinary tract function recommended by the International Continence Society. Br J Obstet Gynaecol 1990;97:1–16.
11. Robinson D, Pearce KF, Preisser JS, et al. Relationship between patient reports of urinary incontinence symptoms and quality of life measures. Obstet Gynecol 1998;91:224–228.
12. Lemack GE, Zimmern PE. Predictability of urodynamic findings based on the Urogenital Distress Inventory-6 questionnaire. Urology 1999;54:161–166.
13. Romanzi LJ, Blaivas JG. Office evaluation of incontinence. In: O'Donnell PD, ed. Urinary Incontinence. St Louis: Mosby-Year Book, Inc.; 1997, pp. 48–54.
14. Harvey MA, Kristjansson B, Griffith D, et al. The Incontinence Impact Questionnaire and the Urogenital Distress Inventory: a revisit of their validity in women without a urodynamic diagnosis. Am J Obstet Gynecol 2001;185:25–31.
15. Smith CP, Chancellor MB. Emerging role of botulinum toxin in the management of voiding dysfunction. J Urol 2004;171:2128–2137.
16. Smith CP, Nushiguchi J, O'Leary M, et al. Single-institution experience in 110 patients with botulinum toxin A injection into bladder or urethra. Urology 2005;65:37–41.

17. Dykstra DD, Sidi AA, Scott AB, et al. Effects of botulinum A toxin on detrusor-sphincter dyssynergia in spinal cord injury patients. J Urol 1988;139:919–922.
18. Dykstra DD, Sidi A. Treatment of detrusor-sphincter dysynergia with botulinum A toxin: A double-blind study. Arch Phys Med Rehabil 1990;71:24–26.
19. Schurch B, Hauri D, Rodic B, et al. Botulinum-A toxin as a treatment of detrusor-sphincter dyssynergia: a prospective study in 24 spinal cord injury patients. J Urol 1996;155:1023–1029.
20. Gallien P, Robineau S, Verin M, et al. Treatment of detrusor sphincter dyssynergia by transperineal injection of botulinum toxin. Arch Phys Med Rehabil 1998;79:715–717.
21. Kuo HC. Effect of botulinum A toxin in the treatment of voiding dysfunction due to detrusor underactivity. Urology 2003;61:550–554.
22. Kuo HC. Botulinum A toxin urethral injection for the treatment of lower urinary tract dysfunction. J Urol 2003;170:1909–1912.
23. Phelan MW, Franks M, Somogyi GT, et al. Botulinum toxin urethral injection to restore bladder emptying in men and women with voiding dysfunction. J Urol 2001;165:1107–1110.
24. Petit H, Wiart E, Gaujard E, et al. Botulinum A toxin treatment for detrusor-sphincter dyssynergia in spinal cord disease. Spinal Cord 1998;36:91–94.
25. MacDiarmid S. Mixed urinary incontinence: effective evaluation and treatment. Cont Urol Feb 2005;10–18.
26. Giannitsas K, Perimenis P, Athanasopoulos A, et al. Comparison of the efficacy of tolterodine and oxybutynin in different urodynamic severity grades of idiopathic detrusor overactivity. Eur Urol 2004;46:776–782.
27. Chapple C, Khullar V, Gabriel Z, et al. The effects of antimuscarinic treatments in overactive bladder: a systematic review and meta-analysis. Eur Urol 2005;48:5–26.
28. Stohrer M, Schurch B, Kramer G, et al. Botulinum A-toxin in the treatment of detrusor hyperreflexia in spinal cord injured patients: a new alternative to medical and surgical procedures? Neurourol Urodyn 1999;18:401.
29. Bagi P, Biering-Sorensen F. Botulinum toxin A for treatment of neurogenic detrusor overactivity and incontinence in patients with spinal cord lesions. Scan J Urol Neph 2004;38:495–498.
30. Schurch B, Stohrer M, Kramer G, et al. Botulinum-A toxin for treating detrusor hyperreflexia in spinal cord injured patients: a new alternative to anticholinergic drugs? Preliminary results. J Urol 2000;164:692–697.
31. Schurch B, De Seze M, Denys P, et al. Botulinum toxin type A is a safe and effective treatment for neurogenic urinary incontinence: results of a single treatment, randomized, placebo controlled 6-month study. J Urol 2005;174:196–200.
32. Reitz A, Stohrer M, Kramer G, et al. European experience of 200 cases treated with botulinum-A toxin injections into the detrusor muscle for neurogenic incontinence. Eur Urol 2004;45:510–515.
33. Schulte-Baukloh H, Michael T, Sturzebecher B, et al. Botulinum-A toxin detrusor injection as a novel approach in the treatment of bladder spasticity in children with neurogenic bladder. Eur Urol 2003;44:139–143.
34. Hajebrahimi S, Altaweel W, Cadoret J, et al. Efficacy of botulinum-A toxin in adults with neurogenic overactive bladder: initial results. Can J Urol 2005;12:2543–2546.
35. Rajkumar GN, Small DR, Mustafa AW, et al. A prospective study to evaluate the safety, tolerability, efficacy and durability of response of intravesical injection of botulinum toxin type A into detrusor muscle in patients with refractory idiopathic detrusor overactivity. BJU Int 2005;96:848–852.
36. Rapp DE, Lucioni A, Katz EE, et al. Use of botulinum-A toxin for the treatment of refractory overactive bladder symptoms: an initial experience. Urology 2004;63:1071–1075.
37. Kessler TM, Danuser H, Schumacher M, et al. Botulinum A toxin injections into the detrusor: an effective treatment in idiopathic neurogenic detrusor overactivity? Neurourol Urodynam 2005;24:231–236.

38. Popat R, Apostolidis A, Kalsi V, et al. A comparison between the response of patients with idiopathic detrusor overactivity and neurogenic detrusor overactivity to the first intradetrusor injection of botulinum-A toxin. J Urol 2005;174:984–989.

39. Giannantoni A, Di Stasi SM, Stephen R, et al. Intravesical resiniferatoxin versus botulinum-A toxin injections for neurogenic detrusor overactivity: a prospective randomized study. J Urol 2005;172:240–243.

40. Ray FR, Moore KH, Hansen MA, et al. Loss or purinergic P2X receptor innervation in human detrusor and subepithelium from adults with sensory urgency. Cell Tissue Res 2003;314:351–359.

41. Chuang YC, Fraser MO, Yu Y, et al. The role of bladder afferent pathways in bladder hyperactivity induced by the intravesical administration of nerve growth factor. J Urol 2001;165:975–979.

42. Szallasi A, Fowler CJ. After a decade of intravesical vanilloid therapy: still more questions than answers. Lancet Neurology 2002;1:167–172.

43. Jasmin L, Janni G. Experimental neurogenic cystitis. Adv Exp Med Biol 2003;539:319–335.

44. Cui M, Khanijou S, Rubino J, et al. Subcutaneous administration of botulinum toxin A reduces formalin-induced pain. Pain 2004;107:125–133.

45. Vemulakonda VM, Somogyi GT, Kiss S, et al. Intravesical botulinum toxin A inhibits the afferent response in the chronically inflamed bladder. J Urol 2005;173:621–624.

46. Chuang YC, Yoshimura N, Huang CC, et al. Inhibitory effect of intravesically applied botulinum toxin A in chronic bladder inflammation. J Urol 2004;172:1529–1532.

47. Gabella G, Davis C. Distribution of afferent axons in the bladder of rats. J Neurocyt 1998; 27:141–155.

48. Huang H, Wu X, Nicol GD, et al. ATP augments peptide release from rat sensory neurons in culture through activation of P2Y receptors. J Pharm Exp Ther 2003;306:1137–144.

49. Rapp DE, Turk KW, Bales GT, et al. Botulinum toxin type A inhibits calcitonin gene-related peptide release from isolated rat bladder. J Urol 2006;175:1138–1142.

50. Apostolidis A, Popat R, Yiangou Y, et al. Decreased sensory receptor P2X3 and TRPV1 in suburothelial nerve fibers following intradetrusor injections of botulinum toxin for human detrusor overactivity. J Urol 2005;174:977–983.

51. Brady CM, Apostolidis A, Harper M, et al. Parallel changes in bladder suburothelial vanilloid receptor TRPV1 and pan-neuronal marker PGP9.5 immunoreactivity in patients with neurogenic detrusor overactivity following intravesical resiniferatoxin treatment. BJU Int 2004;93:770–776.

52. Brady CM, Apostolidis A, Yiangou Y, et al. P2X3-immunoreactive nerve fibres in neurogenic detrusor overactivity and the effect of intravesical resiniferatoxin. Eur Urol 2004;46:247–253.

53. Zermann D, Ishigooka M, Schubert J, et al. Trigonum and bladder base injection of botulinum toxin A (BTX) in patients with severe urgency-frequency syndrome refractory to conservative medical treatment and electrical stimulation. Neurourol Urodyn 2001;20:412.

54. Flynn MK, Webster GD, Amundsen CL. The effect of botulinum-A toxin on patients with sever urge urinary incontinence. J Urol 2004;172:2316–2320.

55. Smith CP, Radziszewski P, Borkowski A, et al. Botulinum toxin A has antinociceptive effects in treating interstitial cystitis. Urology 2004;64:871–875.

56. Maria G, Brisinda G, Massimo I, et al. Relief by botulinum toxin of voiding dysfunction due to benign prostatic hyperplasia: results of a randomized, placebo-controlled study. Urology 2003;62:259–265.

57. Kuo H. Prostate botulinum A toxin injection-an alternative treatment for benign prostatic obstruction in poor surgical candidates. Urology 2005;65:670–674.

58. Reitz A, Schurch B. Botulinum toxin type B injection for management of type A resistant neurogenic detrusor overactivity. J Urol 2004;171:804–805.

59. Doellgast GJ, Brown JE, Koufman JA, et al. Sensitive assay for measurement of antibodies to Clostridium botulinum neurotoxins A, B, and E: use of hapten-labeled-antibody elution to isolate specific complexes. J Clin Microbiol 1997;35:578–583.

60. Dykstra DD, Pryor J, Goldish G. Use of botulinum toxin type B for the treatment of detrusor hyperreflexia in a patient with multiple sclerosis: a case report. Arch Phys Med Rehabil 2003;84: 1399–1400.

61. Dysktra D, Enriquez A, Valley M. Treatment of overactive bladder with botulinum toxin type B: a pilot study. Int Urogynecol J 2003;14:424–426.

62. Pistolesi D, Selli C, Rossi B, et al. Botulinum toxin type B for type A resistant bladder spasticity. J Urol 2004;171:802–803.

63. Gordon PH, Gooch CL, Green PE. Extensor digitorum brevis test and resistance to botulinum toxin type A. Muscle Nerve 2002;26:828–831.

64. Ghei M, Maraj BH, Miller R, et al. Effects of botulinum toxin B on refractory detrusor overactivity: a randomized, double-blind, placebo controlled, crossover trial. J Urol 2005;174:1873–1877.

65. Chancellor MB. Editorial Re: Reitz A and Schurch B. Botulinum toxin type B injection for management of type A resistant neurogenic detrusor overactivity. J Urol 2004;171:804–805.

66. Borodic GE, Joseph M, Fay L, et al. Botulinum A toxin for the treatment of spasmodic torticollis: dysphagia and regional toxin spread. Head Neck 1990;12:392–399.

67. de Paiva A, Meunier FA, Molgo J, et al. Functional repair of motor endplates after botulinum neurotoxin type A poisoning: biphasic switch of synaptic activity between nerve sprouts and their parent terminals. Proc Natl Acad Sci USA 1999;96:3200–3205.

68. Haferkamp A, Krengel U, Reitz A, et al. Are botulinum-A toxin injections into the detrusor of patients with neurogenic detrusor overactivity safe? Ultrastructural data of detrusor biopsies. Neurourol Urodyn 2003;22:499–500.

69. Grosse J, Kramer G, Stohrer M. Success of repeat detrusor injections of botulinum A toxin in patients with severe neurogenic detrusor overactivity and incontinence. Eur Urol 2005;47:653–659.

70. Del Popolo G. Botulinum-A toxin in the treatment of detrusor hyperreflexia. Neurourol Urodyn 2001;20:522.

71. Wyndaele JJ, Van Dromme SA. Muscular weakness as side effect of botulinum toxin injection for neurogenic detrusor overactivity. Spinal Cord 2002;40:599–600.

72. Kim HS, Hwang JH, Jeong ST, et al. Effect of muscle activity and botulinum toxin dilution volume on muscle paralysis. Dev Med Child Neurol 2003;45:200–206.

73. Schurch B, Reitz A, Tenti G. Electromotive drug administration of lidocaine to anesthetize the bladder before botulinum-A toxin injections into the detrusor. Spinal Cord 2004;42:338–341.

74. Smaldone MC, Chancellor MB. Bladder or urethra injection of botulinum toxin type A: one institution's experience. Am J Urol Rev 2005;3:422–426.

# 13

# Gastrointestinal Applications
## *Achalasia, Gastroparesis, and Anal Fissure*

**Shayan Irani and Frank K. Friedenberg**

## INTRODUCTION

The origin, subtypes, physiology and pharmacology of botulinum toxin type A (BTX-A) have been discussed in other chapters. In this chapter, some of the current applications of BTX in gastroenterology are discussed. BTX has been used for a large number of gastrointestinal disorders, however, this chapter is confined to those conditions for which the best data are available (achalasia, gastroparesis, and anal fissure). Other conditions with only preliminary descriptive data are not discussed because widespread use of BTX for these disorders remains unlikely (esophageal spasm, anismus, and sphincter of Oddi dysfunction). This chapter does not address the use of BTX for the treatment of cricopharyngeal spasm because physicians specializing in ears, nose, and throat typically treat this disorder (1,2).

## BTX-A FOR THE TREATMENT OF GASTROPARESIS

Under normal conditions, gastric emptying is a highly regulated process reflecting the integration of propulsive forces generated by proximal fundic tone and distal antral contractions against the resistance of the pyloric sphincter. The motor control of the stomach is dependent on the coordination of neurogenic modulators (central, autonomic, and enteric nervous systems), myogenic control mechanisms (interstitial cells of Cajal), and chemical modulators (excitatory and inhibitory neurotransmitters).

Gastroparesis is the term used to describe delayed stomach emptying. The pathogenesis of this disorder depends on the underlying etiology, but can be broadly categorized as neuropathic or myopathic. Neuropathic processes involving the stomach are characterized by poorly coordinated contractile activity of the stomach (i.e., non-peristaltic), reduced frequency of gastric contractions, but preserved contractile amplitude. On full thickness biopsy, there is a degeneration of axons, dendrites, and/or neurons with preserved circular and longitudinal smooth muscle layers (3). Some neuropathic causes of gastroparesis include endocrine disorders (diabetes mellitus, hypo/hyperthyroidism), post-surgical (e.g., resulting from vagotomy), drug-induced (e.g., anticholinergics and narcotics), post-infectious (e.g., Chagas disease), and complications of systemic neurological disorders (e.g., Parkinson's disease and multiple sclerosis).

A myopathic process, on the other hand, is characterized by coordinated, but low amplitude contractile activity. On full thickness gastric biopsy, there is fibrosis, muscle atrophy, and vacuolar degeneration of the muscularis propria. Some of the myopathic causes of gastroparesis include dermatomyositis, Ehler's-Danlos Syndrome, familial visceral myopathies, metabolic myopathies,

From: *Therapeutic Uses of Botulinum Toxin*
Edited by: G. Cooper © Humana Press Inc., Totowa, NJ

and myotonic dystrophy. Sometimes, a combination of a neuropathic and myopathic process can be seen as in progressive systemic sclerosis and amyloidosis.

Patients with gastroparesis commonly present with recurrent postprandial nausea, vomiting, bloating, early satiety, and abdominal discomfort. Weight loss, vitamin deficiencies, and electrolyte imbalances from chronic vomiting may result if the vomiting and stasis becomes severe. Patients typically have greater difficulty tolerating a solid diet, particularly one composed of a high percentage of long-chain fatty acids. A detailed history and physical examination should be performed to assess the duration of symptoms, the fluid and nutritional status of the patient, and to determine if any other region of the digestive tract is involved *(4)*. The next step should be a structural evaluation of the gastrointestinal tract in the form of an upper endoscopy or upper gastrointestinal radiology series to rule out a mechanical obstruction. The presence of a large amount of retained food in the stomach on endoscopy, especially after an overnight fast, is strongly suggestive of gastroparesis.

The diagnosis of gastroparesis is confirmed with the help of a radionuclide study (i.e., gastric emptying scan). At most institutions, technetium 99m-labeled scrambled eggs are ingested as a marker for solid-phase emptying of a meal. Normal median values for the percentage of meal remaining in the stomach at 120 and 240 minutes are 24 and 1.2%, respectively. Patients with more than 50% retention at 2 hours or 10% at 4 hours are considered to have gastroparesis *(5)*.

A variety of promotility drugs (e.g., metoclopramide) are available, which enhance gastric emptying through differing mechanisms. Unfortunately, the efficacy of these drugs is fair to poor for the neuropathic group and even worse for the myopathic group. In addition, these drugs can have prominent side effects, such as sedation and extrapyramidal symptoms. Domperidone (Motilium®, Janssen-Ortho, Toronto, Canada) may be the most effective for treating symptoms of gastroparesis; however, it is unavailable in the United States *(6)*.

Treatment of gastroparesis through interruption of cholinergic input into the pylorus is an active area of research. Theoretically, relaxation of the pylorus, which acts as a natural resistor to the passage of food, could speed gastric emptying. One study documented that in patients with diabetic gastroparesis, the fasting and postprandial contractile activity of the pylorus is increased above the value found in healthy controls *(7)*. Physiological studies suggest that this abnormality may respond to BTX. A preliminary study using guinea pig pyloric smooth muscle strips demonstrated that BTX inhibits electrical pulse-stimulated responses *(8)*. Others have demonstrated that pyloric BTX injection reduces isolated high-pressure waves in the pyloric region and normalizes antroduodenal peristaltic activity *(9)*. Unfortunately, additional data are unavailable, primarily because of the very difficult task of studying the pyloric sphincter in vivo.

Five open-label studies have been performed to evaluate BTX injection into the pyloric sphincter for the treatment of gastroparesis *(6,10–13)*. These studies have ranged in size from 3 to 63 patients and have included patients with idiopathic, diabetic, and post-surgical gastroparesis. Each study has shown an increase in gastric emptying of a solid meal and corresponding improvements in symptoms for up to 30 weeks. Doses of BTX have ranged from 100 to 200 U injected in all four quadrants of the pyloric sphincter using an injection catheter during a standard upper endoscopy (Fig. 1). In the largest study, performed at Temple University Hospital, 27 of 63 patients who underwent BTX injection into the pylorus showed a symptomatic improvement at 2 months *(13)*. Logistic regression demonstrated that male gender was associated with a response to therapy and patients with vomiting as their major symptom had no response. The results of an ongoing randomized, placebo-controlled trial will be available shortly and may provide more definitive information concerning efficacy of this treatment.

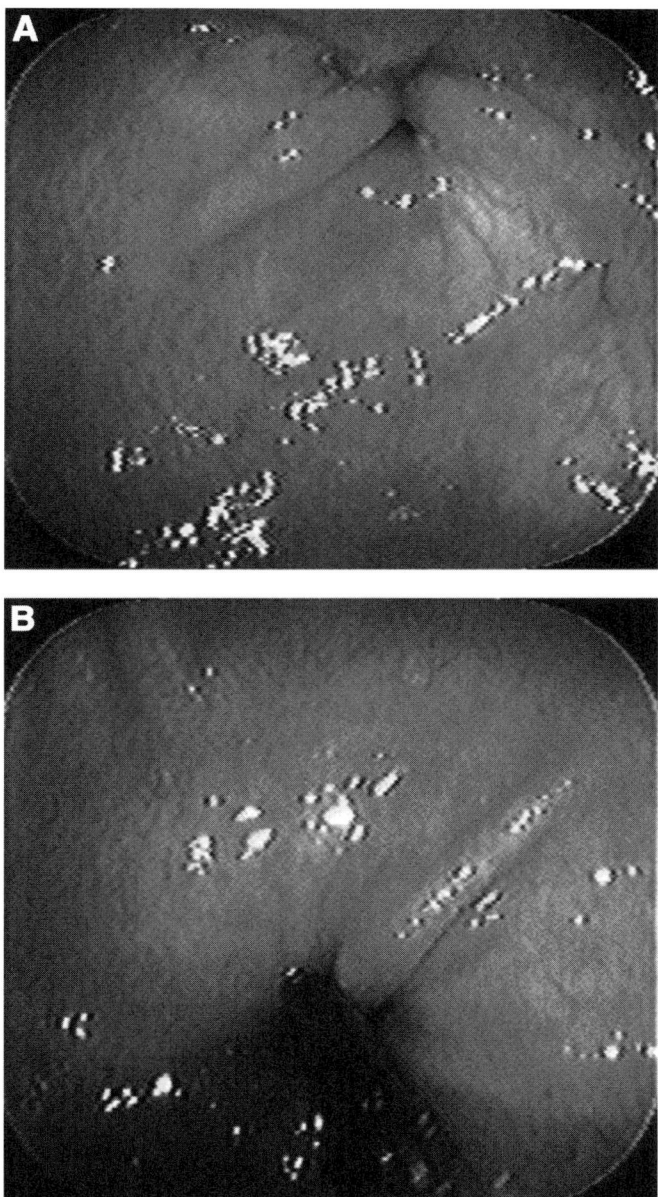

**Fig. 1.** Pyloric muscle injection of botulinum toxin type A in a patient with severe gastroparesis. **(A)** Top panel shows an endoscopic view of the pylorus before injection. **(B)** Bottom panel shows an injection catheter delivering botulinum toxin directly into the sphincter.

## TREATMENT OF ACHALASIA WITH BTX-A

Achalasia is a motor disorder of the esophagus in which the hallmark symptom is dysphagia. Manometrically, it is characterized by aperistalsis in the distal esophagus and failure or incomplete relaxation of the lower esophageal sphincter (LES) upon swallowing *(14)*. The LES is a specialized region of smooth muscle that is tonically contracted. LES relaxation in response to swallowing is precisely regulated by a number of mediators. The excitatory pathway is mediated by cholinergic vagal efferents. Atropine decreases LES pressure significantly in normal subjects and patients with achalasia *(14)*. The inhibitory (i.e., relaxation) pathway is mediated through nitric oxide and vasoactive intestinal peptide *(15)*. Nitric oxide is generated by myenteric neurons utilizing nitric oxide synthase *(16)*. The pathogenesis of achalasia is a degeneration of the inhibitory (nitric oxide) nerves innervating the LES. The loss of inhibitory input allows for failure of the LES to relax and unopposed parasympathetic excitatory input. In the opossum, chemical destruction of the myenteric plexus induces physiological changes compatible with achalasia *(17)*.

The diagnosis of achalasia, like other esophageal motility disorders, is based on a compatible history and characteristic motility abnormalities demonstrated by esophageal manometry. Patients with achalasia classically have solid and liquid food dysphagia that is progressive. They may also have pulmonary complaints (nocturnal cough, recurrent pneumonia) or weight loss. In the past, mechanical disruption of the LES has been the primary treatment for reducing the symptoms of achalasia. Mechanical disruption can be accomplished through vigorous distention of a balloon dilator at the level of the LES (pneumatic dilation) or through surgical myotomy (Heller myotomy). The initial success rate of pneumatic dilation is 60 to 95%; however, symptom recurrence is common and repeat dilation is often necessary *(18)*. Pneumatic dilation is also associated with a 5% risk of perforation *(18)*. Surgical myotomy has become more popular over the past 10 years with the advent of laparoscopic techniques. Surgical failure is rare; however, morbidity is increased in certain patient populations, such as those with morbid obesity or underlying cardiopulmonary disease.

The use of BTX injection directly into the LES represents an alternative, minimally invasive approach to the treatment of achalasia. A preliminary study in piglets suggested that resting LES pressure could be reduced by 60% after BTX injection into the sphincter *(19)*. This reduction occurs through inhibition of acetylcholine. Published in 1994, the first paper to evaluate the treatment of achalasia with BTX was an uncontrolled, pilot study involving 10 patients *(20)*. Pasricha et al. injected the LES with a total of 80 U BTX. In this study and subsequent trials, the LES was identified as the location of the histological squamo-columnar junction (endoscopic gastroesophageal junction) and was visually divided into four quadrants. Equal doses of BTX were injected into each quadrant using an injection sclerotherapy catheter passed through the endoscope. After 7 days, 7 of 10 patients became asymptomatic. Two of three remaining symptomatic patients improved after a second injection and one patient did not improve even with a third injection. In 1996, Fishman and others retrospectively looked at their results in 60 patients with achalasia treated with 80 or 100 U of open-label BTX *(21)*. Responders were defined as those patients with a 50% reduction in symptoms (on a 0-to-12 scoring system) at 1 month post-treatment. At 1 month, 42 of 60 patients were responders and an additional 8 patients had a "mild response." In most patients who responded, response was immediate and was less likely to occur beyond 1 month after injection. Prior failed pneumatic dilation or surgical myotomy did not appear to predict response to BTX. Subsequently, five more uncontrolled trials were reported *(19–23)*. These studies included between 11 and 55 patients and used either 80 or 100 U BTX. Patient follow-up varied but, in general, the majority of patients had sustained improvement through 6 months *(22–26)*. Often, patients who responded to an initial injection had a good response to a second injection once relapse occurred. Those failing to respond to injection usually did not have a successful outcome

**Table 1**
**Randomized Trials of BTX for the Treatment of Achalasia**

| Reference | Year published | n | BTX dose (U) | Alternative treatment | Length of follow-up (months) | Results |
|---|---|---|---|---|---|---|
| 27 | 1995 | 21 | 80 | Saline | 6 | 67% of patients who received BTX in remission at 6 months. No placebo response seen. |
| 29 | 1996 | 16 | 100 | Saline and pneumatic dilation | 12 | Toxin superior to placebo. Improvement at 1 year comparable to dilation. |
| 30 | 1999 | 24 | 80 | Pneumatic dilation | 30 | 100% relapse in BTX group. 40% relapse rate with dilation. |
| 31 | 1999 | 42 | 100 | Pneumatic dilation | 12 | Early failure rates similar. One-year failure rate higher with BTX (68 versus 30%). |
| 32 | 2001 | 40 | 200 | Pneumatic dilation | 12 | Remission rate 53% for dilation and 15% for BTX at 1 year. |
| 33 | 2001 | 17 | 60 and 80 | Pneumatic dilation | 10 | Duration of BTX effect shorter than dilation. BTX useful in tortuous esophagus. |

BTX, botulinum toxin.

with a second treatment. For those responding to a second injection, duration of response was similar to that seen with the initial injection. Patients with vigorous achalasia (a variant of achalasia characterized by high-amplitude contractions in the body of the esophagus in addition to failure of the LES to relax) appeared to respond better to BTX *(24–26)*.

These preliminary studies resulted in the initiation of controlled trials (Table 1). Pasricha and others presented the first data from a randomized, placebo-controlled trial *(27)*. Twenty-one patients with achalasia were randomized to injection with either BTX ($n = 11$) or saline ($n = 10$). In the treatment group, 9 of 11 patients had clinical improvement including 5 who became asymptomatic. No placebo patient responded. The LES pressure dropped by 33% in the BTX arm and rose 12% with placebo ($p = 0.02$). Mean LES diameter and esophageal clearance of barium on upright radiograph were also significantly improved with BTX. In a subsequent study, this group reported the long-term outcome of patients from their two previous trials *(28)*. In BTX responders, the median response time was 16 months (range 5–28 months). Ultimately, 19 of 20 patients from the two studies who responded relapsed and required further BTX injections. Of 15 patients undergoing a second injection, 9 responded with a median duration of response of 10 months.

In the first study to directly compare BTX with pneumatic dilation, 16 patients were randomized to LES injection with 100 U BTX or saline *(29)*. Patients who failed to respond to BTX or received placebo subsequently underwent pneumatic dilation. BTX resulted in improvement in all eight patients who received this therapy, whereas placebo had no effect on symptoms. However, the final data appeared to favor dilation over BTX. BTX decreased LES pressure by 49%, whereas dilation resulted in a 72% reduction. Esophageal retention of barium decreased by 47 and 59% with BTX and dilation, respectively. The beneficial effect of BTX lasted a mean of only 7 months. Another study also compared BTX with pneumatic dilation in 24 patients *(30)*. This study demonstrated that symptomatic improvement from these two treatments was equivalent both 1 week and 1 month after therapy. However, during the 2-year follow-up period, 9 of 12 patients treated with BTX experienced symptom recurrence compared with only 4 of 10 in the dilation group. In the largest randomized study to compare these two treatments, 42 patients were randomized to receive either 100 U BTX ($n = 22$) or pneumatic dilation ($n = 20$; ref. *31*). One year after treatment, 14 of 20 (70%) patients treated with dilation but only 7 of 22 (32%) in the BTX group were in symptomatic remission. Most patients in the BTX group relapsed between 3 and 9 months after injection. Of six patients treated with a second BTX injection, four ultimately relapsed and required dilation. Other parameters of treatment included efficacy in reducing resting LES pressure to less than 12 mmHg and ability to clear barium from the esophagus. Unlike pneumatic dilation, BTX was unable to improve these markers of response above baseline 6 and 12 months post-treatment. The authors determined that age, gender, amplitude of esophageal contractions, and duration of symptoms before treatment did not predict response to BTX. They also found a trend toward enhanced response to BTX in the subset of patients with vigorous achalasia.

Two recent studies have also compared the effects of BTX with pneumatic dilation for the treatment of achalasia. One compared a larger dose of BTX (200 U) with pneumatic dilation in 40 patients *(32)*. All patients had symptoms of dysphagia and esophageal manometry assessed at 1, 6, and 12 months posttreatment. Again, a benefit for both treatments was seen; dilation reduced symptoms in 79% of patients at 1-month assessment compared with 50% for BTX. However, a year after a single BTX treatment, only 14% of patients were in symptomatic remission, whereas 53% undergoing dilation remained asymptomatic. At 12 months, the estimated hazard ratio for relapse and need for retreatment in the BTX group was 2.69 versus the pneumatic dilation group. In the second study, a total of 17 patients were randomized to either BTX or pneumatic dilation *(33)*. In the BTX group, five patients lost response between 8 and 41 weeks after therapy. Only two patients in the dilation group relapsed, 12 and 20 weeks after treatment. The authors concluded that BTX therapy should be reserved as treatment for a select group of patients with achalasia—those with advanced age, serious comorbidities, anatomical variants that make dilation technically difficult or dangerous (e.g., tortuous megaesophagus, epiphrenic diverticulum; ref. *34*), or those with the vigorous achalasia variant. In addition, others have suggested that BTX injection may be useful to clarify difficult clinical situations in which there is doubt concerning the correct diagnosis because of atypical achalasia symptoms or insufficient manometric criteria for definitive diagnosis *(35)*.

Directed, precise injections into the LES potentially could produce improved results. Hoffman and others used endoscopic ultrasound guidance to identify the LES apparatus for precise injection of BTX *(36)*. In a group of four patients, they were able to show that endoscopic ultrasound-guided injection was easily performed. They hypothesized that lower doses of BTX and higher efficacy rates could be achieved by directly visualizing the target site. This hypothesis has not been tested in a controlled trial.

The appropriate dose of BTX remains unknown. In a recent trial, dosages of 50, 100, and 200 U BTX were compared in a large group of patients ($n = 118$; ref. *37*). Patients who underwent injection with 100 U received a second identical dose at 30 days and all groups were followed for 1 year. Interestingly, those patients who received two injections of 100 U faired the best. In the 97 patients who responded, at the end of follow-up, relapse was evident in 47 and 43% of patients in the 50- and 200-U groups respectively, but only in 19% of the double 100-U injection group. Response to BTX was predicted only by the presence of vigorous achalasia and the treatment regimen utilized.

BTX appears to be a safe treatment for achalasia and serious adverse events in clinical trials have rarely been reported. A 77-year-old male developed a pneumoperitoneum immediately after treatment and did well with conservative management *(38)*. A 63-year-old man developed hematemesis 2 weeks after injection of 80 U BTX *(39)*. At endoscopy, distal esophageal ulcerations were seen. During subsequent surgery, the distal esophagus was surrounded by dense adhesions and the entire distal esophageal wall was thickened with loss of normal tissue planes. There has been concern that BTX injection into the LES may, in some individuals, incite a fibrotic response in the submucosal and muscular layers, making subsequent surgical myotomy technically challenging. In a study examining this issue, Patti et al. found the musculature of the LES to be pale, fibrotic, and indurated in several patients who had received BTX before surgical myotomy *(40)*. Ironically, this occurred primarily in patients who initially responded to BTX. Microscopic perforation and inflammation around the esophagus in this group made anatomical dissection difficult and ultimately resulted in a worse outcome from surgery and a longer postoperative hospitalization. Whether these results are representative of the histological changes that occur in most patients is unclear. Interestingly, patients who failed to respond to BTX before surgery had minimal tissue changes. It therefore may be the frequency of injection or differences in endoscopic technique that influence local reactive changes.

The clinical data on the use of BTX is extensive and suggests that this compound is effective for the majority of patients with achalasia. Important uses include those individuals with the vigorous achalasia variant, poor surgical candidates, and in those cases in which it will be used for diagnostic purposes (i.e., where there remains uncertainty about the diagnosis of achalasia). However, it is important to realize that the long-term efficacy of BTX is inferior to both pneumatic dilation and surgery and repeated injection is often needed. Safety appears to be excellent, although there still remains concern about fibrosis around the LES leading to more difficult surgical myotomy.

## BTX-A FOR THE TREATMENT OF ANAL FISSURE

An anal fissure is a break in the epithelial lining (anoderm) of the anal canal. Often, the term *anal ulcer* is used for patients with a chronic (>1 month) anal fissure. A mature ulcer is associated with a sentinel pile (skin tag) and a hypertrophied papilla. A primary anal fissure is one that has no obvious underlying cause. As per Goligher's rule, 90% of anal fissures occur in the midline posteriorly, 10% occur anteriorly, and 1% are both anterior and posterior *(41)*. The most common initiating factor for a fissure is the passage of a large firm bowel movement. Other less common causes include digital insertion, sexual trauma, or foreign body insertion. Any prior anorectal surgery weakens the anoderm increasing the chance for fissure formation. A tear in the anoderm exposes the underlying internal anal sphincter, causing it to spasm and its failure to relax with a bowel movement causes further tearing and spasm. Recurrent spasm of the sphincter (sometimes to pressures >100 mHg) can lead to relative ischemia of the overlying anoderm, which inhibits healing *(42)*. The pain associated with a fissure may cause the patient to ignore the urge to defecate, resulting in the passage of a large hard bowel movement, which further traumatizes the area, leading to a vicious cycle of pain, constipation, and re-injury. The majority of primary anal fissures are painful and may be associated with streaking of the stool with blood or blood on the toilet paper. Secondary anal fissures result from other underlying causes, such as Crohn's disease, anal cancer, HIV, tuberculosis, abscess or fistula, and sexually transmitted diseases. Depending on the cause, some of these may be painless, especially Crohn's disease and anal cancer, and may present as a non-healing ulcer and/or recurrent bleeding. They may also be located away from the midline unlike primary anal fissures. Any suspicion of a secondary cause for a fissure should prompt the physician to get a biopsy to diagnose the above-mentioned secondary causes.

The treatment of anal fissures depends on its duration. Acute fissures (<1 month) can be successfully treated with stool softeners, laxatives, and Sitz baths in up to 90% of patients. Patients with recurrent fissures tend to respond less well to these conservative methods. Chronic fissures (>1 month) should be considered for definitive therapy. The traditional therapy of a primary fissure consists of either open or closed myotomy of the lateral internal anal sphincter, which restores mucosal blood flow and promotes healing of the anoderm. An important complication of this procedure is fecal incontinence, which can occur in 10 to 40% of cases *(43,44)*. Insufficient myotomy, resulting from fear of causing incontinence, leads to fissure recurrence rates of up to 30% *(45)*. Recently, the use of medical therapy to relax the anal sphincter has gained acceptance as an alternative approach. Medications such as glyceryl trinitrate 0.2% ointment *(42,46)* and more recently, BTX injection into the internal sphincter are successful treatments in up to 80% of patients.

Jost, a pioneer in the treatment of anal fissure, presented the first case report on the use of BTX to treat anal fissures in 1993 *(47)*. The following year, Gui and others presented results from the treatment of 10 patients with BTX for anal fissure *(48)*. All patients received 5 U BTX within the contracted internal anal sphincter. At 1 week after treatment, resting sphincter pressure decreased approximately 25%, but healing did not yet occur. At 1 month, 60% of patients had evidence of healing while resting pressure remained reduced by 23.9% ($p < 0.05$ from baseline). At 2 months, eight patients had a healing scar but ultimately two patients relapsed *(48)*. Another small case series looked at five patients with documented anal fissure *(49)*. At day 7, all patients had a fall in resting sphincter pressure ($p < 0.02$). Two of the five patients had sustained healing over the 3-month study period.

In 1997, Jost reported uncontrolled data from the first 100 patients treated with BTX for anal fissure *(43)*. Patients received either 2.5 or 5 U BTX injected into the external anal sphincter on either side of the fissure using a 27-gage needle. At 6 months post-injection, roughly 80% of patients had complete fissure healing and remained asymptomatic. Sphincter pressure normalized in those patients who responded and no cases of incontinence occurred. A follow-up report from this group examined whether BTX injection was efficacious in patients who relapsed. The authors selected 20 patients from the previous study who relapsed after a mean of 12.4 ± 4.1 months *(50)*. By 3 months, after a 2.5-U injection on either side of the recurrent fissure, 14 patients had complete healing.

Minguez and others studied whether higher doses of BTX would be more efficacious in the treatment of anal fissure *(51)*. In a group of 69 patients, study subjects were allocated to three different total dosages. Patients received 10, 15, or 21 U BTX via two injections into the internal sphincter. Bleeding and defecatory difficulty improved in all groups at 3 months

**Table 2**
**Randomized Trials of BTX for the Treatment of Anal Fissure**

| Reference | Year published | n | BTX dose (U) | Alternative treatment | Mean of follow-up (months) | Results |
|---|---|---|---|---|---|---|
| 54 | 1998 | 30 | 20 | Saline | 16 | BTX superior to placebo for healing and symptomatic relief (p = 0.003). |
| 46 | 1999 | 50 | 20 | 0.2% nitroglycerin ointment | 11 | BTX superior to nitrates. Nine patients treated with nitrates eventually responded to BTX. |
| 57 | 2001 | 30 | 20 | BTX 20 U plus topical isosorbide dinitrate | 10 | Nitrates potentiate the beneficial effects of BTX. Unusually low healing rate in toxin alone group (20%). |
| 55 | 2003 | 111 | 20 or 30 (1 or 2 injections) | Lateral sphincterotomy | 12 | Healing rates similar (86% BTX versus 98% surgery). Higher rates of incontinence in surgical group. |

BTX, botulinum toxin.

after injection. However, at 6-month follow-up, there was no meaningful difference in the three groups with regard to healing and requirement for sphincterotomy, although the trend favored the 21-U group. Maria and others evaluated the importance of the location of BTX injection *(52)*. They randomized 50 patients to receive 20 U BTX into the anal sphincter either in the anterior or posterior midline. Patients were allowed to receive a repeat injection of 25 U BTX at 2 months if insufficient healing occurred. Patients receiving an anterior injection had a greater reduction in resting anal sphincter pressure as well as a higher rate of fissure healing (p = 0.025).

Another uncontrolled study of 76 patients looked at a higher dose of BTX (40 U) for the treatment of anal fissure *(53)*. A total of 43 patients responded and 33 had either a partial or no response. These patients received a repeat injection with 40 U and at 3 months a total of 51 patients (67% of all patients) had complete fissure healing. In another study, patients were randomized to receive either 20 U BTX followed by 30 U if the fissure persisted at 2 months (group 1) or 30 U BTX followed by 50 U for unhealed fissures (group 2; ref. *54*). The higher dose was associated with an increased rate of fissure healing, although ultimately nearly all patients were healed by study completion.

In the first randomized, double-blind, placebo-controlled study of BTX for anal fissure, 30 patients were randomized to either 20 U BTX or saline injection into the internal anal sphincter (Table 2; ref. *55*). All patients who did not respond or relapsed at 2 months were given either 20 U (control group) or 25 U (treatment group). By the second month after treatment, 2 of 15 patients in the control group and 11 of 15 in the BTX arm had healed fissures.

All healed patients in the treatment group remained so at a mean of 16 ± 6 months after treatment. Four patients who still had fissures were retreated with 25 U BTX and two had sustained healing at 3-month follow-up. Both resting anal pressure and maximal voluntary squeeze pressures dropped substantially in treated patients ($p = 0.02$; ref. *55*).

Brisinda and others compared the use of 20 U BTX injection with 0.2% nitroglycerin ointment applied twice daily in a group of 50 patients *(56)*. At the 2-month evaluation, 24 patients (96%) in the BTX group but only 15 (60%) in the nitroglycerin group had healed fissures ($p = 0.005$). Furthermore, resting anal pressure was decreased even more among those patients in the BTX group (29 versus 14%, $p = 0.04$; ref. *46*). Response in both groups was durable and no relapses occurred in patients from either group who achieved healing.

Recently, a study comparing the efficacy of BTX with internal anal sphincterotomy was completed *(56)*. In the BTX group, 45 of 61 had initial healing and 10 patients were treated with a second injection. Overall, by 6 months, 53 of 61 patients in the BTX group had complete healing of their anal fissure. Seven patients eventually recurred at 12 months. In the surgery arm, 49 of 50 patients were successfully healed by the second month and there were no relapses ($p = 0.008$ versus BTX) at 12 months. Of concern, there were eight instances of fecal incontinence in the surgery group, whereas this complication was not seen with BTX ($p < 0.001$).

Two studies have looked at the effectiveness of BTX in healing anal fissures in patients who have failed or only partially improved using topical nitroglycerin *(57,58)*. In the first study, 30 patients with chronic anal fissure who failed to respond to topical isosorbide dinitrate were randomized to injection of BTX (20 U) followed by continued daily nitrates, or injection of BTX alone *(57)*. At 6 weeks, the fissure-healing rate was significantly higher in the combination treatment group (66%) versus 20% in the BTX alone group. Subsequently, the second group was given topical nitrates and the healing rates improved over the next 12 weeks to match the original combination therapy group. The authors concluded that topical nitrates augment the healing effects of BTX in patients with refractory anal fissures and that excessive cholinergic tone is at the root of these difficult cases. In a similar study *(58)*, 40 patients failing treatment with glyceryl nitrate were injected with 20 U BTX and assessed for healing. A total of 17 fissures healed (43%) at 8-week follow-up. An additional 12 patients did not have complete healing but experienced a marked improvement in symptoms. Females, and those with fissures of greater than 12 months duration, appeared to derive the most benefit from BTX injection.

In summary, BTX injection into the internal anal sphincter for the treatment of primary anal fissure appears to be effective and long-term sequelae have rarely been seen. Short-term side effects have included incontinence of flatus or feces, which usually resolves quickly, anal hematoma, flu-like syndrome, acute inflammation of hemmorhoids, and hemmorhoidal prolapse *(59)*. In a porcine model, injection of BTX into the anal sphincter was not associated with significant histological changes and muscle atrophy and inflammation were not seen *(60)*.

## CONCLUSION

The treatment of spastic disorders of the gastrointestinal tract remains challenging. Since its pharmaceutical development, BTX has been used for a variety of spastic muscle disorders. Its application for gastrointestinal disorders has been studied over the past 15 years and usage of this therapy has increased. For two disorders in particular, achalasia and anal fissure, BTX represents an efficacious and well-studied treatment. In vigorous achalasia, especially in the elderly, BTX may be the preferred treatment. For gastroparesis, the data remains encouraging; however, controlled trials are needed. In other gastrointestinal disorders, such as esophageal spasm, sphincter of Oddi dysfunction, and anismus, only preliminary data is available. For gastrointestinal disorders, the concern remains that the effects of BTX are relatively short-lived and definitive treatment is delayed. Additional trials are necessary to assess its efficacy, duration of action, and for comparison to other therapeutic agents.

## REFERENCES

1. Shaw GY, Searl JP. Botulinum toxin treatment for cricopharyngeal dysfunction. Dysphagia 2001;16:161–167.
2. Schneider I, Thumfart WF, Pototschnig C, Eckel HE. Treatment of dysfunction of the cricopharyngeal muscle with botulinum A toxin: introduction of a new, noninvasive method. Ann Otol Rhinol Laryngol 1994;103:31–35.
3. Zarate N, Mearin F, Wang XY, Hewlett B, Huizinga JD, Malagelada JR. Severe idiopathic gastroparesis due to neuronal and interstitial cells of Cajal degeneration: pathological findings and management. Gut 2003;52:966–970.
4. Hornbuckle K, Barnett JL. The diagnosis and work-up of patients with gastroparesis. J Clin Gastroeneterol 2000;30:2:117–124.
5. Tougas G, Eaker EY, Abell TL, et al. Assessment of gastric emptying using a low fat meal: establishment of international control values. Am J Gastroenterol 2000;95:1456–1462.
6. Ezzeddine D, Jit R, Katz N, Gopalswamy N, Bhutani MS. Pyloric injection of botulinum toxin for treatment of diabetic gastroparesis. Gastrointest Endosc 2002;55:920–923.
7. Mearin F, Camilleri M, Malagelada JR. Pyloric dysfunction in diabetics with recurrent nausea and vomiting. Gastroenterology 1986;90:1919–1925.
8. James AN, Ryan JP, Parkman HP. Inhibitory effects of botulinum toxin on pyloric and antral smooth muscle. Am J Physiol Gastrointest Liver Physiol 2003;285:291–297.
9. Gupta P, Rao SS. Attenuation of isolated pyloric pressure waves in gastroparesis in response to botulinum toxin injection: a case report. Gastrointest Endosc 2002;56:770–772.
10. Miller LS, Szych GA, Kantor SB, et al. Treatment of idiopathic gastroparesis with injection of botulinum toxin into the pyloric sphincter muscle. Am J Gastroenterol 2002;97:1653–1660.
11. Lacy BE, Zayat EN, Crowell MD, Schuster MM. Botulinum toxin for the treatment of gastroparesis: a preliminary report. Am J Gastroenterol 2002;97:1548–1552.
12. Arts J, Gool SJ, Caenepeel P, Janssens J, Tack J. Effect of intrapyloric injection of botulinum toxin on gastric emptying and meal-related symptoms in gastroparesis. Gastroenterology 2003;124:A53 (Abstract).
13. Bromer MQ, Friedenberg F, Miller LS, Fisher RS, Swartz K, Parkman HP. Endoscopic pyloric injection of botulinum toxin a for the treatment of refractory gastroparesis. Gastrointest Endosc 2005;61:833–839.
14. Holloway RH, Dodds WJ, Helm JF, Hogan WJ, Dent J, Arndorfer RC. Integrity of cholinergic innervation to the lower esophageal sphincter in achalasia. Gastroenterology 1986;90:924–929.
15. Mittal RK, Balaban D. The esophagogastric junction. N Engl J Med 1997;336:924–932.
16. Mearin F, Mourelle M, Guarner F, et al. Patients with achalasia lack nitric oxide synthase in the gastro-esophageal junction. Eur J Clin Invest 1993;23:724–728.
17. Gaumnitz EA, Bass P, Osinski MA, Sweet MA, Singaram C. Electrophysiological and pharmacological responses of chronically denervated lower esophageal sphincter of the opossum. Gastroenterology 1995;109:789–799.
18. Reynolds JC, Parkman HP. Achalasia. Gastroenterol Clin North Am 1989;18:223–256.
19. Pasricha PJ, Ravich WJ, Kalloo AN. Effects of intrasphincteric botulinum toxin on the lower esophageal sphincter in piglets. Gastroenterology 1993;105:1045–1049.
20. Pasricha PJ, Ravich WJ, Hendrix TR, Sostre S, Jones B, Kalloo AN. Treatment of achalasia with intrasphicteric injection of botulinum toxin—a pilot trial. Ann Internal Med 1994;121:590–591.
21. Fishman VM, Parkman HP, Schiano TD, et al. Symptomatic improvement in achalasia after botulinum toxin injection of the lower esophageal sphincter. Am J Gastroenterol 1996;91:1724–1730.

22. Neubrand M, Scheurlen C, Schepke M, Sauerbruch T. Long-term results and prognostic factors in the treatment of achalasia with botulinum toxin. Endoscopy 2002;34:519–523.

23. Cuilliere. C, Ducrotte. P, Zerbib. F, et al. Achalasia: outcome of patients treated with intrasphincteric injection of botulinum toxin. Gut 1997;41:87–92.

24. Annese V, Basciani M, Borrelli O, Leandro G, Simone P, Andriulli A. Intrasphincteric injection of botulinum toxin is effective in long-term treatment of esophageal achalasia. Muscle Nerve 1998;21:1540–1542.

25. Greaves RR, Mulcahy HE, Patchett SE, et al. Early experience with intrasphincteric botulinum toxin in the treatment of achalasia. Aliment Pharmacol Ther 1999;13:1221–1225.

26. Kolbasnik J, Waterfall WE, Fachnie B, Chen Y, Tougas G. Long term efficacy of botulinum toxin in classical achalasia: a prospective study. Am J Gastroenterol 1999;94:3434–3439.

27. Pasricha PJ, Ravich WJ, Hendrix TR, Sostre S, Jones B, Kalloo AN. Intrasphincteric botulinum toxin for the treatment of achalasia. N Engl J Med 1995;332:774–778.

28. Pasricha PJ, Rai R, Ravich WJ, Hendrix TR, Kalloo AN. Botulinum toxin for achalasia: long term outcome and predictors of response. Gastroenterology 1996;110:1410–1415.

29. Annese V, Basciani M, Perri F, et al. Controlled trial of botulinum toxin injection versus placebo and pneumatic dilation in achalasia. Gastroenterology 1996;111:1418–1424.

30. Muehldorfer SM, Schneider TH, Hochberger J, Martus P, Hahn EG, Ell C. Esophageal achalasia: intrasphincteric injection of BTX versus balloon dilation. Endoscopy 1999;31:517–521.

31. Vaezi MF, Richter JE, Wilcox CM, et al. Botulinum toxin injection versus pneumatic dilation in the treatment of achalasia: a randomised trial. Gut 1999;44:231–239.

32. Mikaeli J, Fazel A, Montazeri G, Yaghoobi M, Malekzadeh R. Randomized controlled trial comparing botulinum toxin injection to pneumatic dilatation for the treatment of achalasia. Aliment Pharmacol Ther 2001;15:1389–1396.

33. Ghoshal UC, Chaudhuri S, Pal BB, Dhar K, Ray G, Banerjee PK. Randomized controlled trial of intrasphincteric BTX injection versus balloon dilatation in treatment of achalasia cardia. Dis Esophagus 2001;14:227–231.

34. Wehrmann T, Kokabpick H, Jacobi V, Seifert H, Lembcke B, Caspary WF. Long term results of endoscopic injection of botulinum toxin in elderly achalasia patients with tortuous megaesophagus or epiphrenic diverticulum. Endoscopy 1999;31:352–358.

35. Katzka DA, Castell DO. Use of BTXs a diagnostic/therapeutic trial to help clarify an indication for definitve therapy in patients with achalasia. Am J Gastroenterol 1999;94:637–642.

36. Hoffman BJ, Knapple WL, Bhutani MS, Verne GN, Hawes RH. Treatment of achalasia by injection of botulinum toxin under endoscopic ultrasound guidance. Gastrointest Endosc 1997;45:77–79.

37. Annese V, Bassotti G, Coccia G, et al. A multicentre randomised study of intrasphincteric botulinum toxin in patients with oesophageal achalasia. Gut 2000;46:597–600.

38. Forouzesh A, White KT, Mullin GE. The development of pneumoperitoneum as a result of botox injection for treatment of achalasia. Am J Gastroenterol 2003; 98(Suppl 1): 5–183.

39. Eaker EY, Gordon JM, Vogel SB. Untoward effects of esophageal botulinum toxin injection in the treatment of achalasia. Dig Dis Sci 1997;42:724–727.

40. Patti MG, Feo CV, Arcerito M, et al. Effects of previous treatment on results of laparascopic heller myotomy for achalasia. Dig Dis Sci 1999;44:2270–2276.

41. Hannel N, Gordon PH. Re-examination of clinical manifestations and response to therapy of fissure-in-ano. Dis Colon Rectum 1997;40:229–233.

42. Kennedy ML, Sowter S, Nguyen H, Lubowski DZ. Glyceryl trinitrate ointment for the treatment of chronic anal fissure: results of a placebo-controlled trial and long-term follow-up. Dis Colon Rectum 1999;42:1000–1006.

43. Jost WH. One hundred cases of anal fissure treated with botulinum toxin: early and long-term results. Dis Colon Rectum 1997;40:1029–1032.

44. Oettle GJ. Glyceryl trinitrate vs. sphincterotomy for treatment of chronic fissure-in-ano. Dis Colon Rectum 1997;10:1318–1320.

45. Evans J, Luck A, Hewett P. Glyceryl trinitrate vs. lateral sphincterotomy for chronic anal fissure: prospective randomized trial. Dis Colon Rectum 2001;44:93–97.

46. Brisinda G, Maria G, Bentivoglio AR, Cassetta E, Gui D, Albanese A. A comparision of injections of BTXnd topical nitroglycerin ointment for the treatment of chronic anal fissure. N Engl J Med 1999;34:65–69.

47. Jost WH, Schimrigk K. Therapy of anal fissure using botulin toxin. Dis Colon Rectum 1994; 37:1340.

48. Gui D, Cassetta E, Anastasio G, Bentivoglio AR, Maria G, Albanese A. Botulinum toxin for chronic anal fissure. Lancet 1994: 344:1127–1128.

49. Mason PF, Watkins MJ, Hall HS, Hall AW. The management of chronic fissure in-ano with botulinum toxin. J R Coll Surg Edinb 1996;41:235–238.

50. Jost WH, Schrank B. Repeat botulinum toxin injections in anal fissure in patients with relapse after insufficient effect of first treatment. Dig Dis Sci 1999;44:1588–1589.

51. Minguez M, Melo F, Espi A, et al. Therapeutic effects of different doses of botulinum toxin in chronic anal fissure. Dis Colon Rectum 1999;42:1016–1021.

52. Maria G, Brisinda G, Bentivoglio AR, Cassetta E, Gui D, Albanese A. Influence of botulinum toxin site of injections on healing rate in patients with chronic anal fissure. Am J Surg 2000;179:46–50.

53. Brisinda G, Maria G, Sganga G, Bentivoglio AR, Albanese A, Castagneto M. Effectiveness of higher doses of botulinum toxin to induce healing in patients with chronic anal fissures. Surgery 2002;131:179–184.

54. Maria G, Cassetta E, Gui D, Brisinda G, Bentivoglio AR, Albanese A. A comparison of BTX and saline for the treatment of chronic anal fissure. N Engl J Med 1998;338:217–220.

55. Mentes BB, Irkorucu O, Akin M, Leventoglu S, Tatlicioglu E. Comparision of botulinum toxin injection and lateral internal sphincterotomy for the treatment of chronic anal fissure. Dis Colon Rectum 2003;46:232–237.

56. Lindsey I, Jones OM, Cunningham C, George BD, Mortensen NJ. Botulinum toxin as second-line therapy for chronic anal fissure failing 0.2 percent glyceryl trinitrate. Dis Colon Rectum 2003;46:361–366.

57. Lysy J, Israelit-Yatzkan Y, Sestiery-Ittah M, Weksler-Zangen S, Keret D, Goldin E. Topical nitrates potentiate the effect of botulinum toxin in the treatment of patients with refractory anal fissure. Gut 2001;48:221–224.

58. Cassidy TD, Pruitt A, Perry WB. Permanent fecal incontinence following botulinum toxin injection therapy for chronic anal fissure. Am J Gastroenterol 2003;98:page range.

59. Madalinski MH, Slawek J, Duzynski W, et al. Side effects of botulinum toxin injection for benign anal disorders. Eur J Gastroenterol Hepatol 2002;14:853–856.

60. Langer JC, Birnbaum EE, Schmidt RE. Histology and function of the internal anal sphincter after injection of botulinum toxin. J Surg Res 1997;73:113–116.

# 14

# Blepharospasm

Amir Cohen, Marc J. Spirn, David Khoramian,
and C. Robert Bernardino

## INTRODUCTION

Blepharospasm is a focal dystonia of the orbicularis oculi muscles characterized by chronic intermittent or sometimes persistent involuntary eyelid closure *(1)*. Blepharospasm usually begins in the fifth to sixth decade of life (mean age of 56) and has a slight female preponderance (1.8:1; refs. *2–7*). The prevalence of blepharospasm is estimated at 5 per 100,000 individuals *(3, 8)*, with approximately 50,000 cases occurring in the United States and with nearly 2000 new cases diagnosed annually.

## CLINICAL FINDINGS

Clinically, blepharospasm exists on a continuum. On one end of the spectrum, patients may present with an increased blink rate and intermittent eyelid spasm. On the other end, patients may present with spasmodic eyelid closure during most of the day, resulting in functional blindness and severe debility.

Early on, patients frequently present with increased blinking and photophobia associated with ocular irritants such as wind, sunlight, or dust. These symptoms may precede or occur simultaneously with the development of eyelid spasm *(9)*. During this period, patients often complain of photophobia and foreign body sensation; symptoms that may be exacerbated by concurrent dry eyes or blepharitis. Eventually these symptoms progress to include variably intermittent involuntary eyelid closure, which may be unilateral or bilateral. Patients with longstanding blepharospasm may develop associated ptosis of the eyelid and brow, entropion, dermatochalasis, and abnormalities of the canthal tendon.

## TERMINOLOGY

When the involuntary contractions are limited to the orbital and periorbital muscles, the term *essential blepharospasm* is used. Frequently, however, blepharospasm is associated with other facial dystonias, involving the facial, pharyngeal, oromandibular, laryngeal, or cervical muscles *(10)*. Meige syndrome refers to eyelid spasm occurring in association with midface spasm, particularly those of the perioral and mandibular regions. Spasmodic torticollis, dysphagia, spasmodic dysphonia, and segmental dystonia of the limbs may also be present. Brueghel's syndrome describes eyelid spasms with marked spasms of the lower face and

From: *Therapeutic Uses of Botulinum Toxin*
Edited by: G. Cooper © Humana Press Inc., Totowa, NJ

neck. Segmental cranial dystonia occurs when eyelid and facial spasms occur in conjunction with spasms of cranial nerves other than only the facial nerve. Generalized dystonia describes eyelid and facial spasms with spasms of additional body parts. Hemifacial spasm is typically a unilateral condition in which segmental myoclonus of the facial nerve occurs, causing variable contraction of the orbicularis oculi, corrugator, frontalis, platysma, and zygomaticus muscles *(11)*. Unlike these other dystonias, hemifacial spasm is often caused by a discrete lesion along the facial nerve. As a result, patients with hemifacial spasm should undergo magnetic resonance imaging to rule out a neoplastic, inflammatory, or other process that may require specific treatment. Magnetic resonance imaging is generally not necessary in other types of dystonia, such as benign essential blepharospasm and Meige syndrome.

## DIFFERENTIAL DIAGNOSIS

Multiple disorders may present with blepharospasm as part of their clinical spectrum, including neurological defects such as Parkinson's disease, Huntingtons's disease, Wilson's disease, Creutzfeld-Jacob disease, and postencephalitic syndrome. Psychological causes include habit spasms, Gilles de la Tourette syndrome, and functional spasms. Blepharospasm can occur as a result of medical conditions such as myotonic dystrophy, tetany, tetanus, or seizures. Likewise, it can occur from systemic medications including antipsychotics, antiemetics, anorectics, nasal decongestants, and levodopa. A detailed history and physical exam should help differentiate essential blepharospasm and related dystonias from these other systemic conditions.

Blepharospasm should also be differentiated from other entities, such as apraxia of eyelid opening and blepharoptosis (drooping of the eyelids) because treatment differs. Apraxia of lid opening occurs when patients with otherwise normal eyelids have difficulty opening their eyelids. This can be differentiated from blepharospasm by the fact that both have eyelid closure but only blepharospasm has increased muscular tone. For reasons not entirely understood, apraxia of eyelid opening also frequently occurs in patients with blepharospasm.

## PATHOGENESIS

Blepharospasm is thought to be a defect in neurological circuit activity *(9)*. The circuit has an afferent sensory limb, a central control center, and an efferent motor limb. A defect at any point in the circuit can precipitate blepharospasm. Multiple factors can initiate the afferent limb of the cycle. These include such stimuli as corneal or eyelid irritation, pain, light, emotional stresses, or other factors *(12)*.

The afferent stimuli are transmitted to the central control center. Although its exact location has not been delineated, the central control center is thought to lie in or around the basal ganglia and involve dopaminergic and noradrenergic stimuli. Abnormal stimuli can also originate from this area. Diseases such as Parkinson's and Huntington's, which originate in the basal ganglii, are often associated with blepharospasm because they disrupt the central control center.

From this central location, the signal is transmitted along the efferent limb via the facial nerve and nucleus to the orbicularis oculi, corrugator, and procerus muscles *(12)*. Rarely, abnormal stimuli can arise in the efferent limb. Patients with facial nerve palsies may rarely develop blepharospasm. The blepharospasm may be a result of facial nerve dysfunction itself or a consequence of the dry eyes that occur from facial nerve-induced lagophthalmos and exposure keratopathy.

## TREATMENT

The treatment of blepharospasm is multifactorial. Whenever possible, the treatment should be oriented toward the deficient arm of the neurological circuit. For example, in patients with dry eyes, treatment of the dry eyes should be initiated before more invasive methods. Patients with photophobia should be given tinted glasses in an attempt to resolve symptoms *(13)* and patients with psychological-induced blepharospasm should be referred for counseling and psychological intervention.

If treating the afferent limb is unsuccessful or only partially successful, treatment should be geared toward altering either the central control center or the efferent limb. Multiple pharmacological treatments have been tried. These include Artane® (trihexyphenidyl), Cogentin® (benztropine), Valium® (diazepam), Klonopin® (clonazepam), Lioresal® (baclofen), Tegretol® (carbamazepine), Sinemet® or Modopar® (levodopa), and Symmetrel® (amantadine). These treatments, which aim to regulate the central control center, have attained only mild to moderate success in treating blepharospasm. These treatments are felt to have a secondary role in the treatments of facial dystonias and are discussed later in this chapter.

### Botulinum Toxin Type A

Currently, injection of botulinum toxin type A (BTX-A), which inhibits the efferent limb of the neurological circuit, is the preferred treatment of blepharospasm. There are seven immunologically distinct forms of BTX, each produced by a different *Clostridium* species. Botox® (Allergan, Inc., Irvine, CA), a formulation of BTX-A that is produced by *Clostridium botulinum* (an anaerobic, rod-shaped, Gram-positive bacterium), is the most potent subtype. It interferes with the release of acetylcholine from nerve terminals in the neuromuscular junction. Upon injection of BTX-A into the muscle, the toxin competitively, nearly irreversibly, and rapidly binds to the cholinergic receptor terminals. The toxin is then internalized where it inhibits the release of acetylcholine vesicles from the nerve terminal. By inhibiting acetylcholine release, neuromuscular junction function is decreased and flaccid paralysis occurs locally at the site of action.

The paralytic effect of BTX-A begins approximately 2 to 4 days after injection *(14)*. This delayed action occurs because there may be continued release of acetylcholine from vesicles that have not been blocked by the toxin. Peak effect occurs approximately 3.7 days after injection with a mean duration of action of 12.5 weeks *(15)*. As the drug effect declines, patients typically require repeat injection. However, because responses may vary, some patients may require monthly injections while others may require twice yearly dosing. Treatment must therefore be geared toward the specific individuals needs.

Meticulous technique in the administration and constitution of Botox ensures reliability and consistency. The first step involves reconstituting the Botox with 0.9% non-preserved normal saline. This process must be performed carefully and slowly with a vacuum-sealed vial to prevent frothing. Care should be taken to avoid shaking the solution to prevent denaturing the toxin and thereby decreasing its efficacy. After reconstitution, the solution should be used within a few hours or refrigerated for up to a week *(16,17)*.

One typical reconstitution regimen involves diluting a standard 100-U vial of Botox with 2 mL non-preserved saline, yielding a dilution of 5 U per 0.1 mL. Note that varying the dilution with saline will give more or less concentrated serum per injection volume and this concentration may have an effect on efficacy/diffusion *(18)*. The toxin can then be drawn into a tuberculin syringe and injected with a 30-gauge needle. For the first treatment, a total dose of 25 U or less

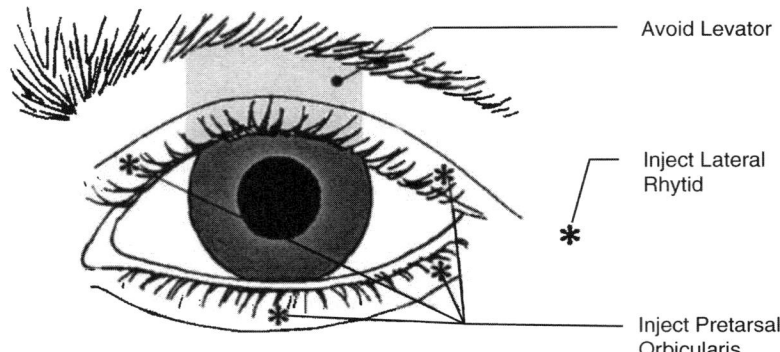

**Fig. 1.** Sketch of the left eye depicting typical injection sites (designated by *) for treating of blepharospasm with Botox. The levator muscle should be avoided (shaded area) because injection here can cause ptosis. (Illustration courtesy of Andreana A. Bernardino.)

per eye, divided among four to six periocular injection sites, is recommended to avoid adverse effects (*see* Fig. 1). Subsequent treatments should be adjusted depending on patient response to the initial doses. At each site, injection of 2.5 to 10 U Botox is recommended. Use of lower volumes (higher concentrations) is suggested to avoid the risk of spread to adjacent areas. The solution should be injected subcutaneously over the orbicularis oculi. Injection into the pretarsal region may be the best part of the orbicularis oculi to inject *(19,15)* and injection into the muscle of Riolan may be particularly effective *(20)*. Intramuscular injection is advocated over the thicker corrugator and procerus muscles when necessary.

Treatment success rate with BTX is estimated at approximately 90% *(21)*. Treatment failures only rarely occur and may result when antibodies to BTX develop. In such patients, re-injection may need to occur more frequently and at higher doses.

The potency of BTX is measured in units. One unit of BTX is the amount that causes 50% chance of death in Swiss Webster mice weighing 18 to 20 g after intraperitoneal injection. In humans, the mean lethal dose is estimated at 39 U/kg *(22)*. Although the doses of BTX are far below these doses, adverse effects can occur and have been reported after injection of BTX-A for blepharospasm. The most common side effect of injection is eyelid swelling with or without bruising. In 2001, Jost reported that the most common adverse effects were dry eyes, ptosis, mid-facial weakness, and diplopia. The side effects most frequently occur when BTX diffuses into an adjacent area that was not intended for treatment. For example, if a rectus muscle is inadvertently treated, diplopia will result. Similarly, if the levator palpebrae superioris is treated, ptosis will ensue. Careful attention to injection site and concentration can avoid many of these untoward outcomes. After the injection, applying ice, elevating the head, and refraining from hot showers may reduce diffusion of the injection and its subsequent untoward effects. Nevertheless, these side effects and others, such as ectropion, entropion, and lagophthalmos, do occur. BTX-A should not be injected if the patient has a known allergy to the drug, has an infection at the site of injection, has a coagulopathy, is pregnant (category C), or is breastfeeding.

*Preparations and Other Injectables*

In the United States, Botox is the only commercially available form of BTX-A. In the United Kingdom, Dysport® (Ipsen, Maidenhead, UK) is the BTX-A alternative. Myobloc®

(Solstice Neurosciences, South San Francisco, CA) is a type of BTX-B and is licensed by the Food and Drug Administration for use in cervical dystonias. Unlike Botox, Myobloc comes in ready-to-use injectable solutions with a shelf life of up to 36 months when refrigerated and up to 9 months when left at room temperature.

### Oral Medications

The symptomatic treatment of blepharospasm is best achieved with BTX. When BTX is either ineffective or poorly tolerated, oral medications are the next best step. A proper trial period for each drug consists of 1 to 2 months. The drug should be administered at the highest tolerated dose. Oral medications may be effective and these drugs may be used alone or in combination with each other.

#### Trihexyphenidyl

Trihexyphenidyl is an oral antimuscarinic drug. It is rapidly absorbed from the gastrointestinal (GI) tract and can cross the blood–brain barrier, making trihexyphenidyl useful in treating parkinsonism. Trihexyphenidyl is an antagonist of acetylcholine and other cholinergic stimuli at muscarinic receptors in the central nervous system (CNS) and in smooth muscle. It has a direct antispasmodic action on smooth muscle, and it has weak mydriatic, antisecretory, and positive chronotropic activities. The onset of action is 1 hour and the drug is renally excreted. Peak effects last 2 to 3 hours and the duration of action is 6 to 12 hours *(23)*.

Anticholinergics are commonly used to treat focal, segmental, and generalized dystonias. About 50% of children and 40% of adults obtain moderate to marked improvement *(24,25)*. Initiating treatment within the first 5 years of symptom onset achieves the best clinical effect *(26)*. A mean dose of 30 mg per day in young patients with a mean age of 18.9 years (range 9–32) is effective for the symptomatic treatment of segmental and generalized dystonia *(27)*. These beneficial results are unfortunately less common in the adult population, possibly owing to poorer efficacy and/or intolerable adverse effects. Central adverse effects, such as forgetfulness, may occur. Children tolerate this effect better than adults, making compliance less problematic in children. Reducing the dosage can minimize this adverse effect *(24)*. Nevertheless, trihexyphenidyl has been shown to be beneficial in adults with acute onset of Meige syndrome following neuroleptic-induced akathisia *(28)*. In fact, one study found trihexyphenidyl to be the most efficient drug for the treatment of craniocervical dystonia *(29)*.

Peripheral adverse effects can be overcome with pyridostigmine. Blurred vision from anticholinergic use may be improved with pilocarpine eye drops.

#### Benztropine

Benztropine is an oral and parenteral muscarinic-receptor antagonist. It is absorbed from the GI tract and may cross the placenta. Benztropine crosses the blood–brain barrier, making it useful in treating all types of parkinsonian syndromes, including antipsychotic-induced extrapyramidal symptoms. Benztropine may be a better drug for geriatric patients who cannot tolerate cerebral-stimulating agents because it produces less CNS stimulation than trihexyphenidyl. Unlike trihexyphenidyl, benztropine does not have a fast onset of action but rather has cumulative effects. Therapeutic benefit can take up to 2 to 3 days, but benztropine has a longer duration of action. Most of the drug is excreted renally *(23)*.

Benztropine competes with acetylcholine at muscarinic receptors in the CNS and in smooth muscle. The muscarinic properties of centrally active anticholinergics are thought to be responsible for the beneficial effects seen in parkinsonism. By blocking muscarinic cholinergic receptors in the CNS, benztropine reduces the excessive cholinergic activity. Benztropine also blocks dopamine reuptake and storage in CNS cells, thus prolonging dopamine's effects.

Several case reports have described improved symptoms in patients with Meige syndrome treated with benztropine *(30,31)*.

*Diazepam*

Diazepam is a long-acting oral and parenteral benzodiazepine. It is well-known for its use in the short-term management of anxiety disorders and acute alcohol withdrawal, as well as a skeletal muscle relaxant. Benzodiazepines act at the level of the limbic, thalamic, and hypothalamic regions of the CNS. γ-Aminobutyric acid (GABA) inhibition of the ascending reticular activating system is potentiated through the allosteric interaction of central benzodiazepine receptors with GABA receptors. The stimulation of the reticular pathways causes cortical and limbic arousal; benzodiazepines block this arousal. Benzodiazepines function as muscle relaxers by inhibiting mono- and polysynaptic pathways, and thus can depress muscle and motor nerve function directly. Studies have shown that benzodiazepines limit the spread of electrical activity by neurons through presynaptic inhibition; the drugs do not actually inhibit the abnormally discharging focus *(23)*.

In its class of drugs, it is the most rapidly absorbed following an oral dose. The onset of action after an intravenous dose is 1 to 5 minutes. Diazepam and its metabolite, desmethyldiazepam, have very long half-lives; the half-life of diazepam is 30 to 60 hours. However, the duration of action for certain clinical effects is much shorter than most would expect. This is partly because of rapid shifts in distribution of diazepam out of the CNS.

Diazepam crosses the placenta and distributes into breast milk. Metabolism is primarily hepatic and it is renally excreted. The drug has three active metabolites: desmethyldiazepam, temazepam, and oxazepam.

Sedatives, especially diazepam, are often used in treating dystonias and blepharospasm *(32)*. However, there have been reports of drug-induced blepharospasm after prolonged administration of etizolam or benzodiazepines *(8)*. This may result from a downregulation of GABA-A receptors involved in the neural circuits *(9)*.

*Clonazepam*

Clonazepam is an oral benzodiazepine used primarily to treat patients with seizure disorder. This drug should be used cautiously in individuals who have a history of seizure disorder. Orally disintegrating tablets of clonazepam are available as Klonopin® wafers *(23)*.

The onset of action is 20 to 60 minutes and the duration of action is 6 to 8 hours in children and up to 12 hours in adults. The half-life of clonazepam is 22 to 33 hours in children and 19 to 50 hours in adults. The drug undergoes hepatic metabolism and renal excretion.

Clonazepam has been shown to be clinically therapeutic in the treatment of blepharospasm *(25,33)*. Among oral medications for the treatment of blepharospasm, one study showed that physicians favored clonazepam most often *(32)*. However, other reports suggest that trihexyphenidyl should be the first-line oral medication and clonazepam a third-line oral agent *(34)*. Clonazepam has also been used for the treatment of parkinsonian dystonia *(35)*, as well as antipsychotic drug-induced dyskinesia with associated anxiety. Low doses of clonazepam are recommended for mild dyskinesia *(36)*. In fact, one study found clonazepam to be the most efficient drug for the treatment of facial hemispasm *(29)*. Intravenous injections of 5.0 mg clonazepam have also been shown to have an increased therapeutic potential for the treatment of patients with Meige syndrome with predominant blepharospasm versus biperiden, haloperidol, and lisuride *(37)*. Doses as low as 1.0 mg intravenously have also been shown to be effective to treat blepharospasm *(38)*.

Clonazepam has been shown to relieve blepharospasm in patients with Meige syndrome as well *(20,39)*. Patients with Meige syndrome who respond to clonazepam show a decrease in plasma levels of homovanillic acid and 3-methoxy-4-hydroxyphenylglycol *(40)*. Plasma homovanillic acid and 3-methoxy-4-hydroxyphenylglycol are surrogate markers of central dopamine and noradrenaline activity, respectively. Central GABA deficiency and increased dopaminergic activity have been implicated in the pathogenesis of this syndrome.

Visual, auditory, and tactile hallucinations as well as paranoia are possible side effects. Reducing the dosage should ameliorate these side effects. In cases in which no other satisfactory treatment is available, dose reduction is recommended as an alternative to drug discontinuation with proper patient monitoring and protection *(41)*.

## Baclofen

Baclofen is an oral skeletal muscle relaxant. It is a structural analog of the inhibitory neurotransmitter GABA. Baclofen is best known for its ability to decrease the number and severity of spasms and relieve associated pain, clonus, and muscle rigidity. Baclofen is also available in an orally-disentegrating tablet formulation (Kemstro™), as well as for intrathecal administration (Lioresal) for the treatment of spasticity of cerebral origin *(23)*.

It is thought that the drug blocks both polysynaptic and monosynaptic afferent pathways at the level of the spinal cord, inhibiting the transmission of impulses through these pathways as a GABA agonist. Baclofen may function either as an inhibitory neurotransmitter itself or by hyperpolarizing the primary afferent nerve terminals. This causes a decreased release of the neurotransmitters aspartate and glutamate from afferent nerve terminals, and therefore causes decreased excitatory input into alpha motor neurons. Large doses of baclofen cause CNS depression, suggesting that the drug also works at supraspinal sites.

Baclofen is rapidly absorbed following an oral dose, and has a half-life of 2.5 to 4 hours. Baclofen minimally crosses the blood–brain barrier, crosses the placenta, and is excreted into breast milk. A small percentage of each dose undergoes hepatic metabolism, with both renal and fecal excretion. Onset of action following intrathecal administration occurs within 0.5 to 1 hour. Peak antispasmodic effect is seen 4 hours after administration and duration of action is 4 to 8 hours *(23)*.

Baclofen may be considered as a second-line oral medication after trihexyphenidyl for the treatment of blepharospasm *(34)*. Generalized dystonias should be treated with anticholinergic agents; however, baclofen can also be used as a first-line agent in some cases *(42)*.

Baclofen has also been used in the treatment of Meige syndrome. An increase in dopaminergic activity may be a cause for dystonic symptoms. The synthesis of dopamine by nigral neurons in the nigrostriatal pathway is dependent on GABA through one of the retrograde loops in its feedback control. GABA agonists that cross the blood–brain barrier could result in a decreased dopaminergic action in the nigro-striatal pathway, thus ameliorating the dystonic symptoms. In one study, five patients were treated with a dose of 20 mg per day, with an increase in dose by 10 mg each 3 days, reaching a maximum dose of 70 mg per day. Forty percent of the patients experienced improvement in their blepharospasm *(43)*. The use of sodium valproate with baclofen can also provide a physiological means of reducing dopaminergic predominance in the striatum *(44)*. In fact, one patient with idiopathic blepharospasm had complete and sustained remission of symptoms and signs after treatment with this GABA-mimetic combination.

## Carbamazepine

Carbamazepine is an oral anticonvulsant drug used for treatment of partial seizures, both simple and complex, and for tonic-clonic seizures. Carbamazepine is also used to treat pain of neurological origin, such as trigeminal neuralgia. Carbamazepine is available in two extended-release dosage forms, Tegretol-XR tablets and Carbatrol® capsules. It is also available as Equetro™, an extended-release (multi-phasic) formulation for the treatment of bipolar I disorder *(23)*.

Carbamazepine inhibits the repetitive firing of neurons by blocking use-dependent sodium channels. The drug reduces post-tetanic potentiation of synaptic transmission in the spinal cord. This effect may explain its ability to limit the spread of seizures. Pain relief is believed to be associated with blockade of synaptic transmission in the trigeminal nucleus.

Possible adverse effects should be reviewed with the patient. Side effects may arise from the drug's anticholinergic, central antidiuretic (syndrome of inappropriate antidiuretic hormone), antiarrhythmic, muscle relaxant, antidepressant, sedative, and neuromuscular-blocking properties. Carbamazepine is also a potent enzyme inducer and can induce its own metabolism, probably through its effects on the hepatic CYP3A4 isoenzyme.

Carbamazepine is administered orally, and GI absorption is slow and variable. Because of its lipophilic properties, the drug is present in cerebrospinal fluid, bile, and saliva. Carbamazepine crosses the placenta with accumulation in the fetus and it is excreted into breast milk.

Carbamazepine undergoes hepatic metabolism and forms the active metabolite, carbamazepine 10,11-epoxide. Both renal and fecal excretion occurs. Carbamazepine is a potent enzyme inducer. It has a half-life of 25 to 65 hours initially and 12 to 17 hours after repeated dosing.

Carbamazepine may be effective in some cases of hemifacial spasm *(34)*. The availability of anticholinergic and dopaminergic oral medications precludes the use of carbamazepine for blepharospasm. It may be considered as an alternative oral medication if the others are ineffective or not tolerated by the patient. However, carbamazepine may be a drug of choice in Schwartz-Jampel syndrome with blepharospasm *(45)*.

## Levodopa/Carbidopa

The combination of levodopa and carbidopa is used in the treatment of Parkinson's disease. Levodopa is the metabolic precursor of dopamine. Carbidopa is a noncompetitive decarboxylase inhibitor added to inhibit the peripheral destruction of levodopa, increasing the availability of levodopa for transport to the brain. In fact, less than 1% of levodopa would reach the CNS if given without carbidopa. Only the combination drug product is available; levodopa by itself has been discontinued in the United States. Combination therapy allows lower doses of levodopa to be used owing to higher availability of drug. It also minimizes adverse reactions such as the dopaminergic side effects of nausea and vomiting. The dosage of carbidopa–levodopa should be individualized to provide the maximum relief of symptoms with the least amount of side effects *(23)*.

An orally disintegrating formulation of carbidopa–levodopa (Parcopa™) is available, as well as a tablet intended for oral suspension before administration (Carbilev™), which is considered bioequivalent to the reference-listed drug Sinemet® tablets.

Levodopa is converted to dopamine in the CNS by L-aromatic amino acid decarboxylase and 3-*O*-methyldopa. The increase in dopamine and resulting decrease in acetylcholine is believed to improve nerve impulse control and to be the basis of the drug's antiparkinsonian activity.

The combination drug is administered orally as regular- and extended-release tablets. Amino acid transport mechanisms carry levodopa across the membrane of the GI tract. High concentrations of amino acids in the GI tract from a high-protein diet may interfere with absorption of levodopa.

Therapeutic effects of the combination drug can be appreciated 2 to 3 weeks after therapy is initiated. Maximal response to a given dosage may be seen up to 6 months following initiation of therapy in some patients. The plasma half-life of levodopa is 1 to 2 hours. The duration of action is 5 hours after administration of the regular-release dosage; however, this varies between individuals and their disease process, so treatment regimens should be individualized. The drug is renally excreted.

Differing amounts of dopamine, either high or low, can disrupt the normal balance between the dopamine system and another neurotransmitter system, which interferes with smooth and continuous movement. Because dopamine deficiency may be one etiology for blepharospasm, improvement in blepharospasm has been seen with levodopa and dopaminergic agonist use *(2,23)*. Patients with striatal lesions and dopaminergic denervation demonstrate blepharospasm as well as a pallido-pyramidal syndrome. Levodopa treatment can improve this blepharospasm *(46)*. A reduction in dosage of carbidopa–levodopa in a patient with Parkinson's disease can also precipitate a sustained blepharospasm that prevents the eyelid from opening. A significant improvement should be expected with an increase in the dosage of carbidopa–levodopa *(47)*. Sustained blepharospasm, also common in progressive supranuclear palsy, can occur without any motor deficits and may respond to levodopa therapy *(48)*. Although the mechanisms and pathogenesis of dystonia are not fully understood, basal ganglia activity and levodopa levels are considered to play important roles. Adjusting levodopa doses and adding a dopamine agonist, anticholinergics, baclofen, or clonazepam are medical options for the improvement of blepharospasm in these patients *(49)*. However, induced blepharospasm by levodopa has been documented in progressive supranuclear palsy patients *(50,51)*. Dopaminergic medication should be adjusted to rule out the possibility of treatment-induced symptoms.

## Amantadine

Amantadine is an antiviral agent first introduced for prophylaxis of influenza A and later found to cause symptomatic improvement in parkinsonism *(52)*.

The drug may function to potentiate CNS dopaminergic responses, increasing the amount of dopamine and norepinephrine. Amantadine is not as effective as levodopa but can be considered in patients experiencing maximal or waning effects from levodopa. Amantadine also has anticholinergic actions, however, there are no reports documenting its therapeutic significance.

Amantadine is administered orally, with rapid and complete absorption from the GI tract. The drug crosses the blood–brain barrier and the placenta, and distributes into tears, saliva, and nasal secretions. It is excreted into breast milk and through the kidneys. Acidifying the urine increases the rate of excretion.

There has been only one published article documenting the use of amantadine for blepharospasm. Amantadine was not shown to ameliorate the symptoms of blepharospasm *(53)*.

## Surgery

Surgical treatments can be entertained if BTX and oral medication therapy fail to provide relief. Surgical indication is dependent on the patient's functional disability and therefore relies on the patient's quality of life and ability to function. A protractor myectomy may be considered if all pharmacological treatment attempts fail and the patient is too disabled to remain untreated. The functional disability assessment scale grades functional disability and provides a way to quantify the disability from the patient's point of view, to determine surgical indication, and to predict the efficacy of surgery *(54)*.

Most patients are extremely satisfied with their functional improvement after surgery. A recent study of 138 patients diagnosed with essential blepharospasm, apraxia of eyelid opening, and intermediate forms was performed to assess surgical outcome *(54)*. Surgical procedures consisted of orbicularis myectomy alone, frontalis suspension alone, or both procedures concomitantly. The functional disability score was assessed pre-operatively and 3 months postoperatively, showing a significant decrease in functional disability postoperatively.

### Myectomy

Myectomy is the major surgical treatment for benign essential blepharospasm. It is usually reserved for individuals who respond poorly to more conservative therapy or for those who need correction of anatomical problems, such as ptosis *(55)*. The pretarsal, preseptal, and orbital portions of upper eyelid orbicularis oculi muscles are removed. Extended myectomy also includes removal of the procerus and corrugator muscles. A modified or limited myectomy involves the removal of only the orbicularis muscle in the upper lid. Advantages to the limited myectomy are a quicker recovery and less morbidity *(55)*. Upper and lower eyelid myectomy surgery should not be performed together in order to avoid chronic lymphedema *(56)*.

Although most patients are extremely satisfied with their functional improvement following surgery, the aesthetic outcomes may be of concern to individuals considering this procedure. Limited extirpation of only the orbicularis oculi muscle and the corrugator supercilii muscle through an eyelid crease incision may still result in irregular contours and a hollow and excavated appearance in the periorbital region. Recent studies using a muscle graft as an adjunct to myectomy has been shown to improve aesthetic outcomes for patients *(57)*.

### Chemomyectomy

Doxorubicin chemomyectomy is a recently studied treatment that has been used for both facial spasm and blepharospasm. Injection of doxorubicin had sustained improvement in blepharospasm over 8 years of follow-up *(45,58)*. However, side effects, including skin erythema, edema, and ulceration, caused up to one-third of initial study participants to discontinue treatment *(59)*. A newer liposome-encapsulated form of doxorubicin called DOXIL® (Sequus Pharmaceuticals, Menlo Park, CA) has shown some promise in alleviating the skin changes.

### Selective Destruction or Differential Section of the Facial (Seventh) Nerve

Differential section of the seventh nerve has been shown to be a reasonable alternative in patients with persistent disability from blepharospasm. This procedure may be considered after failed treatment with BTX injections and eyelid protractor myectomy. It is rarely performed because of the therapeutic benefits of BTX and myectomy, as well as a high incidence of paralytic complications that may result *(60)*.

## CONCLUSION

In summary, blepharospasm and other focal facial dystonias can range from mildly to severely debilitating. Their causes may be multifactorial and they may occur in isolation or as part of a related systemic condition. Treatment is best geared toward the underlying defect but when the defect occurs idiopathically, BTX-A is frequently highly effective and often the mainstay of treatment.

## REFERENCES

1. Costa J, Espirito-Santo C, Borges A, Ferreira et al. Botulinum toxin type A therapy for blepharospasm. Cochrane Database Syst Rev 2005;1:CD004900.
2. Frueh BR, Callahan A, Dortzbach RK, et al. A profile of patients with intractable blepharospasm. Trans Sect Ophthalmol Am Acad Ophthalmol Otolaryngol 1976;81:591–594.
3. Grandas F, Traba A, Alonso F, Esteban A. Blink reflex recovery cycle in patients with blepharospasm unilaterally treated with botulinum toxin. Clin Neuropharmacol 1998;21:307–311.
4. Henderson JW. Essential blepharospasm. Trans Am Ophthalmol Soc 1956;54:453–520.
5. Jankovic J, Ford J. Blepharospasm and orofacial-cervical dystonia: clinical and pharmacology findings in 100 patients. Ann Neurol 1983;13:402–411.
6. Marsden CD. Blepharospasm-oromandibular dystonia syndrome. J Neurol Neurosurg Psychiatry 1976;390:1204–1209.
7. Tolosa ES. Clinical features of Meige's disease (idiopathic orofacial dystonia): a report of 17 cases. Arch Neurol 1981;36:147–151.
8. Nutt JG, Muenter MD, Melton LJIII, Aronson A, Kurland LT. Epidemiology of focal and generalized dystonia in Rochester, Minnesota. Mov Disord 1988;3:188–194.
9. McCann JD, Gauthier M, Morschbacher R, et al. A novel mechanism for benign essential blepharospasm. Ophthal Plast Reconstr Surg 1999;15:384–389.
10. Tolosa ES, Klawans HL. Meige's disease: a clinical form of a facial convulsion, bilateral and medial. Arch Neurol 1979;36:635–637.
11. Costa J, Espirito-Santo C, Borges A, et al. Botulinum toxin type A therapy for hemifacial spasm. Cochrane Database Syst Rev 2005;1:CD004899.
12. Anderson FL, Patel BCK, Holds JB, Jordan DR. Blepharospasm: past, present, future. Ophthal Plast Reconstr Surg 1998;15:305–317.
13. Herz NL, Yen MT. Modulation of sensory photophobia in essential blepharospasm with chromatic lenses. Ophthalmology 2005;112:2208–2211.
14. Harrison AR. Chemodenervation for facial dystonias and wrinkles. Curr Opin Ophthalmol 2003;14:241–245.
15. Aramideh M, Ongerboer de Visser BW, Vrans JW, Koelman JH, Speelman JD. Pretarsal application of botulinum toxin for treatment of blepharospasm. J Neurol Neurosurg Psychiatry 1995;59:309–311.
16. Klein AW. Dilution and storage of botulinum toxin. Dermatol Surg 1998;24:1179–1180.
17. Lowe NJ. Botulinum toxin A for facial rejuvenation: United States and United Kingdom Perspectives. Dermatol Surg 1998;24:1216–1218.
18. Hsu TS, Dover JS, Arndt KA. Effect of volume and concentration on the diffusion of botulinum exotoxin A. Arch Dermatol 2004;140:1351–1354.
19. Kowal L. Pretarsal injections of botulinum toxin improve blepharospasm in previously unresponsive patients. J Neurol Neurosurg Psychiatry 1997;63:556.
20. Mackie IA. Riolan's muscle: action and indications for botulinum toxin injection. Eye 2000;14: 347–352.
21. Jost WH, Kohl A. Botulinum toxin: evidence-based medicine criteria in blepharospasm and hemifacial spasm. J Neurol 2001;248:21–24.
22. Osako, Keltner JL. Botulinum A toxin (Oculinum) in ophthalmology. Surv Ophthalmol 1991; 36:28–46.

23. Katzung B. Basic & Clinical Pharmacology. Ninth ed. New York: McGraw-Hill;2004.
24. Fahn S. Systemic therapy of dystonia. Can J Neurol Sci 1987;14:528–532.
25. Defazio G, Lamberti P, Lepore V, et al. Facial dystonia: clinical features, prognosis and pharmacology in 31 patients. Ital J Neurol Sci 1989;10:553–560.
26. Fahn S. High dosage anticholinergic therapy in dystonia. Neurology 1983;33:1255–1261.
27. Burke RE, Fahn S, Marsden CD. Torsion dystonia: a double-blind, prospective trial of high-dosage trihexyphenidyl. Neurology 1986;36:160–164.
28. Hayashi T, Furutani M, Taniyama J, et al. Neuroleptic-induced Meige's syndrome following akathisia: pharmacologic characteristics. Psychiatry Clin Neurosci 1998;52:445–448.
29. Astarloa R, Morales B, Penafiel N, et al. Craniocervical dystonia and facial hemispasm: clinical and pharmacological characteristics of 52 patients. Rev Clin Esp 1991;189:320–324.
30. Ortiz A. Neuropharmacological profile of Meige's disease: overview and a case report. Clinic Neuropharmacol 1983;6:297–304.
31. Duvoison RC. Meige syndrome: relief on high dose anti-cholingergic therapy. Clinic Neuropharmacol 1983;6:63–66.
32. Mezaki T, Hayashi A, Nakase H, et al. Therapy of dystonia in Japan. Rinsho Shinkeigaku 2005; 45:634–642.
33. Jankovic J, Ford J. Blepharospasm and orofacial-cervical dystonia: clinical and pharmacological findings in 100 patients. Ann Neurol 1983;13:402–411.
34. Boghen DR, Lesser RL. Blepharospasm and Hemifacial Spasm. Curr Treat Options Neurol 2000;2:393–400.
35. Dowsey-Limousin P. Parkinsonian dystonia. Rev Neurol 2003;159:928–931.
36. Tarsy D. Tardive Dyskinesia. Curr Treat Options Neurol 2000;2:205–214.
37. Ransmayr G, Kleedorfer B, Dierckx RA, et al. Pharmacological study in Meige's syndrome with predominant blepharospasm. Clin Neuropharmacol 1988;11:68–76.
38. Hipola D, Mateo D, Gimenez-Roldan S. Meige's syndrome: acute and chronic responses to clonazepan and anticholinergics. Eur Neurol 1984;23:474–478.
39. Jankovic J, Orman J. Botulinum A toxin for cranial-cervical dystonia: a double-blind, placebo-controlled study. Neurology 1987;37:616–623.
40. Yoshimura R, Kakihara S, Soya A, et al. Effect of clonazepam treatment on antipsychotic drug-induced Meige syndrome and changes in plasma levels of GABA, HVA, and MHPG during treatment. Psychiatry Clin Neurosci 2001;55:543–546.
41. White MC, Silverman JJ, Harbison JW. Psychosis associated with clonazepam therapy for blepharospasm. J Nerv Ment Dis 1982;170:117–119.
42. Papaterra Limongi JC. Dystonia: therapeutic aspects. Arq Neuropsiquiatr 1996;54:147–155.
43. De Andrade LA, Bertolucci PH. Treatment of Meige disease with a GABA receptor agonist. Arq Neuropsiquiatr 1985;43:260–266.
44. Wirtschafter JD. Clinical doxorubicin chemotherapy: an experimental treatment for benign essential blepharospasm and hemifacial spasm. Ophthalmology 1991;98:357–366.
45. Sandyk R. Blepharospasm—successful treatment with baclofen and sodium valproate. A case report. S Afr Med J 1983;64:955–956.
46. Srivastava T, Goyal V, Singh S, et al. Pallido-pyramidal syndrome with blepharospasm and good response to levodopa. J Neurol 2005;252:1537–1538.
47. Lee KC, Finley R, Miller B. Apraxia of lid opening: dose-dependent response to carbidopa-levodopa. Pharmacotherapy 2004;24:401–403.
48. Dewey RB Jr, Maraganore DM. Isolated eyelid-opening apraxia: report of a new levodopa-responsive syndrome. Neurology 1994;44:1752–1754.
49. Dowsey-Limousin P. Parkinsonian dystonia. Rev Neurol 2003;159:928–931.
50. Barclay CL, Lang AE. Dystonia in progressive supranuclear palsy. J Neurol Neurosurg Psychiatry 1997;62:352–356.
51. Lamberti P, De Mari M, Zenzola A, et al. Frequency of apraxia of eyelid opening in the general population and in patients with extrapyramidal disorders. 2002;23:S81–S82.

52. Grandas F, Elston J, Quinn N, et al. Pharmacologic, surgical and infiltration of botulin toxin treatment in blepharospasm. Neurologia 1989;4:194–199.

53. Arthurs B, Flanders M, Codere F, et al. Treatment of blepharospasm with medication, surgery and type A botulinum toxin. Can J Ophthalmol 1987;22:24–28.

54. Grivet D, Robert PY, Thuret G, et al. Assessment of blepharospasm surgery using an improved disability scale: study of 138 patients. Ophthal Plast Reconstr Surg 2005;21:230–234.

55. Yanoff M, Duker JS. Ophthalmology. Second ed. St. Louis, MO: Mosby;2004.

56. McCann JD, Ugurbas SH, Goldberg RA. Benign essential blepharospasm. Int Ophthalmol Clin 2002;42:113–121.

57. Yen MT, Anderson RL, Small RG. Orbicularis oculi muscle graft augmentation after protractor myectomy in blepharospasm. Ophthal Plast Reconstr Surg 2003;19:287–296.

58. Topaloglu H, Serdaroglu A, Okan M, et al. Improvement of myotonia with carbamazepine in three cases with the Schwartz-Jampel syndrome. Neuropediatrics 1993;24:232–234.

59. Wirtschafter JD, McLoon LK. Long-term efficacy of local doxorubicin chemomyectomy in patients with blepharospasm and hemifacial spasm. Ophthalmology 1998;105:342–346.

60. Fante RG, Frueh BR. Differential section of the seventh nerve as a tertiary procedure for the treatment of benign essential blepharospasm. Ophthal Plast Reconstr Surg 2001;17:276–280.

61. Wakakura M, Tsubouchi T, Inouye J. Etizolam and benzodiazepine induced blepharospasm. J Neurol Neurosurg Psychiatry 2004;75:506–507.

62. Klein RL, Harris RA. Regulation of GABAA receptor structure and function by chronic drug treatments in vivo and with stably transfected cells. Jpn J Pharmacology 1996;70:1–15.

63. Pikielny RT, Micheli FE, Fernandez Pardal MM, et al. Treatment of blepharospasm with botulinum toxin. Medicina 1990;50:129–134.

64. McLoon LK, Wirtschafter JD. Doxil-induced chemomyectomy: effectiveness for permanent removal of orbicularis oculi muscle in monkey eyelid. Invest Ophthalmol Vis Sci 2001; 42:1254–1257.

# 15

# Economics, Immunity, and Future Directions

## Victoria Chan Harrison and David Lin

## INTRODUCTION

Similar to other fields of medicine in which promising new developments have emerged at an accelerated pace during the past 10 years, therapeutic uses of botulinum toxin (BTX) for the treatment of neurological, cosmetic, urinary, gastrointestinal, and pain-related conditions continue to develop. Currently, the Food and Drug Administration has approved the use of BTX type A (BTX-A; Botox®, Allergan Inc., Irvine, CA) for treating cervical dystonia, strabismus, blepharospasm, hemifacial spasm, axillary hyperhidrosis, and glabellar wrinkles. The Food and Drug Administration also has approved BTX-B (Myobloc®, Solstice Neurosciences, South San Francisco, CA) for the treatment of cervical dystonia. In 1990, The National Institutes of Health issued a consensus statement reviewing the safety and efficacy of using Botox in connection with additional disorders, including spasmodic dysphonia, stuttering and vocal tremors, and focal dystonias. There are many other published uses of BTX, including the treatment of achalasia, anismus, detrusor-sphincter dyssynergia, myofascial pain syndromes, migraine headaches, and piriformis syndrome.

## ECONOMIC CONSIDERATIONS

Because BTX is very expensive, it is primarily used in patients who can afford the high costs associated with, or have an insurance policy that will cover, these procedures. As the use of BTX becomes more commonplace, it should become more accessible to the general population. To justify such expense, publication and research, including large-scale randomized trials supporting its clinical efficacy, are necessary. Insurance companies are now utilizing evidence-based medicine to justify such expenditures.

Off-label uses of BTX may not be reimbursed by insurance companies. The amount of insurance coverage varies by the disorder and by physician documentation of medical necessity. The complexities and logistics of insurance coverage often limit patient access to optimal health care. Because the current available neurotoxins are very expensive, reimbursement will require knowledge and attention to the rules and requirements of each individual payer source.

Immunological issues are associated with long-term use of neurotoxins. Many patients who have benefited from BTX will need multiple injections or long-term maintenance, especially patients who are being treated for chronic conditions. In these patients, immunological issues often develop, limiting the efficacy of repeated treatments. Patients who have been

From: *Therapeutic Uses of Botulinum Toxin*
Edited by: G. Cooper © Humana Press Inc., Totowa, NJ

benefiting from repeated BTX treatments may require increased dosages for similar results. As the population of long-term BTX users increases, resistance and antibody formation will become a greater issue in the future. When increasing the dosage fails to elicit the desired response because of immunity, using a different BTX subtype may be an alternative. Although various strains of *Clostridium* BTX antigen serotypes have been produced and named from types A to G, only two types of BTX complex proteins are widely available in the United States: Botox and Myobloc.

Risk factors associated with antibody formation to BTX are increased chronicity and frequency of use and the quantity of protein load administered *(1–3)*. Before assuming antibody formation as the cause of resistance to treatment, other concomitant factors that can limit treatment response must be ruled out, such as the progression of the disease being treated, muscle selection, and adequate therapeutic dosage. Current recommendations are to deliver the lowest effective amount of the neurotoxin complex protein and to attempt to prolong injection intervals to once every 3 months to reduce the risk of antibody formation in patients.

Preserving treatment response to BTX in patients who require multiple injections will become a priority because the number of individuals developing antibody formation will increase as those living with these disorders age. In addition to the established risk of developing antibodies to a neurotoxin serotype from overexposure, there is evidence suggesting the development of an immunological cross-reaction between different BTX serotypes. When chronic overexposure to a neurotoxin serotype triggers antibody production, the immune system becomes primed for future exposures to any new neurotoxin serotype by relatively quickly producing antibodies to the second serotype. Laboratory studies comparing the amino acid sequences of different BTX serotypes with tetanus toxin have found that the percentage of identical amino acids shared is 31% of light chains and 51% of heavy chains *(4,5)*. The higher percentage of identical amino acids shared between neurotoxin serotypes would imply a greater number of common epitopes shared to stimulate antibody formation between neurotoxin serotypes, creating molecular mimicry.

Additional studies examining cross-reactivity between botulinum serotypes have demonstrated a primed immunological response forming antibodies between exposures of BTX-A followed by other serotypes in mice *(6)*. Subjects exposed to fragments of BTX-A aimed at forming antibodies had their serum collected and subsequently exposed to another serotype. Measured titer levels revealing all protein fragments tested stimulated the production of antibodies that cross-reacted with at least one of the other serotypes. Theoretically, there are concerns for BTX-A-resistant patients who change to treatments using BTX-B and then develop a resistance to treatment from cross-reactivity. In the future, immunological work needs to examine the phenomenon of cross-reactivity in humans with BTX-A resistance to other serotypes.

In anticipation of BTX-A resistance, clinical trials are beginning to investigate clinical uses of other BTX serotypes such as types C, E, and F. Trials of BTX-F in humans reveal a short duration of efficacy, lasting 5 weeks, compared with BTX-A *(7,8)*. In 2002, Eleopra et al. performed a small trial of BTX-C and BTX-E in comparison with BTX-A in humans for the treatment of focal dystonia *(9)*. BTX-E was also found to be inferior because of short duration of efficacy. However, BTX-C was found to have efficacy similar to BTX-A without evidence of motor neuron destruction. In a small pilot trial, patients with blepharospasm or cervical dystonia with established antibody formation to BTX-A were given BTX-C (WAKO, Japan) and demonstrated symptomatic improvement of up to 4 weeks. BTX-C may be a viable alternative to treatment for those with BTX-A resistance, but further large-scale trials are needed for additional data on safety and long-term efficacy.

For those who currently have BTX resistance, the use of chemodenervation with phenol or carboxylic acid has been traditionally used but limited by the side effect profile. The most common side effects are pain and injury to nearby structures. Electromyography or nerve stimulation-guided intramuscular injection of phenol is strongly suggested to selectively administer the agents as close to the motor point as possible. This technique also enables patients to receive the maximum benefit with minimal side effects. However, because of the painful dysesthesias that may be experienced, most individuals will not tolerate repeat injections and this method should be used only as a last resort. Overall, BTX is superior to chemodenervation in the treatment of various chronic disorders associated with involuntary muscle contractions with respect to patient tolerance. Judicious use of BTX in the treatment of chronic disorders must be adhered to in order to avoid the development of resistance.

## THE DEVELOPING ROLE OF BTX

When cosmetic BTX injections were first used to diminish forehead wrinkles, practitioners observed that their patients also had fewer episodes of migraine headaches *(10)*. This serendipitous observation instigated clinical trials examining the efficacy of neurotoxin use for the treatment of migraine headaches. Initially, the efficacy of Botox injections for migraine prophylaxis was thought to be related to muscle relaxation. However, the level of efficacy of pain relief from injections did not significantly correlate with the level of weakness or muscle relaxation. Traditionally, migraines were thought to be caused by vasoconstriction followed by vasodilatation. Although the exact pathophysiology of migraines remains elusive, many clinicians now believe that migraines arise from increased sensitivity of cerebral structures in the dorsal raphe area of the brainstem. These sensitized cerebral structures, when reacting to stimuli, can trigger a cascade of responses that activate the trigeminal nerve to release proinflammatory neuropeptides. The neuropeptides released produce local vasodilatation and perivascular inflammatory reactants that bind to nociceptors, causing pain perception *(11)*. Once this localized response begins, a cascade of central sensitization occurs in which the brainstem is sensitized followed by the thalamus. The brain becomes hyperexcitable to all sensory stimuli, causing benign stimuli to exacerbate headache symptoms and pain *(12)*.

The mechanism of action of BTX-A in the treatment of migraine is now believed to have anti-nocicpetive properties that block pain receptors at the nerve fiber level *(13)*. BTX-A also has the action of inhibiting the efferent muscle spindle fibers. The blocked neuromuscular junction of the γ-motor neuron fibers diminishes muscle spindle output, thereby decreasing the sensory feedback centrally *(14)*. Altering the sensory feedback to the structures in the brainstem is thought to prevent cerebral central sensitization and arrest the inflammatory cascade associated with migraines.

Encouraged by the treatment of migraine headaches with neurotoxin, many clinicians have also examined the use of neurotoxin in the treatment of myofascial pain. Although there may be a wide variety of underlying etiologies, all myofascial pain syndromes are characterized by muscle, soft tissue, and fascia tightening. Muscle trigger points may develop that involve localized static shortening of muscle fibers and stiffening of surrounding connective tissue. The prevention of uncontrolled muscle fiber contractions has been postulated as a potential mechanism for pain relief.

The action of BTX-A injected into trigger points is believed to block the release of acetylcholine presynaptically at the motor end plates inhibiting muscle contraction. Studies have indicated that muscle trigger points are hypercontracted muscle fibers located and produced by a region of abnormal motor end plate discharges. The abnormal spontaneous firing at the neuromuscular junction is also associated with an excessive continuous release of acetylcholine, possibly by muscle spindles *(15–17)*. Furthermore, end plate spikes are more likely to appear in more active muscle trigger points using electromyography techniques. If abnormal end plate activity is responsible for active muscle trigger points, then the use of a neuromuscular blocking agent, such as BTX, would effectively decrease the spontaneous firing and muscle tension observed.

Local hypercontracted muscle fibers associated with trigger points are thought to limit local circulation, causing localized tissue hypoxia. This can lead to the release of substances that sensitize local nociceptors, creating the referred pain patterns characterized by trigger points. Histological examination of rabbit muscle identified with active trigger points found small C afferent nerve pain fibers in the immediate vicinity *(18)*. These findings suggest myofascial pain from trigger points is mediated by not only local muscle hypercontractility, but also some component of hypersensitization of local nociceptors. BTX has been theorized to not only diminish muscle contraction, but also to inhibit the release of neuropeptides associated with myofascial pain. Indeed, in vitro studies of embryonic rat dorsal root ganglia neurons treated with BTX demonstrated decreased neuropeptide release *(19,20)*. Furthermore, in vitro examination of rabbit ocular tissue treated by BTX-A revealed inhibited release of acetylcholine and substance P *(21)*. BTX may reduce the release of nociceptive neuropeptides whether from cholinergic neurons or from C or A delta fibers, preventing local sensitization associated with chronic pain.

Excited by the promising results of BTX use in the treatment of pain syndromes by blocking the release of nociceptive neuropeptides, researchers have begun to look at intra-articular use of BTX for chronic refractory joint pain. Five patients with chronic knee or ankle joint pain who did not respond to intra-articular injections of corticosteroids were administered 20 to 50 U Botox into the knee or ankle. Overall outcomes were a 50% pain reduction lasting for 2 to 6 months. Patients did not have any local or systemic adverse effects *(22)*. These same investigators also examined the efficacy of intra-articular injections of BTX-A for the treatment of chronic shoulder pain in six elderly patients. Patients were administered 50 to 100 U BTX-A via intra-articular injection into the shoulder. Subjects post-treatment had a 33 to 50% pain reduction in their symptoms and some improvements in shoulder range of motion in flexion and abduction. Improvements were reported to last from 6 to 11 weeks *(23)*. The findings from these case series are preliminary and will require additional investigation to examine the anti-nociceptive properties of intra-articular BTX to determine efficacy.

Concomitant with the expanding role of BTX in the treatment of various pain conditions, the toxin has already helped a plethora of other conditions, as outlined in this book. With the discovery of a new tool have come new applications, new treatments, and ultimately better patient care. As we continue to understand the precise mechanism of BTX's efficacy, more applications may emerge.

## CONCLUSION

With BTX, we have found a new, potent tool that can be used across a wide array of medical specialties for an even broader array of medical conditions, leading to an overall improved quality of life for patients. In general, BTX injections are well tolerated. Still, certain important considerations apply, such as economic costs that can be prohibitive. Future research is likely to demonstrate that for certain conditions, BTX injections are more cost-effective in the long run than more invasive procedures. For now, however, insurance companies remain reluctant to reimburse for many off-label treatments. Immunity remains a concern and should prompt further moderation in the dosage and frequency of use of the toxin. Finally, physicians must remember that although BTX injection is a relatively safe procedure, it must only be done in the hands of experienced, expert clinicians to avoid potential complications and give the patient his or her best chance for maximal benefit.

The future of the utility of BTX injections helping patients remains bright. Further research will help convince insurance companies that it is in their best interests, as well as those of their patients, to reimburse in appropriate cases. The role of BTX in various treatment algorithms will continue to become better elucidated. Certainly, BTX has its limitations. The effects are only temporary, but then this, too, mitigates adverse reactions. Because of the positive effects experienced for so wide a range of patients, there is a temptation and tendency to want to use BTX for increasingly diverse applications. Certainly, exploration of novel uses for BTX is admirable. This is, after all, how science is advanced. However, BTX should not be used where it is not indicated and has no concept validity for efficacy. As the mechanism of action of the toxin continues to be tested and explored, new valuable applications are likely to continue to emerge.

## REFERENCES

1. Goschel H, Wohlfarth K, Frevert J, Dengler R, Bigalke H. Botulinum A toxin therapy: neutralizing and nonneurtralizing antibodies: therapeutic consequences. Exp Neurology 1997;147:96–102.
2. Jankovic J, Schwartz K. Response and immunoresistance to botulinum toxin injections. Neurology 1995;45:1743–1746.
3. Rosenberg JS, Middlerook JS, Atassi MZ. Localization of the regions on the C-terminal domain of the heavy chain of botulinum toxin A recognized by T lymphocytes and by antibodies after immunization of mice with pentavalent toxiod. Immunol Invest 1997;26:491–504.
4. Whelan SM, Elmore MJ, Bodsworth NJ, Brehm JK, Atkinson T, Minton NP. Molecular cloning of the Clostridum botulinum structural gene encoding the type B neurotoxin and determination of its entire nucleotide sequence. Appl Environ Microbiol 1992;58:2345–2354.
5. Hutson RA, Collins MD, East AK, Thompson DE. Nucleotide sequence of the gene coding for non-proteolytic Clostridium botulinum type B neurotoxin: comparison with the other clostridial neurotoxins. Curr Microbiol 1994;28:101–110.
6. Dertzbaugh MT, West MW. Mapping of protective and cross reactive domains of the type A neurotoxin of Clostridium botulinum toxin. Vaccine 1996;14:1538–1544.
7. Chen R, Karp BI, Hallett M. Botulinum toxin type F for the treatment of dystonia: long-term experience. Neurology 1998;51:1494–1496.
8. Mezaki T, Kaji R, Kohara N, et al. Comparison of therapeutic efficacies of type A and F botulinum toxins for blepharospasm: a double blind, control study. Neurology 1995;45:506–508.
9. Eleopra R, Tugnoli V, Quatrale R, et al. Botulinum toxin serotypes C and E clinical trials. In: Scientific and Therapeutic Aspects of Botulinum Toxin, Brin MF, Hallett M, Jankoric J, eds. Philadelphia: Lippincott Williams & Wilkins; 2002, p. 441–450.
10. Binder W, Brin M, Blizer A, Schenrock L, Diamond B. Botulinum toxin type A for treatment of migraines: an open label assessment. Mov Disorder 1998;13:241.
11. Aurora SK, Welch KMA. Brain excitability in migraine: evidence from transcranial magnetic stimulation studies. Curr Opin Neurolo 1998;11:205–209.
12. Mathew NT, Mullani N. Migraine with persistent visual aura and sustained metabolic activation in the medial occipital cortex measured by PET [abstract]. Neurology 1998;50:A350–A351.
13. Aoki KR. Pharmacology and immunology of botulinum toxin serotypes. J Neurol 2001;248:3–10.

14. Gilio F, Curra A, et al. Effects of botulinum toxin type A on intracortical inhibition in patients with dystonia. Ann Neurology 2000;48:20–26.
15. Hong CZ, Yu J. Spontaneous electrical activity of rabbit trigger sot after transaction of spinal cord and peripheral nerve. J Musculoskeletal Pain 1998;6:45–58.
16. Hubbard DR, Berkoff GM. Myofascial trigger points show spontaneous needle EMG activity. Spine 1993;18:1803–1807.
17. Simmons DG, Hong CZ, Simons LS. Endplate potentials are common to midfiber myofascial trigger points. Am J Phys Med Rehabil 2002;81:212–222.
18. Hong CZ, Simons DG. Pathophysiologic and electrophysiologic mechanisms of myofascial trigger points. Arch Phys Med Rehabil 1998;79:863–872.
19. Purkiss J, Welch M, Doward S, Foster K. Capsaicin-stimulated release of substance P from cultured dorsal root ganglion neurons: involvement of two distinct mechanisms. Biochem Pharmacol 2000;59:1403–1406.
20. Welch MJ, Purkiss JR, Foster KA. Sensitivity of embryonic rat dorsal root ganglia neurons to clostridium botulinum neurotoxins. Toxicon 2000;28:245–258.
21. Ishikawa H, Mitsui Y, Yoshitomi T, et al. Presynaptic effects of botulinum toxin type A on the neuronally evoked response of albino and pigmented rabbit iris sphincter and dilator muscles. Jpn J Opthalmol 2000;44:106–109.
22. Mahowald ML, Singh JA. Dykstra: repost on intra-articular botulinum toxin type A for refractory joint pain. J Invest Med 2004;52:S379.
23. Singh JA, Mahowald ML. Dykstra: intra-articular botulinum A toxin for chronic shoulder pain in the elderly. J Invest Med 2004;52:S380.

# Index

## A

Acetaminophen
  migraine, 98
Acetylcholine, 4, 123, 154
Achalasia
  BTX-A, 197–201, 199t
  diagnosis, 198
  pneumatic dilation, 200
Achilles tendon
  contracture release, 14
Acupuncture
  hyperhidrosis, 156
Age
  LBP, 40
Alkaloids
  migraine, 98
Amantadine
  blepharospasm, 217–218
Amitriptyline
  migraine, 99
Anal fissure
  BTX-A, 201–204, 203t
Analgesics
  migraine, 98
Ankle dorsiflexion stretch, 79f
Ankylosing spondylitis
  LPB, 44
ANS. See Autonomic nervous system (ANS)
Anthropomorphic factors
  LBP, 40
Anticholinergic therapy
  DO, 174–175
Antiperspirants
  hyperhidrosis, 156
Apocrine glands, 155
Apoeccrine glands, 155
Ashworth scales, 9
Aspirin
  migraine, 98, 99
Autonomic nervous system (ANS), 123

## B

Baclofen
  blepharospasm, 215
  MS, 12–13

Barbiturates
  migraine, 98
Benign prostatic hypertrophy
  BTX, 178–179
Benzodiazepines
  MS, 13
Benztropine
  blepharospasm, 213–214
Biofeedback therapy
  hyperhidrosis, 156
  TTH, 99
Blepharoptosis
  BoNT-A, 103–104
Blepharospasm, 209–219
  BTX-A, 211–213
    injection site, 212f
    preparations, 212–213
  BTX-C, 224–225
  chemomyectomy, 218
  clinical findings, 209
  differential diagnosis, 210
  essential, 209–210
  facial nerve destruction or differential
      section, 218
  myectomy, 218
  oral medications, 213–218
  pathogenesis, 210
  surgery, 218–219
  terminology, 209–210
  treatment, 211–218
BoNT-A. See Botulinum toxin type A (BTX-A)
BoNT-B. See Botulinum toxin type B (BTX-B)
Botox. See Botulinum toxin type A (BTX-A)
Botulinum toxin (BTX), 1–5. See also spe-
      cific types
  antibody formation, 224
  benign prostatic hypertrophy, 178–179
  developing role, 225–226
  discoverers, 5t
  economics, 223–225
  immunological issues, 223–224
  LUT clinical application, 171–182
  mechanism of action, 4–5
  normal neuromuscular junction, 4–5

229